ABDOMINAL WALL HERNIAS

AN ATLAS OF **ANATOMY** AND **REPAIR**

Upper Left

The inferior segment of the fascia of the right posterior inguinal wall, held in tissue forceps, is retracted upward to show the arched turn-in as it courses to insert into Cooper's ligament.

Upper Right

This intraoperative photograph, complementary to the upper left figure, shows "live" the turn-in of the inferior fascial segment and its continuity laterally as the anterior femoral sheath. The relationship of this segment to the underlying pyriform fossa and inguinal ligament is also visible.

Center

Artist's illustration of the completed one-layer fascial reconstruction of the posterior inguinal wall and its relationship to the pyriform fossa.

Lower Left

Another intraoperative photograph complementary to the upper left figure, shows the pyriform fossa in relation to the surrounding structures that form its boundaries. These are, superiorly, the inferior segment of the fascia of the posterior inguinal wall, held in clamps; inferiorly, the inguinal ligament; laterally, the medial wall of the femoral sheath; and medially, the confluence of the paddle-shaped tendinous expansion of the inguinal ligament (Gimbernat's) and the medial angle of the fascia of the posterior inguinal wall. The "floor" of the pyriform fossa is formed by the fascial or lateral portion of Gimbernat's ligament. The distance between the inferior segment of the fascia of the posterior inguinal wall and the inguinal ligament is noteworthy.

Lower Right

Photograph of a cadaver dissection by W. J. Lytle of the normal right groin in a man. The medial segment of the tansected inguinal ligament is forcibly retracted downward to expose the lateral and fixed crescentic margin of the fascial portion of Gimbernat's ligament that forms the medial boundary (border) of the femoral sheath. Also, the paddle-shaped expansion of the tendinous portion of Gimbernat's ligament medially, and its insertion into the pubic tubercle and adjacent medial portion of Cooper's ligament, may be seen.

Forcible upward traction on the rake retractor attached to the inferior segment of the fascia of the posterior inguinal wall has avulsed its attachment to Cooper's ligament. Its continuation laterally as the medial wall of the femoral sheath and the anterior femoral sheath, respectively, is demonstrated.

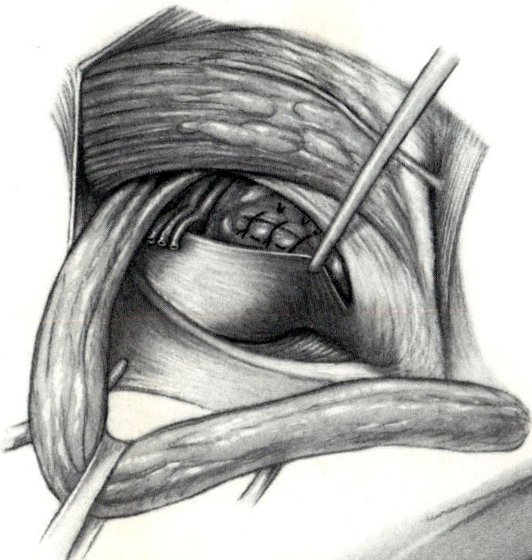

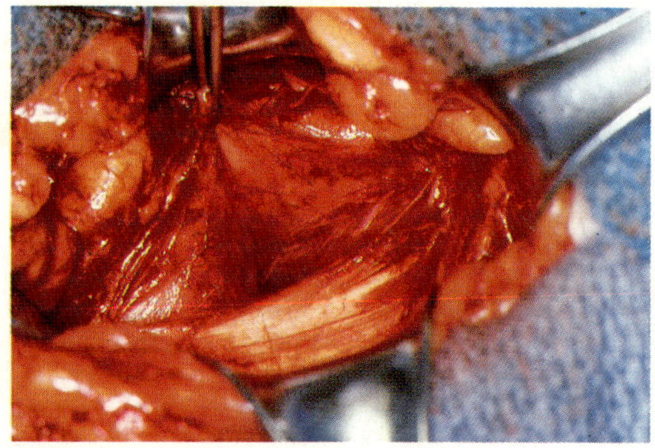

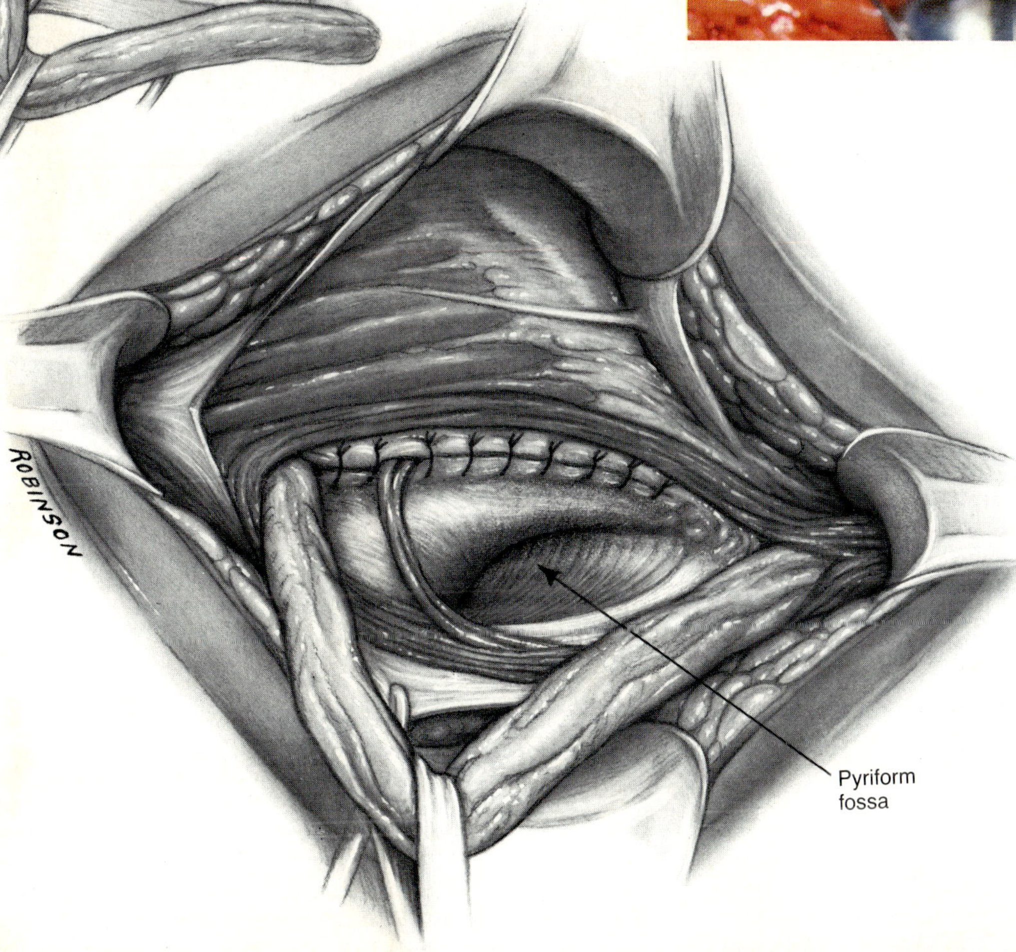
ROBINSON
Pyriform
fossa

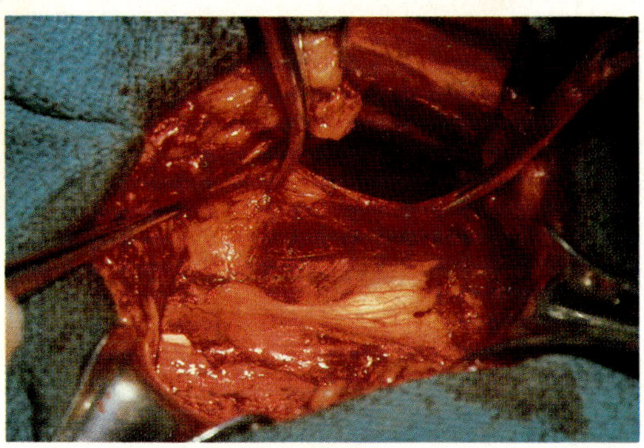

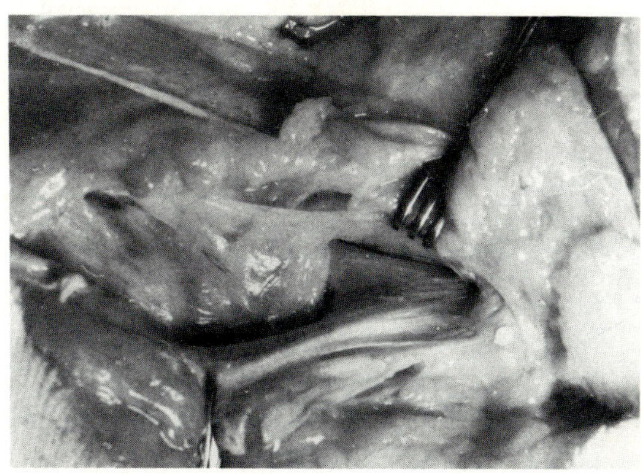

ABDOMINAL WALL HERNIAS

AN ATLAS OF **ANATOMY** AND **REPAIR**

JOHN L. MADDEN, M.D.

1989
W.B. SAUNDERS COMPANY
Harcourt Brace Jovanovich, Inc.
Philadelphia London Toronto Montreal Sydney Tokyo

W. B. SAUNDERS COMPANY
Harcourt Brace Jovanovich, Inc.

The Curtis Center
Independence Square West
Philadelphia, PA 19106

Library of Congress Cataloging-in-Publication Data

Madden, John P. L. (John Patrick Leo), 1912–
Abdominal wall hernias.

1. Hernia—Surgery—Atlases. I. Title. [DNLM: 1. Hernia, Femoral—surgery—atlases. 2. Hernia, Inguinal—surgery—atlases. 3. Hernia, Ventral—surgery—atlases. WI 17 M179a]

RD621.M25 1989 617.5′59059 89–10160

ISBN 0–7216–1288–1

Editor: W. B. Saunders Staff
Designer: Paul Fry
Production Manager: Carolyn Naylor
Manuscript Editor: Tom Gibbons
Illustration Coordinator: Brett MacNaughton
Page Layout Artist: Paul Fry
Indexer: Ellen Murray

ABDOMINAL WALL HERNIAS:
An Atlas of Anatomy and Repair ISBN 0-7216–1288–1

Last digit is the print number: 9 8 7 6 5 4 3 2 1

DEDICATION

To my wife "Birdie" and our children Pam, John, Brian, Michael, Tommy, and Kathy.

To the resident in surgery, in the hope that the illustrated intraoperative surgical anatomy and related surgical techniques for the repair of groin hernias will enhance his or her knowledge of a subject that, for centuries, has intrigued surgeons throughout the world.

CONTRIBUTORS

John L. Madden, M.D., F.A.C.S.
Attending Surgeon, Doctors Hospital; Clinical Professor of Surgery, New York Medical College, New York

Chester B. McVay, M.D., F.A.C.S.
Late Emeritus Professor of Surgery and Chairman of the Department of Surgery, University of South Dakota School of Medicine, Sioux City, South Dakota

William P. Mikkelsen, M.D., F.A.C.S.
Clinical Professor of Surgery, University of Southern California Medical School and Los Angeles County Hospital, Los Angeles, California

Lloyd M. Nyhus, M.D., F.A.C.S.
Warren H. Cole Professor and Head, Department of Surgery, University of Illinois at Chicago; Surgeon-in-Chief, University of Illinois Hospital, Chicago, Illinois

Joseph L. Ponka, M.D., F.A.C.S.
Consultant in Surgery, Henry Ford Hospital, Detroit, Michigan; Clinical Professor of Surgery, University of Michigan Medical School, Ann Arbor, Michigan

René Stoppa, M.D., F.A.C.S.
Professor of Surgery and Chairman, Department of Surgery, Centre Hospitalier Regional et Universitaire d'Amiens, Amiens Cedex, France

George E. Wantz, M.D., F.A.C.S.
Attending Surgeon, New York Hospital; Clinical Associate Professor of Surgery, Cornell University Medical School, New York

Christian R. Warlaumont
Chief Clinical Assistant, Department of Surgery, Centre Hospitalier Regional et Universitaire d'Amiens, Amiens Cedex, France

PREFACE

The treatment of groin hernias has been an ongoing challenge from the earliest civilization to the present. It has evolved slowly through the unscientific and empirical use of taxis, intensive purgations, opiates, emollient fomentations, leeches, tobacco glysters, bloodletting, hot and cold poultices and prolonged bed rest, to a science that is founded on a thorough knowledge of anatomy and the rigid principles of surgical antisepsis and asepsis.

During the preceding two centuries, recognition of the importance of the study of anatomy as the basis for the surgical treatment of hernia resulted in the publication of classic treatises of anatomy, whose authors could best be described as Surgical Anatomists. They include Pieter (Petrus) Camper of Holland, Jules Cloquet of France, Astley Cooper and John Gay of England, Antonio de Gimbernat of Spain, Franz Hesselbach of Germany, and Antonio Scarpa of Italy. Collectively they provided the foundation for our present knowledge of applied surgical anatomy in the treatment of groin hernias. The evolution of this progress continued with advances in surgical techniques and culminated with their unification in the Listerian era of antisepsis and asepsis.

Subsequent to Joseph Lister's initial publication in 1867, one of his early visitors in London was Henry O. Marcy of Cambridge (Massachusetts), who in 1871 was the first to establish the two basic concepts in the repair of an inguinal hernia—high ligation and excision of the sac and suture reconstruction of the defect in the posterior inguinal wall. Interestingly, these two concepts, espoused by Marcy more than a century ago, constitute the basic principles for the modern-day surgical treatment of inguinal hernias.

The expression "The more things change, the more they remain the same" is epitomized in the following quotations, 150 years apart, from Sir Astley Cooper of England and Chester B. McVay of the United States. In 1804 Cooper wrote, "No disease of the human body . . . requires in its treatment a greater combination of accurate anatomical knowledge, with surgical skill, than hernia in all its varieties." Similarly, McVay in 1954 stated, ". . . a hernia is an anatomic derangement and to understand . . . the repair of a hernia, a detailed knowledge of the anatomy . . . is absolutely essential." Elaborating on this statement, he remarked that "Nowhere in the field of surgery is there such a multiplicity of operations for a given anatomic defect; this not only reflects basic misunderstanding . . . but is most confusing to the young surgeon."

Since the study of anatomy is a prime essential in the surgical management of groin hernias, it was thought that a selection of illustrations from the original published works of the master surgical anatomists, which generally are not easily available to the inquiring scholar, would be instructive (see the Appendix). The author, therefore, is indebted to Brett Kirkpatrick, Librarian of the New York Academy of Medicine, and in particular to Inge DuPont, Librarian in charge of the Rare Book Room, for the many courtesies extended in making possible the publication of these treasured illustrations. It is hoped that they will provide an ease of reference for both the surgeon and the anatomist, sparing them what otherwise would be a difficult research task.

In the same spirit, Astley Cooper's descriptions of the transversalis fascia and the ligament that bears his name are found in Section I. Also included are the English translations by Thomas Beddoe (1795) of selected portions of Antonio de Gimbernat's original Spanish monograph of 1793. This is done to stimulate and facilitate scholarly pursuit by the interested student.

To convey anatomic realism and for clarity of surgical description, intraoperative color photographs are reproduced as a complement to the illustrations. Comparison of the two serves as an immediate anatomic guide for the practicing surgeon and demonstrates the importance of having both the artist and the photographer as eye witnesses to the operations performed. Otherwise, artistic liberties may be taken that result in "scissors and glue" illustrations, which through the years have been the prime cause of the perpetuation of errors in anatomic fact. The ultimate result of such errors is the inability of the surgeon to identify during the operation the anatomic structures that are labeled in the various illustrated surgical techniques. This applies in particular to the iliopubic tract, which has been depicted in so many false anatomic guises as to preclude its intraoperative recognition. In fact, most frequently the only anatomic clue to its identity is the label "iliopubic tract."

The importance of a one-on-one relationship between the artist and the surgeon cannot be overemphasized. In support of this statement, the artist, Frank Robinson,* was commissioned to visit Chester McVay,* Lloyd Nyhus, Francis Usher,* and Joseph Ponka in the United States and W. J. Lytle* in Sheffield, England, to be an eyewitness to and illustrator of their operative techniques in the treatment of groin hernias. Since the same artist executed all of the illustrations, a uniform standard of excellence has been maintained. I am indebted to these surgeons and to the artist for their expressed kindnesses.

Furthermore, I wish to sincerely thank George Wantz for his illustrated technique of the Shouldice method of hernial repair and R. E. Stoppa and C. R. Warlaumont for their contributions regarding the use of giant preperitoneal mesh prostheses in the repair of groin hernias.

Thanks are also due to Grant Lashbrook for his eyewitness illustrations and the touch-ups required to complete several of Frank Robinson's unfinished drawings, and to Mrs. Ada Gams, the Reference Librarian of the New York Academy of Medicine, whose untiring efforts in tracing both antiquated and current references is deeply appreciated. Also, with the utmost admiration and appreciation, thanks to my secretary, Mrs. Consorcia ("Connie") Camacho, for her unstinting support in the preparation of the many preliminary drafts and, ultimately, the final manuscript of this book.

Finally, and importantly, I wish to thank Carroll Cann, former Medical Editor of W. B. Saunders Co., whose patience, guidance, and counsel helped to make the publication of this book possible. In addition, an expression of sincere gratitude to his successor, Edward H. Wickland, Jr., whose editorial talents and suggestions made possible the ease of transition in the uninterrupted completion of the book.

---

*Deceased.

INTRODUCTION

Admittedly, there are many excellent published texts and atlases pertaining to the anatomy and surgical treatment of groin hernias. The provocation for the writing of this atlas was the fact that during the operations performed for groin hernias, an anatomic structure was repeatedly demonstrated that could not be properly identified by name. This stimulated an intensive search for its identity in current and old texts and atlases of anatomy and surgical techniques, but to no avail.

The search continued through frequent discussions with surgical colleagues about this unnamed anatomic structure. The suggestions that it might be the innominate fascia of Gallaudet or possibly the pectineus fascia proved to be incorrect. Subsequently, during an operation for a hernia it was observed that this structure extended from the inguinal ligament to Cooper's ligament and by definition should be the lacunar or Gimbernat's ligament. The reason for the failure to recognize this ligament previously was the false perception of its true anatomic structure. *Gray's Anatomy* (35th edition, 1973) states that the length of Gimbernat's ligament is 1.25 cm, but the structure seen at operation is longer and has a different anatomic configuration.

In all subsequent operations, this "new" Gimbernat's ligament was readily demonstrated. In fact, the desire to document its surgical anatomic identity led to an association with Frank Robinson, a consummate medical artist, who observed more than 50 operations performed by the author for the repair of groin hernias. In his completed illustrations, which represent a composite of the operations witnessed, the artist has captured the "eyes of the surgeon" in what is a truly remarkable portrayal of the surgical anatomy of the groin, and particularly that of the posterior inguinal wall. The illustrations "breathe" and convey a genuine "feel" of living tissues. In studying them carefully, the reader may readily conclude from their feel and anatomic detail that these drawings are truly original and unique.

The primary purpose of this book is to present the concepts of the author as they pertain to the intraoperative surgical anatomy observed during the operations performed for groin hernias. These observations, though frequently contrary to generally accepted tenets, are complemented by those of the artist and photographer, whose eyewitness intraoperative illustrations and complementary color photographs, respectively, are a totally accurate rendition of the surgical anatomy of the groin as perceived by the author. These illustrations and photographs have served as the anatomic basis for the illustrated step-by-step surgical techniques that have evolved in the repair of groin hernias and that are presented here. They also possess an anatomic realism that is an indispensable guide for the practicing surgeon.

In introducing the subject of hernia, I should like to define some of the descriptive terms commonly applied to groin hernias. Although they may be considered elementary, these definitions are included because of the frequently observed inability of the surgical intern or resident to define such terms clearly and succinctly.

An *inguinal hernia* is an abnormal protrusion of a viscus through the abdominal parieties, the protruding portion being covered by a sac (peritoneum).

An *incarcerated hernia* is simply an irreducible hernia, which may or may not be associated with varying symptoms of bowel obstruction.

A *strangulated hernia* is an irreducible hernia in which there is a compromise of the circulation, either reversible or irreversible, in the herniated viscus.

A *"sliding" hernia* is an incompletely reducible hernia in which a portion of the wall of the sac is formed by the protruding viscus. This viscus may be the cecum on the right side, the sigmoid colon on the left side, and the urinary bladder on either side. A large direct inguinal hernia is invariably associated with a sliding hernia of the bladder.

Richter's hernia is a hernia of a portion of the circumference of the bowel wall; it may be simply incarcerated (irreducible) or strangulated.

A *spigelian* hernia* is a relatively rare lateral ventral hernia. It occurs just below at the junction of the semicircular line (arcuate line of Douglas) and semilunar line, superiorly and laterally, and above the inferior epigastric vessels, medially and inferiorly.

Reductio en masse refers to the forcible pseudoreduction of an incarcerated or strangulated inguinal hernia, either interparietal or intraperitoneal, with persistence of the clinical symptoms of bowel obstruction.

---

*Named after Adriaan van der Spieghel (1578–1625) who, like Andreas Vesalius (1514–1564), was Flemish born. Both studied anatomy at the University of Padua.

CONTENTS

SECTION

SURGICAL ANATOMY

DESCRIPTIVE TEXT

In the study of the anatomy of the groin, the surgeon is confronted with terminology that is frequently confusing and with artist's illustrations depicting anatomic structures that, at operation, are not discernible. Furthermore, the commonplace artistic license results in gross misrepresentation of anatomic fact. Similarly, the study of cadaver dissections may prove a further hindrance, because the anatomy perceived may be at variance with applied surgical anatomy. In this atlas the illustrated surgical anatomy is based on the observations of the surgeon, the artist, and the photographer during the operations performed for the repair of groin hernias. It represents, therefore, a concept of the surgical anatomy of the groin that is both seen and recorded in the operation room.

The posterior inguinal wall comprises two intimately adherent fascial layers. The superficial layer, which is the thicker and stronger of the two, is formed by the aponeurosis of the transversus abdominis muscle (the transversalis muscle in the old terminology). Immediately beneath this aponeurosis is the thinner layer, the transversalis fascia. Therefore, to refer to the fascia of the posterior inguinal wall simply as the transversalis fascia is anatomically incorrect. For clarity of presentation, these combined fascial layers are depicted as a single layer and referred to as the fascia of the posterior inguinal wall.

An inguinal hernia, whether indirect or direct, is defined as a protrusion of a viscus through the abdominal parietes, the protruding portion being covered by a peritoneal sac. Accordingly, it represents a defect in the fascia of the posterior inguinal wall that separates the fascia into two segments—a superior ("medial") and an inferior ("lateral"). The degree of separation of these segments varies in direct ratio to the size of the hernia. For the surgeon, the anatomic essential in the repair of the hernia is to close the defect in the unified fascial layer of the posterior inguinal wall. This is accomplished by suture approximation of the superior segment to the inferior segment. In some patients a complete reconstruction of the fascia of the posterior inguinal wall may be required, because of the large size of the hernial defect. Therefore, a knowledge of the surgical anatomy of the groin is basic to the treatment of hernias.

There is universal agreement when one speaks of the superior segment of the fascia of the posterior inguinal wall. However, confusion exists concerning the inferior segment. Heretofore, this segment has been variously named the iliopubic tract, Thomson's ligament (see Figs. 1 to 5), the deep crural or femoral arch (in England), and the *bandelette iliopubienne* (in France). To recognize the superior segment of the fascia of the posterior inguinal wall but refer to its inferior counterpart by a multiplicity of names is both confusing and anatomically illogical.

Figures 1 to 5. The "Journal des Connaissances Médicales Pratiques" (Fig. 1), in which Alexandre Thomson's article "Cause Anatomique de la Hernie Inguinale Externe" was published in 1836.[13] Because of its length, the article appeared in two parts in separate issues of the Journal. On the title page of the first part (Fig. 2), the author's surname is listed as "Thomson." However, on the title page of the second part (Fig. 3), published in the succeeding issue of the Journal, the author's name is spelled "Thompson." This spelling is repeated in the concluding page of the second part of the article (Fig. 4) and in the index, the "Table des Matières" (Fig. 5). Thus it appears that the insertion of the letter "p" in "Thomson" is a typographic error that has been perpetuated.

JOURNAL

DES

CONNAISSANCES MÉDICALES

PRATIQUES

ET DE PHARMACOLOGIE,

PUBLIÉ PAR UN COMITÉ COMPOSÉ DE:

MM. BEAUDE, inspecteur des établissemens d'eaux minérales, membre du conseil de salubrité;
CAFFE, chef de la clinique ophthalmologique des hôpitaux de Paris;
CAPITAINE, docteur en médecine;
CARRON DU VILLARDS, directeur du dispensaire ophthalmique;
LEROY D'ÉTIOLLES, docteur en médecine;
LESUEUR, professeur agrégé à la faculté de médecine de Paris;
MARTINS, docteur en médecine, ancien Aide naturaliste à la faculté de médecine;
TANCHOU, docteur en médecine;
TAVERNIER, docteur en médecine;
VÉE, pharmacien, membre de la société de pharmacie.

TOME QUATRIÈME.

1836—1837.

SIX FRANCS PAR AN,

HUIT FRANCS POUR LES DÉPARTEMENS.

Fig. 1

On s'abonne à Paris,

AU BUREAU DU JOURNAL, RUE FEYDEAU, N. 22.

1836.

CONNAISSANCES MÉDICALES. 137

CAUSE ANATOMIQUE

DE LA HERNIE INGUINALE EXTERNE.

Par M. Alexandre THOMSON, D. M.

Présenté à l'Académie de Médecine, 23 *nov*. 1835;

A l'Académie des Sciences, 17 *nov*. 1835.

(1er article.)

DE SON ÉCHAPPEMENT A TRAVERS L'ANNEAU INGUINAL INTERNE.

Fig. 2

CONNAISSANCES MÉDICALES. 169

CAUSE ANATOMIQUE

DE LA HERNIE INGUINALE EXTERNE.

Par M. le Docteur Alexandre THOMPSON.

(2e article.)

§ 4. *De son échappement d'en dessous ou d'en arrière du ventrier, ou couvercle fibreux de l'anneau inguinal externe.*

Fig. 3

CONNAISSANCES MÉDICALES. 176

13° Tout ce qu'on vient de lire est également applicable chez la femme dans les hernies labiales complètes et volumineuses, à l'exception que la résistance offerte par la partie interne de l'ouverture herniaire composée sera moindre chez elle, puisque les fibres inférieures des deux muscles transverse et petit oblique étant dilatées et poussées en avant du sac, ne sauraient, comme chez l'homme, augmenter cette résistance en se recourbant de dedans en dehors en bas du collet du sac.

A. THOMPSON.

Fig. 4

TABLE DES MATIÈRES. 383

Thompson (sur un nouveau mode d'essai des manganèses. 60.
→Thompson (A.) (cause anatomique de la hernie inguinale externe, par M. le docteur). 137 et 169.
Tœnia multiple (sur un cas remarquable de), par M. Potèse. 27.
Tophen (de l'extraction du placenta après l'accouchement, par M.). 120.

Fig. 5

The term "iliopubic tract," which has attained common usage, is primarily responsible for the confusion concerning the surgical anatomy of the posterior inguinal wall. Those who favor its use, except for Fruchaud in Egypt, have failed to illustrate its surgical anatomy clearly and accurately; its only surgical identity is its label. This has resulted in the publication of numerous and disparate anatomic concepts pertaining to the iliopubic tract, which precludes its recognition during the operative repair of a groin hernia. The simplest way for the surgeon to identify the iliopubic tract is to refer to it by its correct anatomic and surgical name: the inferior segment of the fascia of the posterior inguinal wall. This name has a better surgical connotation and a more practical anatomic meaning relative to the closure of the hernial defect. Simply restated, the hernial defect is closed by suture of the superior segment of the fascia of the posterior inguinal wall to its inferior segment. This new name for the iliopubic tract will be used throughout this atlas.

The inferior prolongation of the fascia of the posterior inguinal wall and its insertion into Cooper's ligament are hidden by the "shelving" border of the inguinal ligament and are only exposed by surgical dissection. In fact, the intimate adherence by contiguity of the inferior segment of the fascia of the posterior inguinal wall to the ligament's shelving border is probably the basis for the long held and commonly accepted belief that the inguinal ligament forms its inferior boundary. This belief underlies the universally accepted surgical practice of using the shelving border to anchor sutures in the repair of inguinal hernias.

The key to the complete anatomic definition of the inferior segment of the fascia of the posterior inguinal wall is the pyriform fossa (Fig. 6). This fossa, so named because of its anatomic similarity to the pyriform fossa of the larynx, is a potential space only, being filled by a loose matrix of fibroareolar tissue. Surgical dissection of this tissue exposes the fossa and defines the full extent of the anatomy of the posterior inguinal wall.

To expose the pyriform fossa, the inguinal or crural ligament is identified as it crosses over the anterior femoral (crural) sheath. Dissection is then begun in a plane medial to the sheath and deep to the inguinal ligament and is continued toward the pubic tubercle until the fossa is exposed and its boundaries are defined.

The fossa is bounded superiorly by the inferior segment of the fascia of the posterior inguinal wall; inferiorly, by the shelving border of the inguinal ligament; medially, by the paddle-shaped tendinous portion of Gimbernat's ligament and its expansion onto the adjacent medial extension of the fascia of the posterior inguinal wall; and laterally, by the medial wall of the femoral sheath. The concave floor of the fossa is formed by the fascial portion of Gimbernat's ligament.

Exposure of the pyriform fossa confirms the fact that the inguinal ligament forms the inferior boundary of the fossa and not the inferior boundary of the posterior inguinal wall. Heretofore, Fruchaud[6] (Fig. 7) is the only author to have demonstrated the pyriform fossa* and its relation to the inferior segment of the fascia of the posterior inguinal wall, as described and illustrated here.

The primary reason for the failure to clearly understand the surgical anatomy of the posterior inguinal wall is an incomplete anatomic dissection, either at operation or on the cadaver. Most of the difficulty lies in the representation of the inferior segment of the fascia of the posterior inguinal wall in relation to the following anatomic structures: (1) the iliopectineal line (pecten of the pubis or Cooper's ligament); (2) the shelving border of the inguinal ligament; and (3) the lacunar or Gimbernat's ligament and the medial wall of the femoral sheath. Since these are the neighboring structures that form the anatomic boundaries of the pyriform fossa, a description of each will clarify the surgical anatomy of the posterior inguinal wall.

---

*Apparently unknowingly, since there is neither an identifying label on the illustration nor a description in his text.

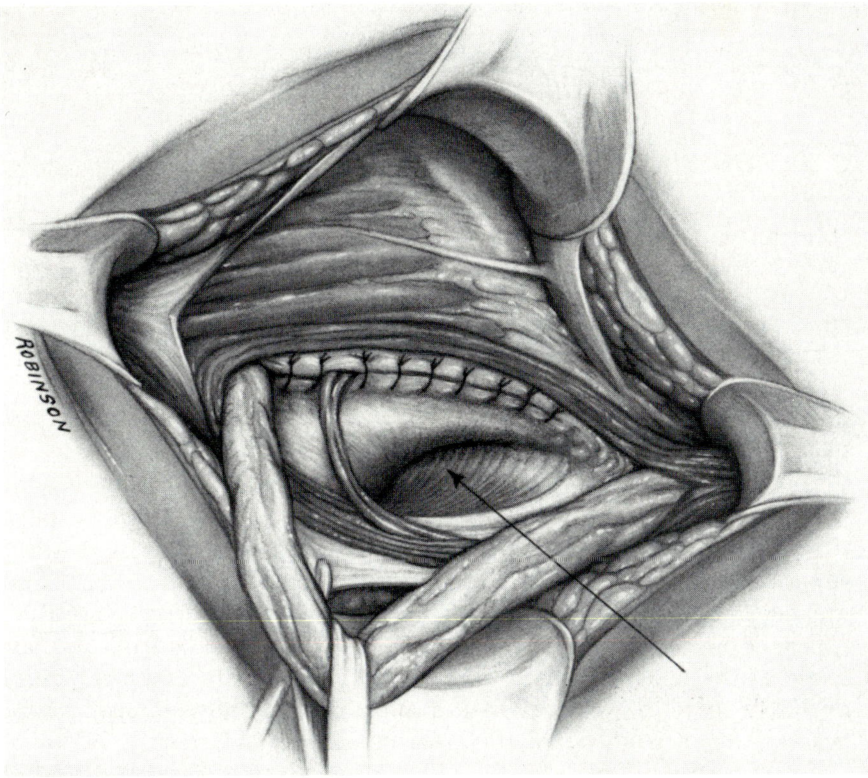

Figure 6. The completed reconstruction of the fascia of the posterior inguinal wall by suture of the superior segment to the inferior segment ("iliopubic tract"). Its relation to the adjacent structures, particularly the "pyriform fossa" (*arrow*), is shown.

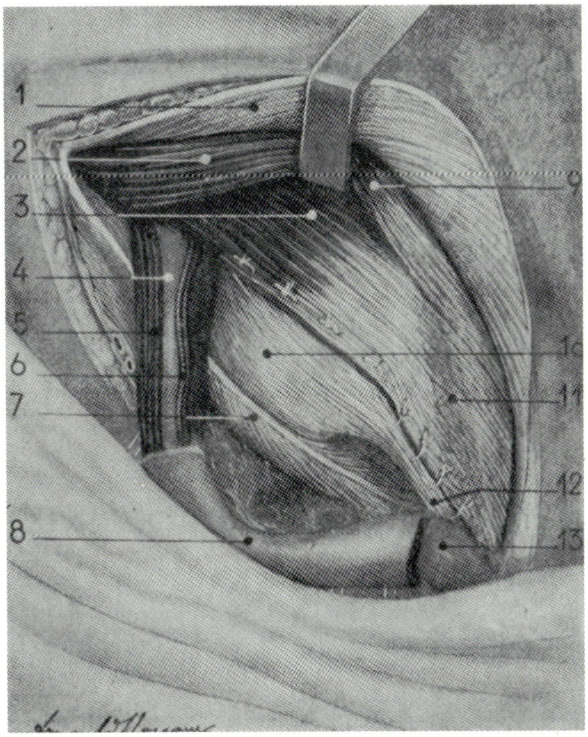

Figure 7. The fossa. The numbers 10 and 12 indicate the *bandelette iliopubienne*, which corresponds to the inferior segment of the fascia of the posterior inguinal wall (iliopubic tract). (From Fruchaud H: *Anatomie Chirurgicale des Hernies de l'Aine*. Paris: C Doin & Cie, 1956, p 169.)

The inferior segment of the fascia of the posterior inguinal wall, which forms the superior boundary of the pyriform fossa, turns down and then inward in a rolled or arched fashion to insert at approximately a 45-degree angle into the iliopectineal line (Cooper's ligament) (see Fig. 16). This insertion extends from the pubis to the medial angle of the femoral sheath. From this angle, it curves acutely outward to form the medial wall of the femoral sheath and then continues laterally to cover the femoral vessels; thus it is known as the anterior femoral sheath.

The inguinal ligament, the inferior boundary of the pyriform fossa, courses down and medially from its origin, the anterosuperior iliac spine, and passes over the anterior femoral sheath to form the crural arch—so named, according to Gimbernat, because of its ". . .resemblance to an arch or vault." It then continues medially to insert, as a paddle-shaped longitudinal expansion of its fibers, into the pubic tubercle, the adjacent medial angle of the fascia of the posterior inguinal wall, and the anterior part of Cooper's ligament, and forms the superficial or tendinous component of Gimbernat's ligament.

Between the crural arch and its tendinous insertion, the inguinal ligament and its accompanying portion of the fascia lata turn abruptly in on a horizontal plane (Gimbernat's "duplicature of the crural arch") to form a concave, triangular fascial expansion of radiating fibers that insert into Cooper's ligament as the deep or fascial component of Gimbernat's ligament (Fig. 8). Its lateral crescent-shaped base forms the medial boundary of the femoral sheath.

Accordingly, Cooper's ligament provides a conjoint line of insertion for the inferior segment of the fascia of the posterior inguinal wall superiorly and the fascial part of Gimbernat's ligament inferiorly. Although these two structures have a common line of insertion, they lie in separate directional and anatomic planes of origin (superior and inferior, respectively) (Fig. 9*A*). Also, Cooper's ligament is the site of origin of the pectineus muscle and fascia. This fascia, as it descends from its origin, lies in close apposition to the overlying fascial segment of Gimbernat's ligament as it ascends to insert into Cooper's ligament (Fig. 9*B*, *C*). These anatomic relationships are depicted semidiagrammatically for clarity. (Figure 9 is complemented by Plate LII, Figures 4 and 5.)

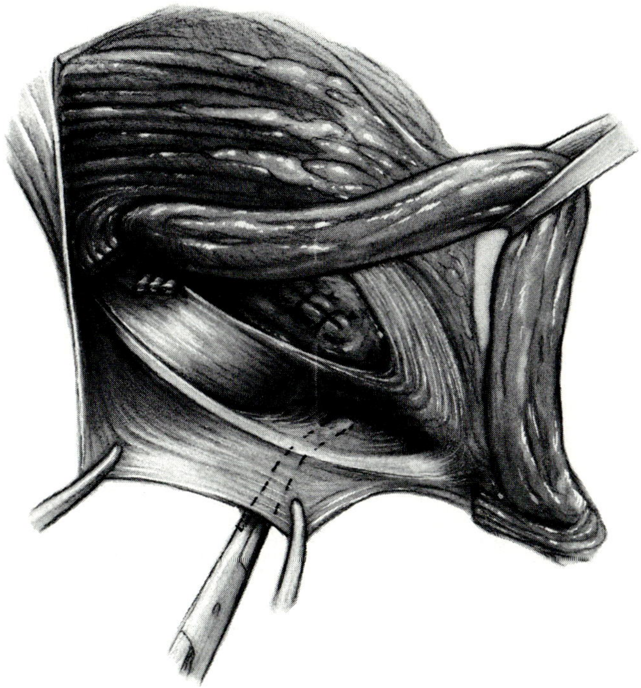

Figure 8. The deep or fascial part of Gimbernat's ligament is elevated on the tip of a curved clamp. Its superficial part inserts as a paddle-shaped tendinous expansion into the pubic tubercle, the adjacent medial angle of the fascia of the posterior inguinal wall, and the hidden, subjacent anterior part of Cooper's ligament.

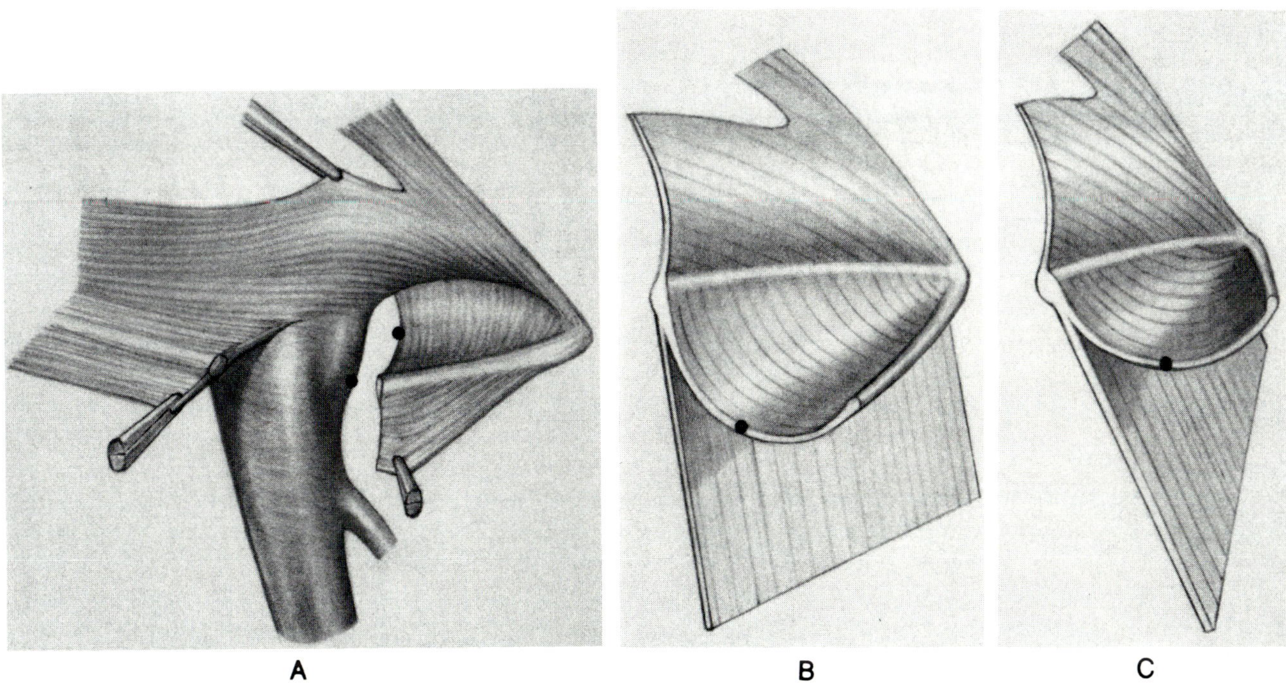

Figure 9. *A*, Semidiagrammatic representation of the conjoint line of insertion of the inferior segment of the fascia of the posterior inguinal wall (superior plane) and the deep fascial part of Gimbernat's ligament (inferior plane) into Cooper's ligament. The black dots indicate the site of the femoral hernial orifice (Lytle). *B, C*, Superior oblique and end-on views show the intimate adherence of the fascial part of Gimbernat's ligament and the pectineus fascia as they insert into and rise from Cooper's ligament, respectively. The black dots indicate the site of apposition of the concave crescentic base of Gimbernat's ligament with the fascial covering of the adjacent lower portion of the femoral canal. (These illustrations are complemented by Plate LII, Figs. 4 and 5.)

The tendinous component of Gimbernat's ligament often is perceived by the surgeon to represent the full extent of its insertion. This false image, which precludes complete surgical dissection of the inferior segment of the fascia of the posterior inguinal wall, has resulted in the mistaken belief that the shelving border of the inguinal ligament forms its inferior boundary. The fascial or fan-shaped component of Gimbernat's ligament is only visible when the pyriform fossa is completely exposed; it is then seen that this fascial component forms the floor of the fossa, which is the normal anatomic barrier between the peritoneum (cephalad) and the upper portion of the thigh (caudad).

Lytle[7] repeatedly stressed this composite anatomic origin of Gimbernat's ligament and declared it to be a confirmation of the previous anatomic studies of ". . .the two Antonio's; Gimbernat (1793) and Scarpa (1823)." It is unfortunate, however, that the two illustrations in Gimbernat's original article (Fig. 10*A, B*) are poorly done and do not agree with the text.[4] In contrast, Lytle's illustrated anatomy and descriptive text pertaining to the dual origin of Gimbernat's ligament are exemplary.[8] Furthermore, Lytle's cadaver dissection of the right inguinal region (see Fig. 22) clearly depicts the component parts of Gimbernat's ligament.[9] The longitudinal splaying of the fibers of the tendinous component as they insert into the anterior portion of Cooper's ligament is visible. The concave, triangular fascial component that inserts into Cooper's ligament can also be seen. Its base or lateral crescentic margin, so clearly visible, forms the medial boundary of the femoral sheath.

Lytle[10] also emphasized the anatomic fact that in an incarcerated or strangulated femoral hernia, the obstruction is not at the femoral ring but below it, at the site of a defect in the medial wall of the femoral sheath that is in juxtaposition to the unyielding lateral crescentic margin of Gimbernat's ligament. To release the obstruction requires a partial transection of this ligament, as described originally by Gimbernat.

This hernial defect in the femoral sheath, named the "femoral hernial orifice" by Lytle[8] (Fig. 11), is approximately 1.5 cm below or caudad to the femoral ring. Subsequent to Lytle's description, the precise location of the femoral hernial orifice and its consistent relation to the concave crescentic margin of Gimbernat's ligament has been repeatedly confirmed at operation. Furthermore, simple closure of this orifice is the anatomic essence of the "low" or femoral approach for the elective repair of a femoral hernia. It may also complement an emergency operation performed through an inguinal or "high" approach for an acutely strangulated or incarcerated femoral hernia. The phrase "closure of the femoral ring" is actually a semantic anomaly, since the anatomic configuration of this "ring" precludes its surgical closure.

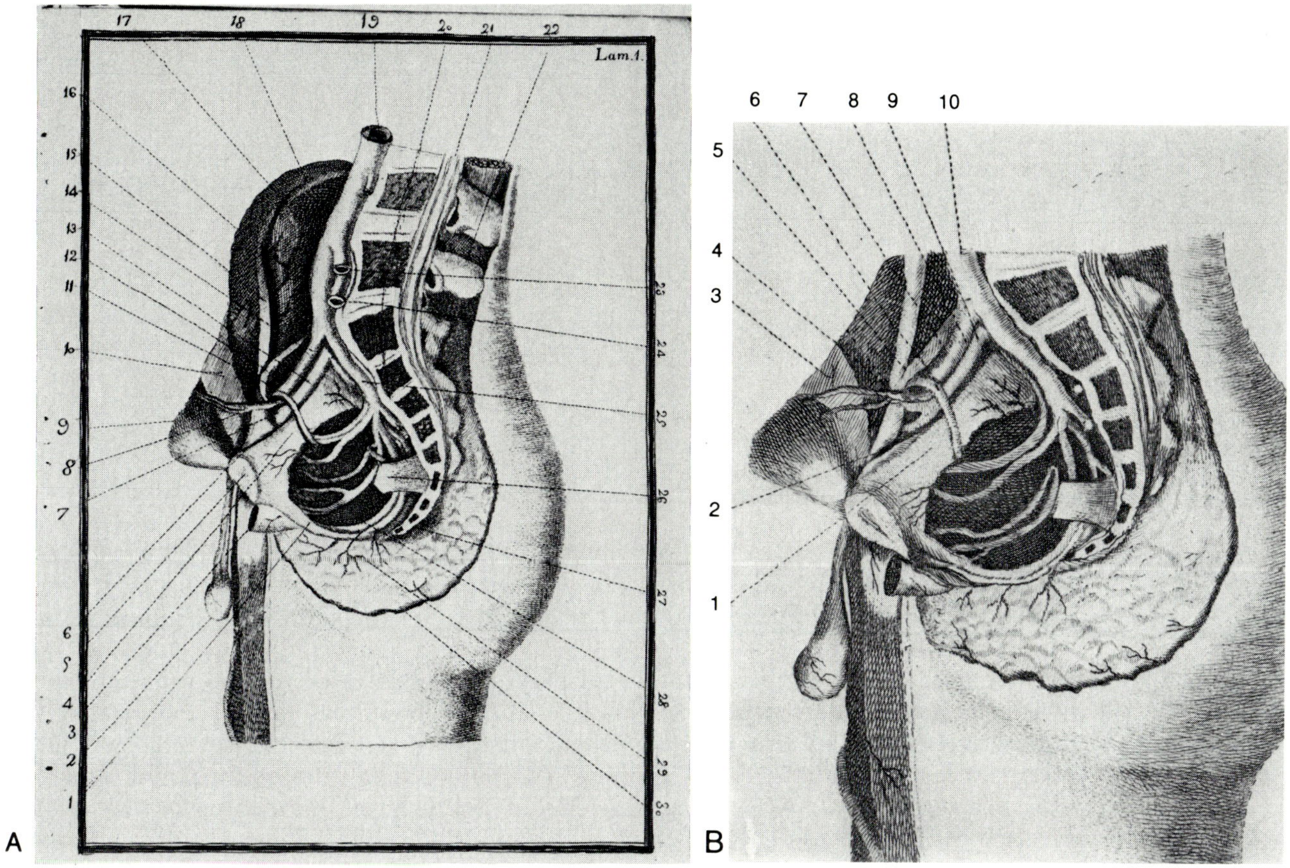

Figure 10. The original illustrations of the "duplicature of the crural arch" (Gimbernat's ligament), before (*A*, No. 6) and after (*B*, No. 2) its severance. They do not, however, provide a practical anatomic orientation for the surgeon, and furthermore, they are not in conformity with the descriptive text.

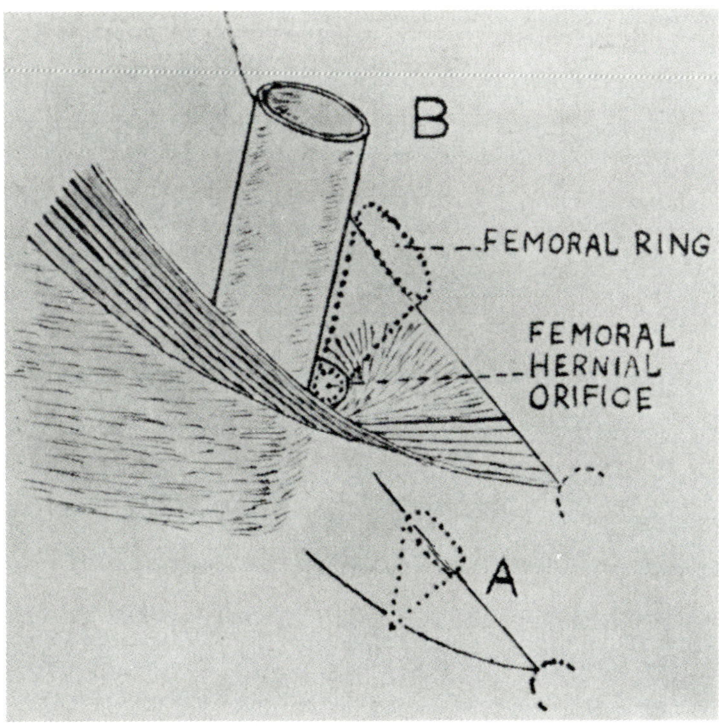

Figure 11. The "femoral hernial orifice" (Lytle). *A* shows in dashed lines the intact femoral canal; *B* shows the canal breached by a femoral hernia. The curved edge of Gimbernat's ligament lies at the site of the orifice. (From Lytle WJ: Anatomy and function in hernia repair. Proc R Soc Med *54*:967–970, 1961.)

In support of Gimbernat's concept of the "duplicature of the crural arch" is the striking semidiagrammatic illustration of Testut (Fig. 12), which depicts a broad fascial structure extending in continuity from a highly mobilized inguinal ligament to its insertion into the iliopectineal line.[12]

Additional support for this concept may be demonstrated at operation. Following the exposure of the external oblique aponeurosis, mobilization and elevation of the characteristic abrupt turn-in of the external border of the inguinal ligament will make apparent its continuation and ultimate insertion into the iliopectineal line (Cooper's ligament) (Fig. 13). Also, since the site of the femoral hernial orifice is exposed concomitantly, the presence of a femoral hernia in the initial stages of the repair of an inguinal hernia may be detected. In fact, it is specifically for this purpose that the technique is routinely used.

Further surgical confirmation of Gimbernat's concept is obtained after exposure of the pyriform fossa. Two clamps are applied to the cut margin of the inferior leaflet of the aponeurosis of the external oblique muscle, and strong outward retraction is applied. The continuity of the aponeurosis with the internal fascial expansion of the inguinal (Gimbernat's) ligament and its insertion into the iliopectineal line are demonstrated (see Fig. 8).

Sir Astley Cooper of London apparently was fully cognizant of Gimbernat's original work in Spanish (1793) and its English translation (1795), since he referred to Gimbernat in his own publications in 1804[2] and 1807. In the latter Cooper wrote, ". . .a fascia is attached to the posterior edge of the crural arch and extends. . .over the iliacus and psoas muscles. It has been particularly described by Gimbernat, and should be called from its situation, the '*fascia iliaca.*' "[3]

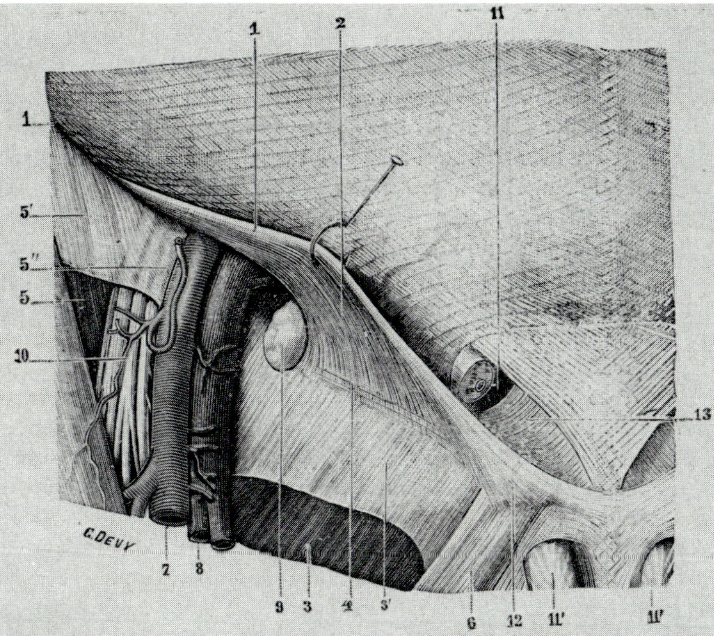

Fig. 663.
La partie interne de l'arcade crurale, érignée en haut pour montrer la partie réfléchie de cette arcade ou ligament de Gimbernat.

Figure 12. Semidiagrammatic illustration of the right inguinal region (Testut), showing the mobilized crural arch held upward by a hook (1). Its relation to the underlying Gimbernat's ligament (2) and the iliopectineal line (4) is depicted.

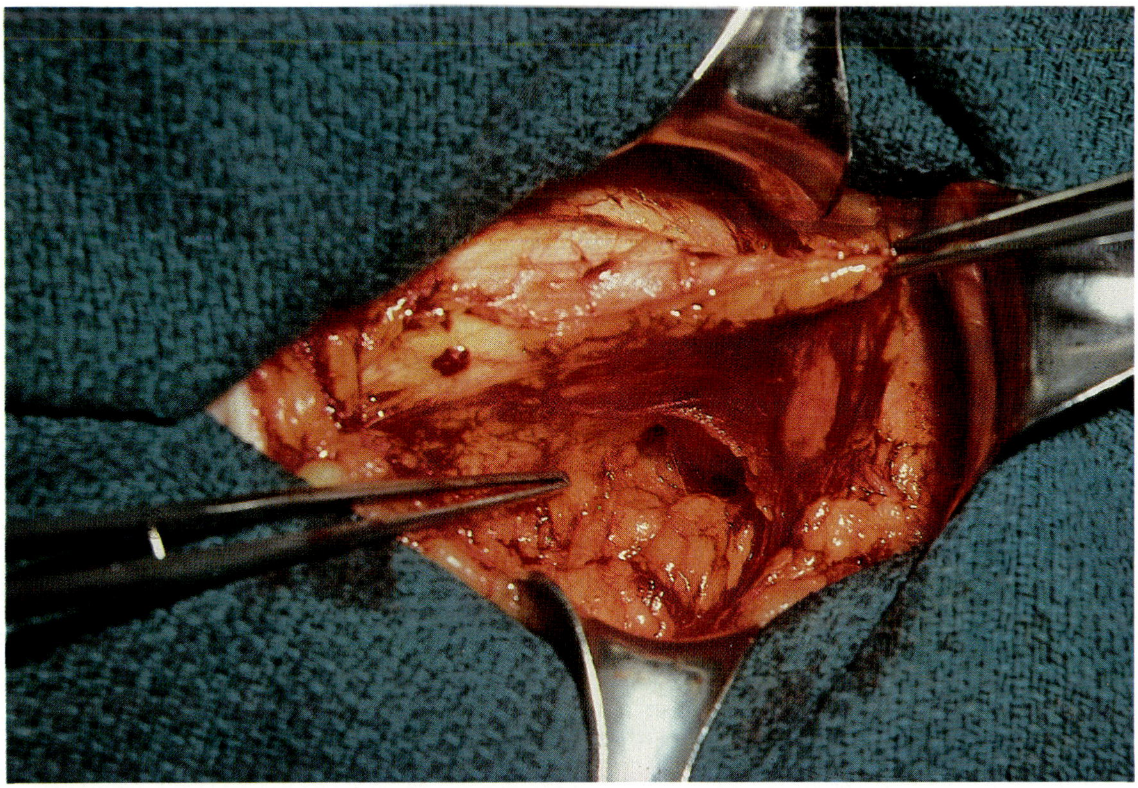

Figure 13. Intraoperative color photograph, complementary to Figure 12 but on the left side, demonstrating the turn-in of the inguinal ligament. The tip of the tissue forceps is the directional line to the oval opening in the pectineus fascia that juxtaposes the femoral hernial orifice. This technical maneuver, in an early stage of the operation, rules out the presence of a concomitant femoral hernia.

However, Gimbernat described not only the fascia iliaca but also the ligament that bears his name, to which Cooper never referred. This is difficult to understand since on the page immediately preceding the "Description of the Crural Arch," Gimbernat noted that "That part. . .had been little examined. . .till I demonstrated it for the first time in 1768."[5] (This, incidentally, was the year in which Cooper was born.) Furthermore, the English translation of Gimbernat's monograph was entitled "New Method of Operating for the Femoral Hernia." Its primary purpose was to describe and illustrate the surgical technique for the severance of the crescentic margin of Gimbernat's ligament in the treatment of the incarcerated or strangulated crural (femoral) hernia. It is ironic, therefore, that Cooper would link Gimbernat's name to the fascia iliaca and not to the ligament referred to by his contemporaries, and since then by all surgeons, as Gimbernat's ligament.

Describing the crural arch, Gimbernat stated that "In the lower abdomen, the external oblique muscle forms a strong and broad aponeurosis. The fibers are parallel; they descend obliquely from without inwards, and the lower extend from the anterior superior spine of the ilium to the os pubis. . . ." In his description of the duplicature of the crural arch he wrote: "The particular disposition of this duplicature, extending from below upwards, and its insertion from the spine to the end of the crest [ileopectineal line], which makes more than an inch in some subjects, is highly worthy of our consideration, for without it, we should all probably suffer large and dangerous protrusions of the abdomen. In consequence of this structure, the crural arch [inguinal ligament] has two edges, one external. . .; to this adheres the expansion of the fascia lata; . . . The other. . .internal, is the termination of the edge of the aponeurosis. . . ."

The "internal edge" represent the lateral crescentic margin of the fascial portion of Gimbernat's ligament that forms the medial boundary of the femoral sheath. Interestingly, this edge was later described by Cooper as the third insertion of the aponeurosis of the external oblique muscle that ". . .forms a crescent shaped edge which is turned towards the crural vein. . . ."

Another controversy pertaining to Gimbernat's ligament concerns its base or lateral crescentic margin. Both McVay[11] and Condon[1] have stated that the iliopubic tract, and not the lateral crescentic margin of Gimbernat's ligament, forms the medial boundary of the femoral sheath. Admittedly, this tract (the inferior segment of the fascia of the posterior inguinal wall) in its acute angulation laterally forms the medial wall of the femoral sheath and the anterior femoral sheath, respectively. It is believed, therefore, to be an intrinsic fascial component rather than a true anatomic boundary of the femoral sheath. Furthermore, in the surgical treatment of femoral hernias McVay observed attrition of the insertion of the fascia of the posterior inguinal wall into Cooper's ligament, the extent of which varied in direct ratio to the size of the hernia. Accordingly, he postulated that a femoral hernia, as it enlarges, ultimately abuts against the unyielding lateral crescentic margin of Gimbernat's ligament and creates the false impression that this ligament forms the medial boundary of the femoral sheath.

For this to occur, however, it would seen an absolute necessity that the insertion of the fascia of the posterior inguinal wall into Cooper's ligament and the crescentic margin of Gimbernat's ligament be on the same anatomic plane. Yet in Figure 9 and in the photograph of the cadaver dissection by Lytle (see Fig. 22), the fascia of the posterior inguinal wall is on a plane superior to that of its inferior counterpart, the fascial portion of Gimbernat's ligament. It would be anatomically impossible, therefore, for an enlarging femoral hernia to abut against the lateral crescentic margin of Gimbernat's ligament, regardless of the extent of attrition of the insertion of the fascia of the posterior inguinal wall into Cooper's ligament. In fact, even a total attrition of its insertion by excision (see Fig. 21) would not terminate in such an abutment, since it is on a plane superior to that of Gimbernat's ligament.

Furthermore, the unyielding crescentic margin of Gimbernat's ligament constitutes the anatomic reason why the acutely strangulated femoral hernia is almost invariably small. Owing to its small size, it is frequently unrecognized as the cause of an existing acute small bowel obstruction. Interestingly, in this regard Gimbernat observed, "If the particular structure of the crural arch and its tension are kept up by the expansion of the fascia lata. . .we shall clearly see the reason why the crural [femoral] seldom obtains so great a bulk as the inguinal hernia."

It appears, then, that these anatomic and clinical observations negate the attritional postulate of McVay. In addition, since the lateral crescentic margin of Gimbernat's ligament maintains a relatively fixed and unyielding anatomic relationship with the femoral sheath (see Fig. 22), it represents its true medial boundary. This agrees with the "old" rather than the "new" anatomic concept expressed by McVay and Condon.

REFERENCES

1. Condon RE: The anatomy of the inguinal region and its relationship to groin hernias. In Nyhus LM and Harkins H (eds): *Hernia.* Philadelphia: JB Lippincott, 1964, pp 34–35.
2. Cooper AP: *The Anatomy and Surgical Treatment of Inguinal and Congenital Hernia.* London: Longman & Co, 1804, p 5.
3. Cooper AP: *The Anatomy and Surgical Treatment of Crural and Umbilical Hernia, Part II.* London: Longman & Co, 1807, p 3.
4. De Gimbernat DA: *Nuevo Método De Operar En La Hernia Crural.* Madrid: Ibarra, 1793.
5. De Gimbernat DA: *New Method of Operating for the Femoral Hernia* (English translation from Spanish). London: J. Johnson, 1795.
6. Fruchaud H: *Anatomie Chirurgicale des Hernies de l'Aine.* Paris: C Doin & Cie, 1956, p. 301.
7. Lytle WJ: Femoral hernia. Brit J Hosp Med *4*(1):17–22, 1970.
8. Lytle WJ: Femoral hernia. Ann R Coll Surg Engl *21*:244–262, 1957.
9. Lytle WJ: The inguinal and lacunar ligaments. J Anat *118*(2):241–251, 1974.
10. Lytle WJ: Anatomy and function in hernia repair. Proc R Soc Med *54*:967–970, 1961.
11. McVay CB: *Hernia.* Springfield: Charles C Thomas, 1954.
12. Testut L: *Traité D'Anatomie Humaine.* Quatrième Edition. Tome Premier. Paris: Octave Doin, 1899, p 818.
13. Thomson A: Cause anatomique de la hernie inguinale externe. Journal des Connaissances Médicales, Tome quatrième (1836–1837), 137–164 (1er article), 169–176 (2e article).

INTRAOPERATIVE ILLUSTRATIONS AND COMPLEMENTARY PHOTOGRAPHS

Figure 14 The large peritoneal sac of a direct hernia has been excised and its wide base closed with interrupted sutures, mattress and simple, of 4-0 silk. The hernial defect in the fascia of the posterior inguinal wall and its relationship to the pyriform fossa (caudad) and the surrounding structures are visible. The basic principle in the repair of a groin hernia is closure of the fascial defect by suture of the superior segment of the fascia of the posterior inguinal wall to the inferior segment (iliopubic tract), using interrupted sutures of 3-0 silk.

Figure 15 A clamp is applied to the cut margin of the inferior segment of the fascia of the posterior inguinal wall at the site where it angulates acutely outward and continues laterally as the anterior femoral sheath. Upward traction on the clamp demonstrates the turn-in of the inferior fascial segment as it courses to insert into the iliopectineal line (Cooper's ligament).

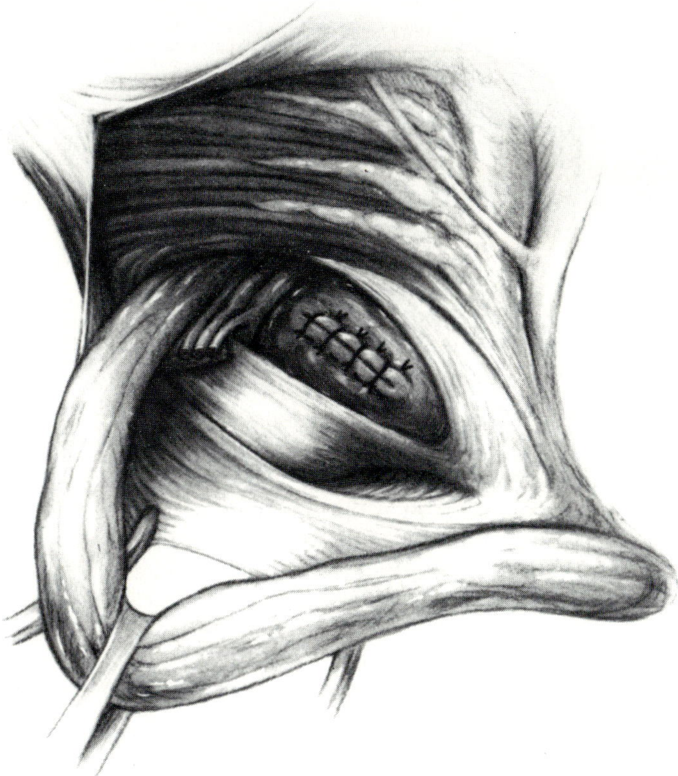

14

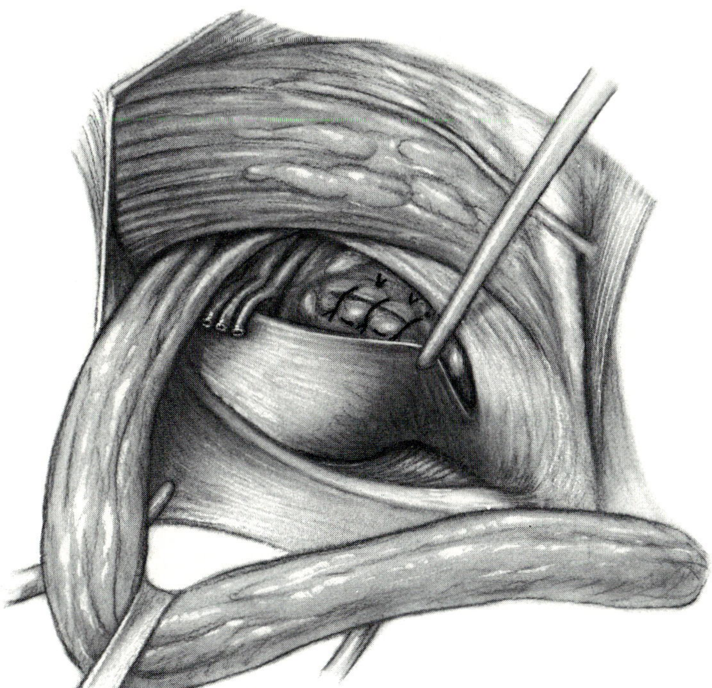

15

INTRAOPERATIVE ILLUSTRATIONS AND COMPLEMENTARY PHOTOGRAPHS

Continued

Figure 16 An intraoperative photograph, complementary to Figure 15, shows the same turn-in of the inferior fascial segment and its continuation laterally as the anterior femoral sheath. The relationship of this segment to the underlying pyriform fossa and inguinal ligament can also be seen.

Figure 17 A second intraoperative photograph complementary to Figure 15 clearly depicts the pyriform fossa in relation to the surrounding structures that form its boundaries. These boundaries are superiorly, the inferior segment of the fascia of the posterior inguinal wall (held in clamps); inferiorly, the inguinal ligament; laterally, the medial wall of the anterior femoral sheath; and medially, the convergence of the paddle-shaped tendinous expansion of the inguinal ligament (Gimbernat's) and the medial angle of the fascia of the posterior inguinal wall. Subjacent and hidden is the anterior part of the "linea ileopectinea" (Cooper's ligament). The floor of the pyriform fossa is formed by the fascial or lateral part of Gimbernat's ligament.

The inferior segment of the fascia of the posterior inguinal wall is retracted upward by two clamps to show the turn-in of its insertion, at approximately a 45-degree angle, into the iliopectineal line (Cooper's ligament). This insertion occurs conjointly with the approximate 90-degree angle of insertion of the fascial or deep part of Gimbernat's ligament, but on an anatomic plane superior to it.

The location of the lateral clamp corresponds to the site of completion of the "transition" suture of McVay[3] in the surgical reconstruction of the medial wall of the femoral sheath. Between this clamp and the tissue forceps lateral to it, the inferior segment of the fascia of the posterior inguinal wall continues laterally over the femoral vessels to form the anterior femoral sheath.

Figure 17A In this intraoperative photograph complementary to Figure 17, the cut margin of the inferior segment of the fascia of the posterior inguinal wall is retracted up and held taut with tissue forceps showing the turn-in as it courses at an angle of about 45 degrees to insert into the pecten pubis (iliopectineal line).

The tips of the forceps laterally correspond to the site of the acute outward angulation of the inferior segment of the fascia of the posterior inguinal wall to form the medial wall of the femoral sheath, and its continuation laterally as the anterior femoral sheath. The relationship of its medial portion to the underlying pyriform fossa and tendinous expansion of the inguinal ligament is visible.

The existence of an inferior segment of the fascia of the posterior inguinal wall is often questioned. Its recognition at operation, however, varies in direct ratio to the extent of the surgical dissection. The key to this recognition is the exposure of the pyriform fossa. When identified, it invariably demonstrates excellent "holding power," as is evident in the photograph.

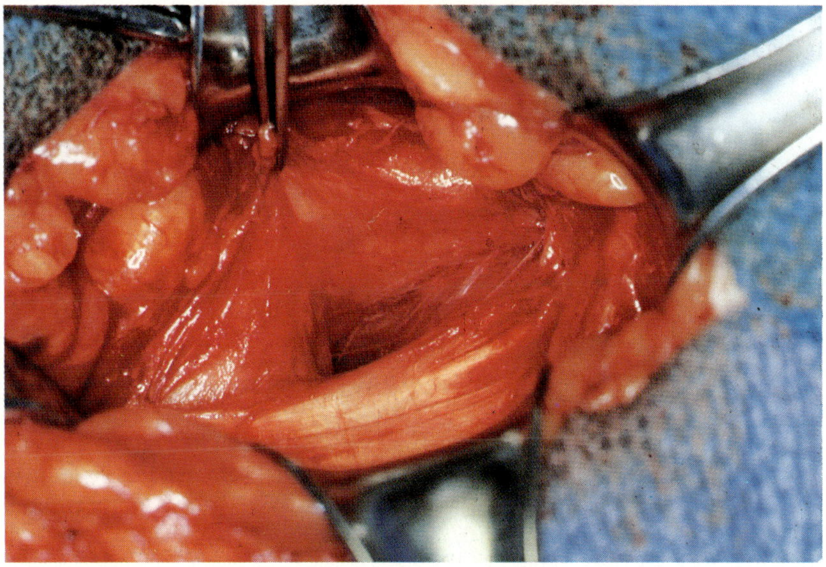

16

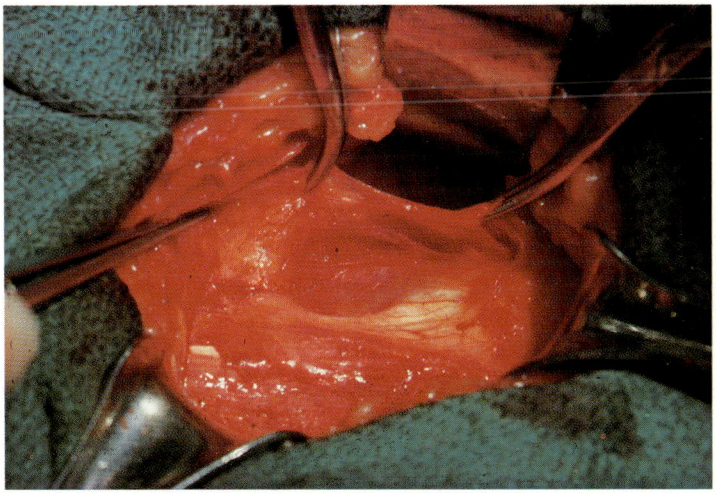

17

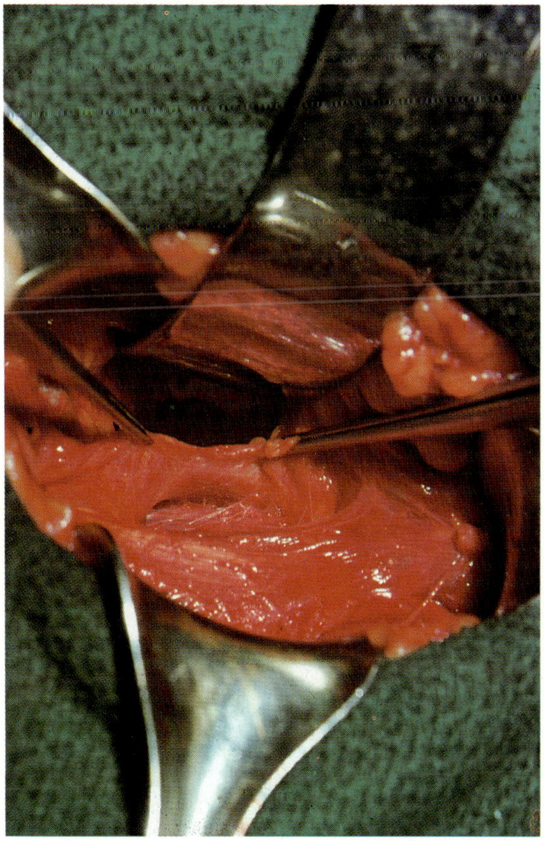

17A

Figures 18, 18A An intraoperative photograph (Fig. 18), showing the tip of a Mixter clamp inserted between the inguinal ligament (crural arch) and the underlying anterior femoral sheath, demonstrates that the inguinal ligament has only a contiguous anatomic relationship in the repair of a groin hernia.

The extent of the distance between the inguinal ligament and the inferior segment of the fascia of the posterior inguinal wall, held taut in clamps, is visible. Therefore, in repairing the hernial defect, it is anatomically more effective to suture the superior segment of the fascia of the posterior inguinal wall to its inferior segment than to the more distant inguinal ligament.

This photograph is complemented by the artist's illustration (Fig. 18A).

Figure 19 The right posterolateral wall of the peritoneum and subjacent intraperitoneal viscera are retracted inward, and the inferior segment of the fascia of the posterior inguinal wall (held in a clamp) is retracted down and out to show the turn-in of its insertion into Cooper's ligament. The posterior extension of this ligament is visible beneath the tip of the retractor.

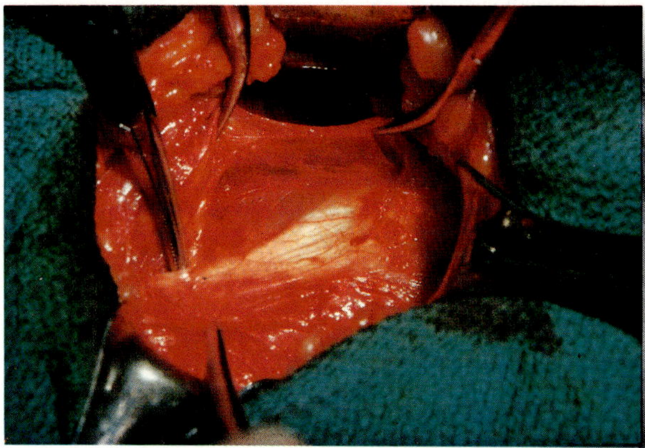

18

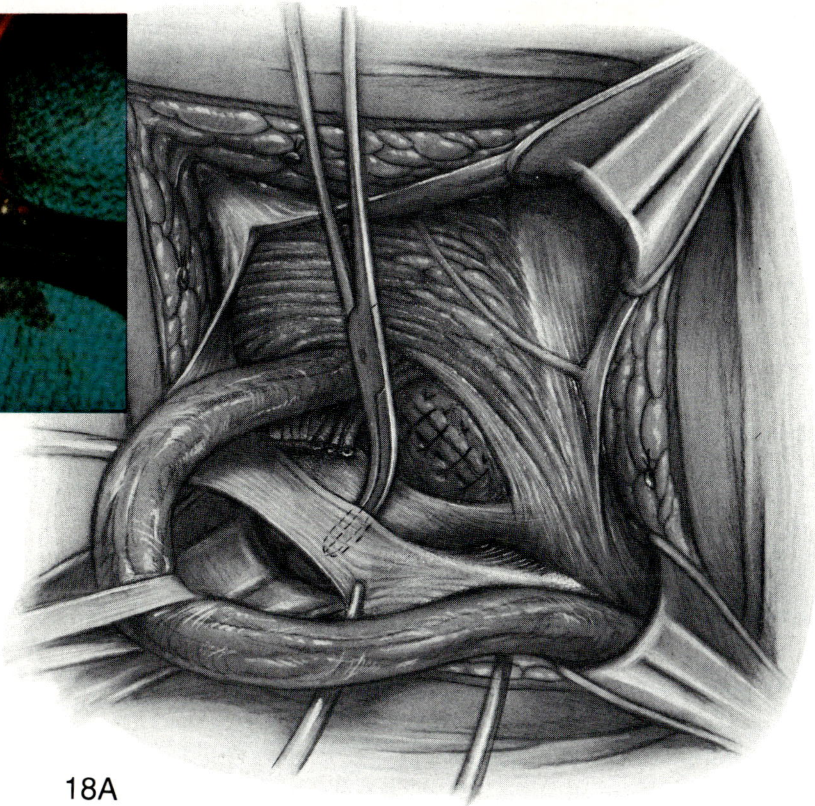

18A

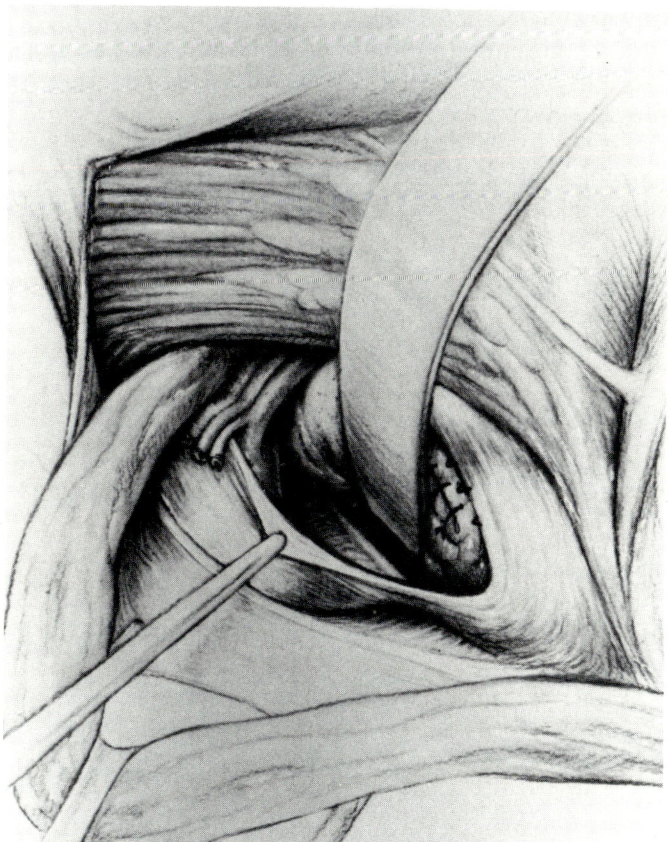

19

Figures 20, 20A These intraoperative photographs are complementary to Figure 19. The inferior segment of the fascia of the posterior inguinal wall is elevated to show its insertion into Cooper's ligament, as indicated by the tips of the tissue forceps (Fig. 20).

The inferior fascial segment is retracted down and out to demonstrate Cooper's ligament (oblique white line), into which it inserts (Fig. 20A).

Figure 21 For clarity of illustration, the inferior segment of the fascia of the posterior inguinal wall and its lateral extension as the medial and anterior walls of the femoral sheath have been excised. Medially, the origin of Cooper's ligament and the juxtaposed insertion of the paddle-shaped expansion of the inguinal ligament (tendinous portion of Gimbernat's ligament) are clearly visible. The medial angle of the expansion of the superior segment of the fascia of the posterior inguinal wall also may be seen.

Extending laterally from the medial angle, between the inguinal and Cooper's ligaments, is the concave, triangular fascial expansion of Gimbernat's ligament, the base of which terminates in a crescentic margin that forms the unyielding medial boundary of the femoral sheath. The intimate apposition of the fibers of this crescentic fascial margin and the underlying pectineus fascia at their insertion and origin, respectively (relative to Cooper's ligament), is visible.

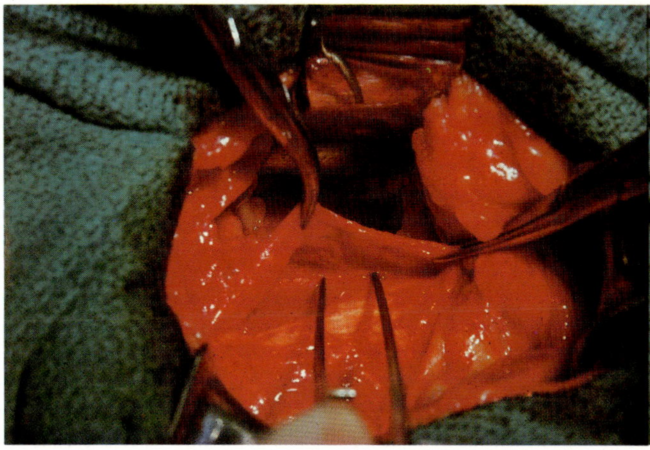

20

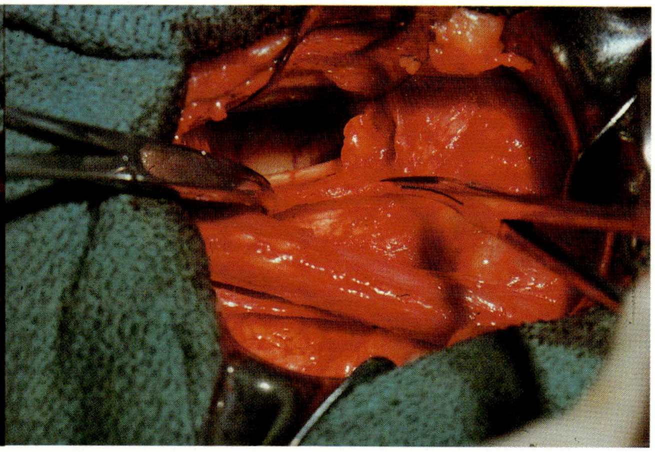

20A

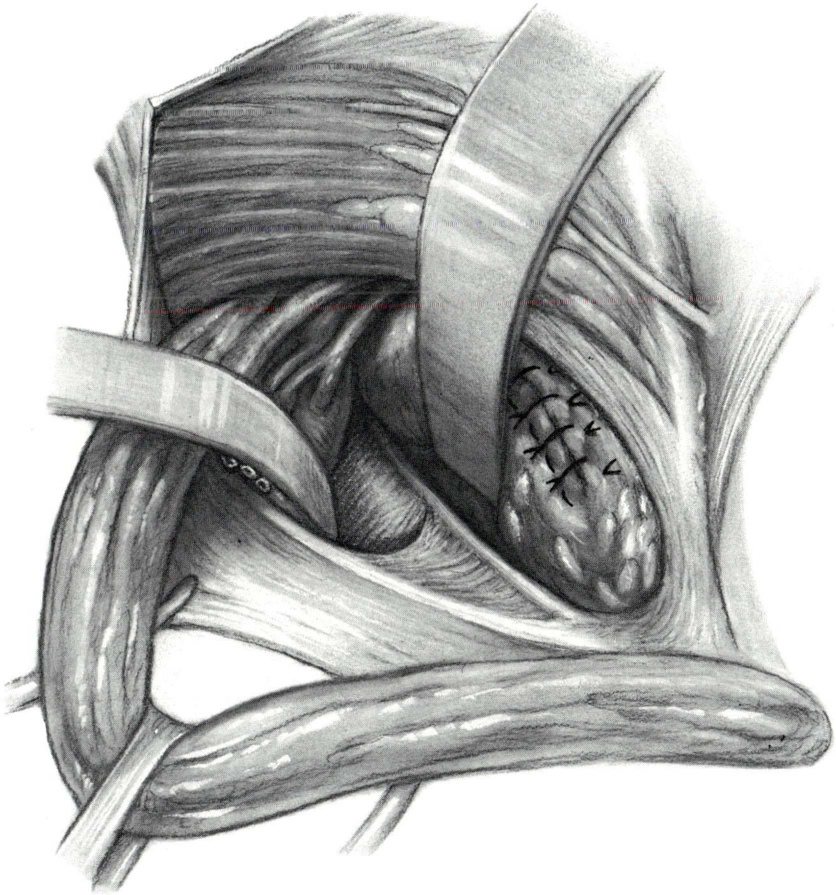

21

Figure 22 In this photograph of a cadaver dissection by Lytle[2] of a normal right groin of a male, the inguinal ligament has been transected at the level of the central portion of the femoral sheath; its medial segment, grasped in a clamp, is retracted down to expose the lateral, and fixed, crescentic margin of the fascial part of Gimbernat's ligament, which forms the medial boundary or border of the femoral sheath.

Despite the retraction force applied to the medial transected end of the inguinal ligament, the cleft between the medial wall of the femoral sheath and the crescentic margin of Gimbernat's ligament is disproportionately narrow. In both the intact cadaver specimen and the "living" state, this cleft would not be as wide. This agrees with the generally held opinion that the crescentic margin of Gimbernat's ligament constitutes a fixed and unyielding boundary (border) of the medial wall of the femoral sheath. Such a relationship would explain why the acutely strangulated femoral hernia is invariably small and, therefore, frequently undetected as the cause of an existing acute small bowel obstruction.

The upward traction on the "rake" retractor, attached to the inferior segment of the fascia of the posterior inguinal wall, has avulsed its fascial attachment to Cooper's ligament, as is shown by the space visible between these two structures. The continuation laterally of the inferior segment of the fascia, first as the medial wall of the femoral sheath and then as the truncated funnel-shaped anterior femoral sheath, is clearly depicted. In fact, this cadaver dissection is in complete accord with the surgical anatomy, as portrayed both in the illustrations and in the intraoperative photographs.

Figure 23 The superior and inferior segments of the fascia of the posterior inguinal wall are drawn taut to expose the medial angle of the hernial defect. The thickness of the fascial segments and the adequacy of their "holding power" for sutures are apparent. The relation of the inferior segment to the underlying paddle-shaped tendinous expansion of the inguinal ligament is readily seen.

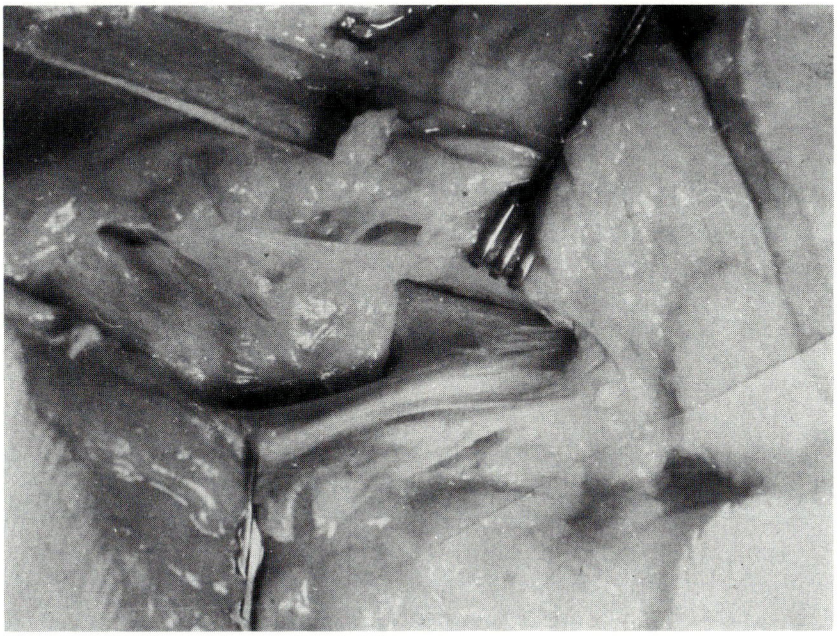

22

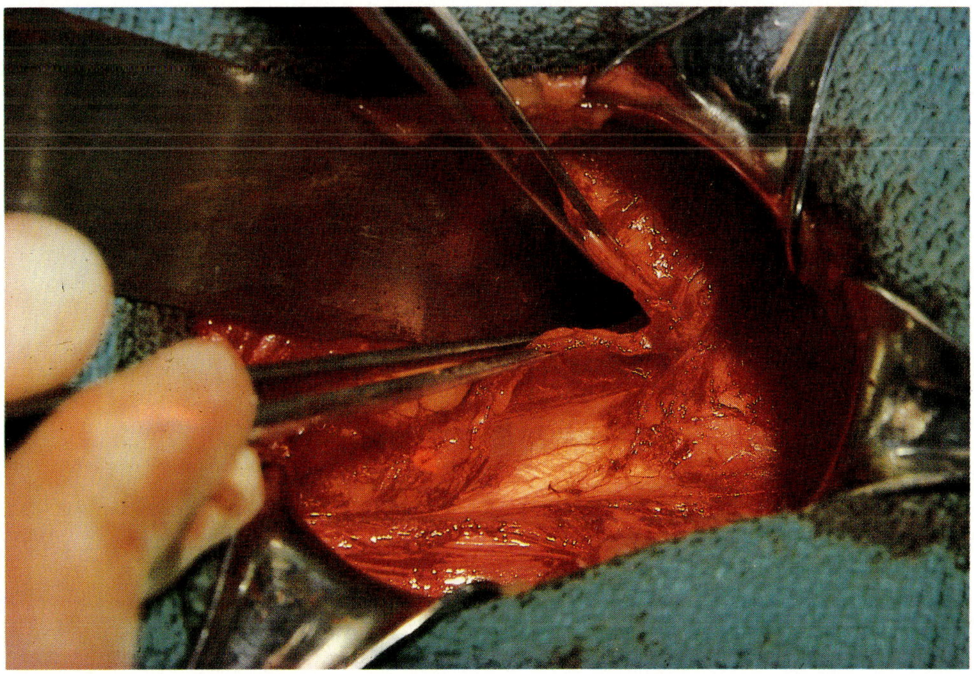

23

Figures 24, 24A The closure of the fascial defect in the posterior inguinal wall ("floor") is begun by the insertion of the medial-angle or "crown" suture of 3-0 silk. The suture is inserted through the superior fascial segment and then continued, from below, through this fascial layer at its medial angle (Fig. 24). A good "bite" in this angle is essential to preclude a recurrence of the hernia. The suture is then drawn through the inferior fascial segment to complete its insertion, as shown in the intraoperative photograph (Fig. 24A).

Figure 25 The completed insertion of the crown suture is indicated by the direction of the arrows. The relationship of the inferior segment of the fascia of the posterior inguinal wall, both to Cooper's ligament (subjacent to the retractor) and to the femoral sheath and vessels laterally, may be seen.

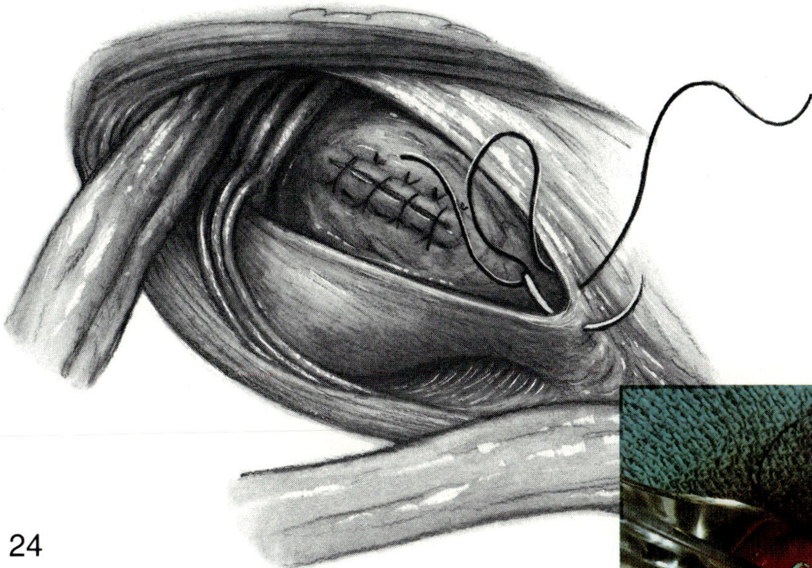

24

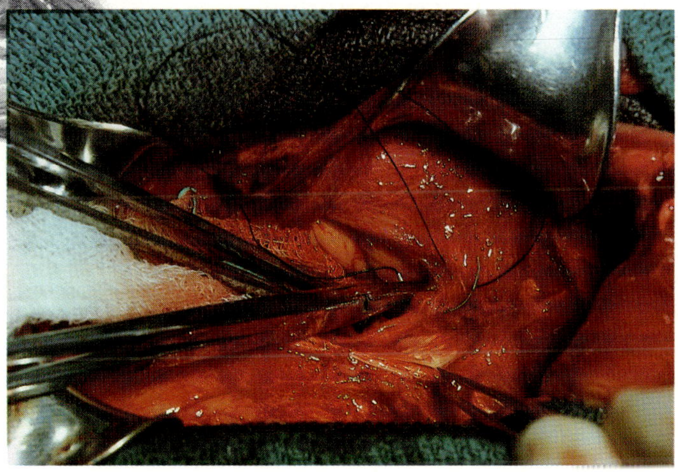

24A

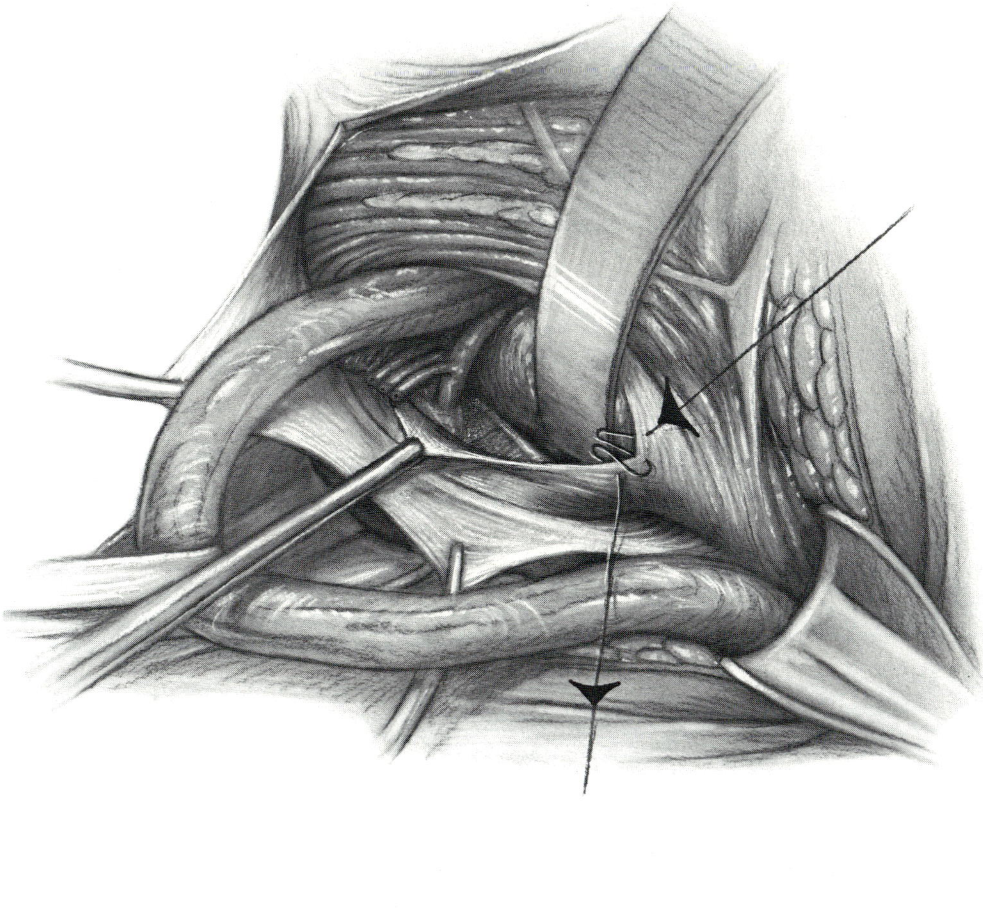

25

INTRAOPERATIVE ILLUSTRATIONS AND COMPLEMENTARY PHOTOGRAPHS
Continued

Figure 26 The illustration depicts the normal in-continuity closure of the fascia of the medial portion of the posterior inguinal wall. The lateral suture being inserted is in the same site as the "transition" suture of McVay.[3] It differs, however, in that it effects a normal anatomic fascial restoration, without either a mandatory "relaxing" incision in the rectus sheath or a resulting trough deformity.

Figure 27 In this intraoperative photograph, the "transition" suture has been tied and its strands have been retracted down to expose the completed in-continuity closure of the medial wall of the femoral sheath and the fascial reconstruction of the medial portion of the fascia of the posterior inguinal wall. The relationship of the suture line to the underlying pyriform fossa and inguinal ligament is visible.

The lateral portion of the superior segment of the fascia of the posterior inguinal wall is elevated with forceps to show its relationship to the transected funnel-shaped margin of the anterior femoral sheath below.

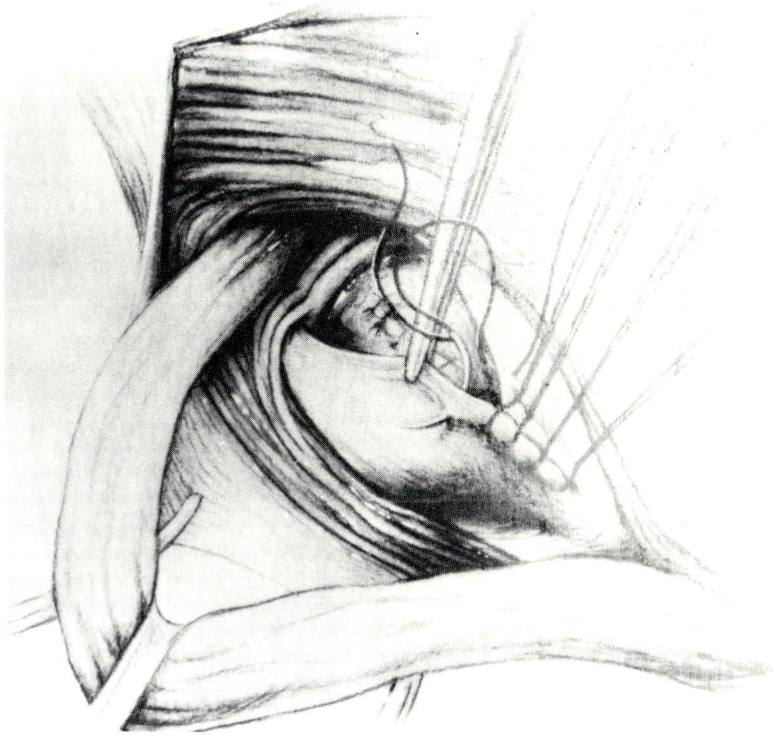

26

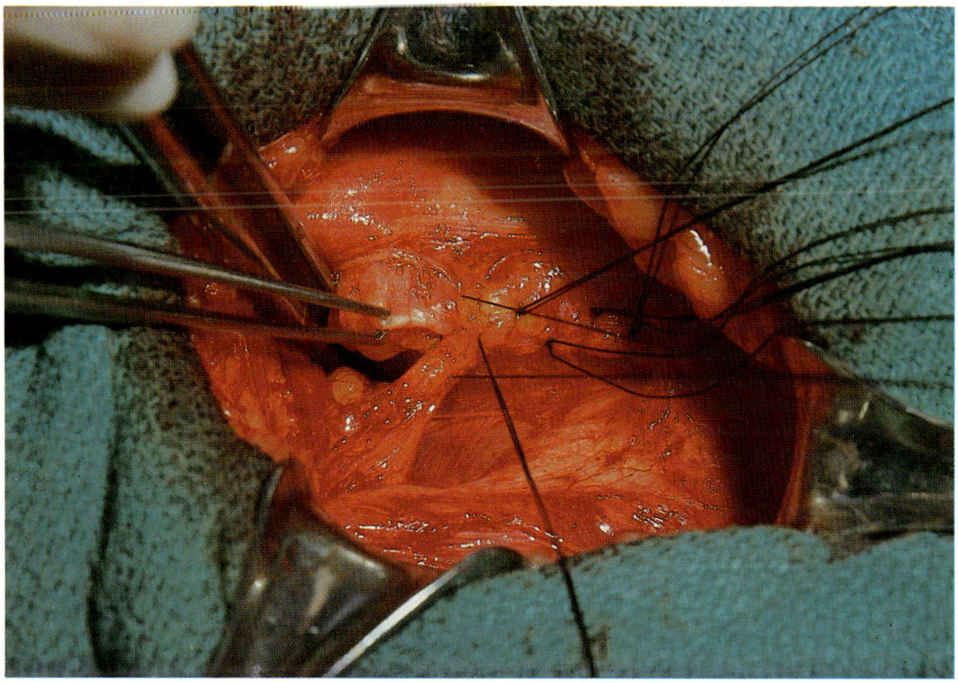

27

Figure 28 The reconstruction of the hernial defect in the fascia of the posterior inguinal wall is completed. The tied strands of the suture, lateral to the strands of the transition suture (retracted down), effect a snug closure of the internal ring around the exit of the spermatic cord. The internal oblique muscle superiorly and the inguinal ligament inferiorly have a proximate anatomic relationship only in the repair of an inguinal hernia.

Figure 29 The spermatic cord is elevated preparatory to being repositioned on the underlying one-layer fascial reconstruction of the posterior inguinal wall.

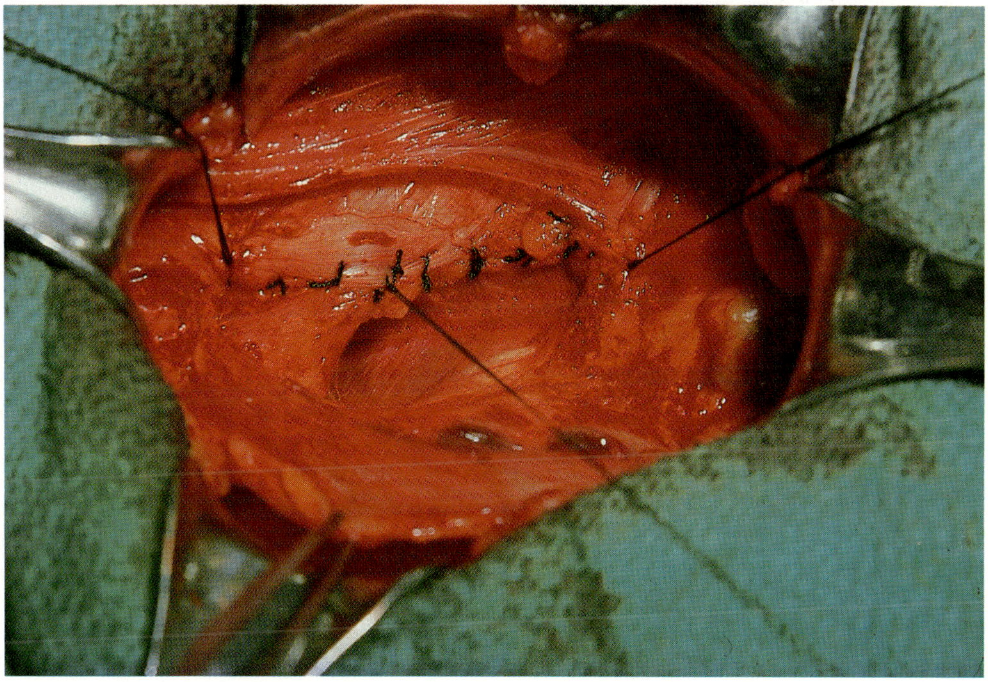
28

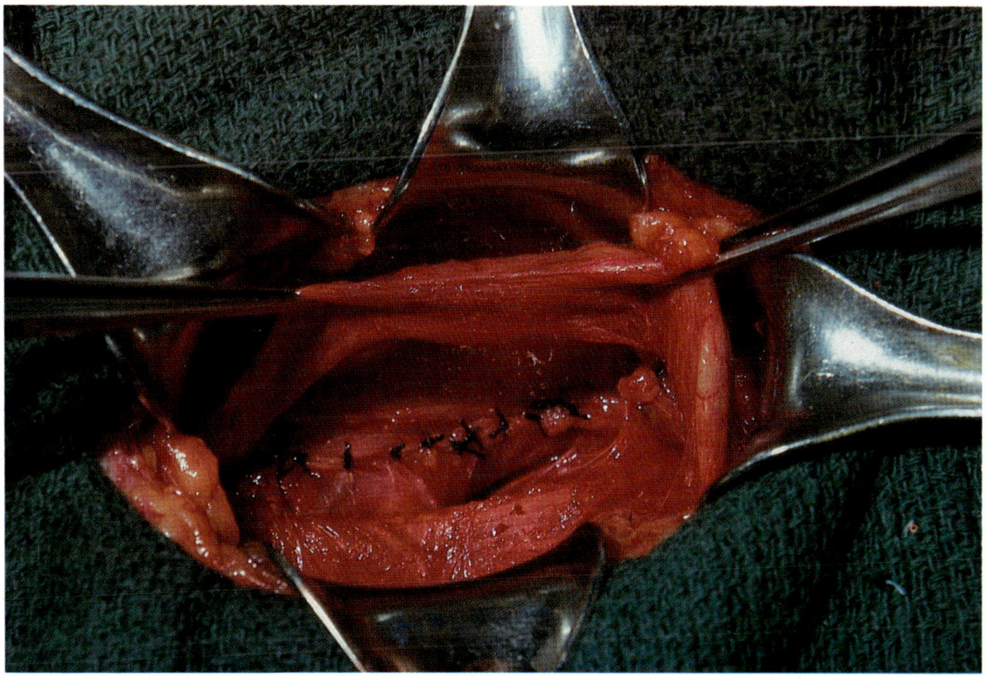
29

Figure 30 To emphasize the anatomy of repair, the surgical technique is demonstrated in a second patient, a 76-year-old man with a large right direct inguinal hernia and sliding hernia of the bladder.

The reconstruction of the fascia of the posterior inguinal wall is begun by the approximation medially of its superior and inferior segments, using interrupted sutures of 3-0 silk. The medial angle suture is tied, and for technical expediency the subsequent sutures are inserted, preparatory to being tied. The suture that is farthest lateral, when tied, will restore the medial wall of the femoral sheath. Its position corresponds to the site of the transition suture of McVay,[3] but on a normal rather than abnormal anatomic plane.

Figure 31 The sutures are tied to reconstruct the medial portion of the fascia of the posterior inguinal wall. The relationship of the suture line to the juxtaposed femoral sheath and underlying pyriform fossa is again evident. The inguinal ligament courses anterior to the femoral sheath (crural arch) and continues medially to its insertion into the pubic tubercle, thereby forming the inferior boundary of the pyriform fossa.

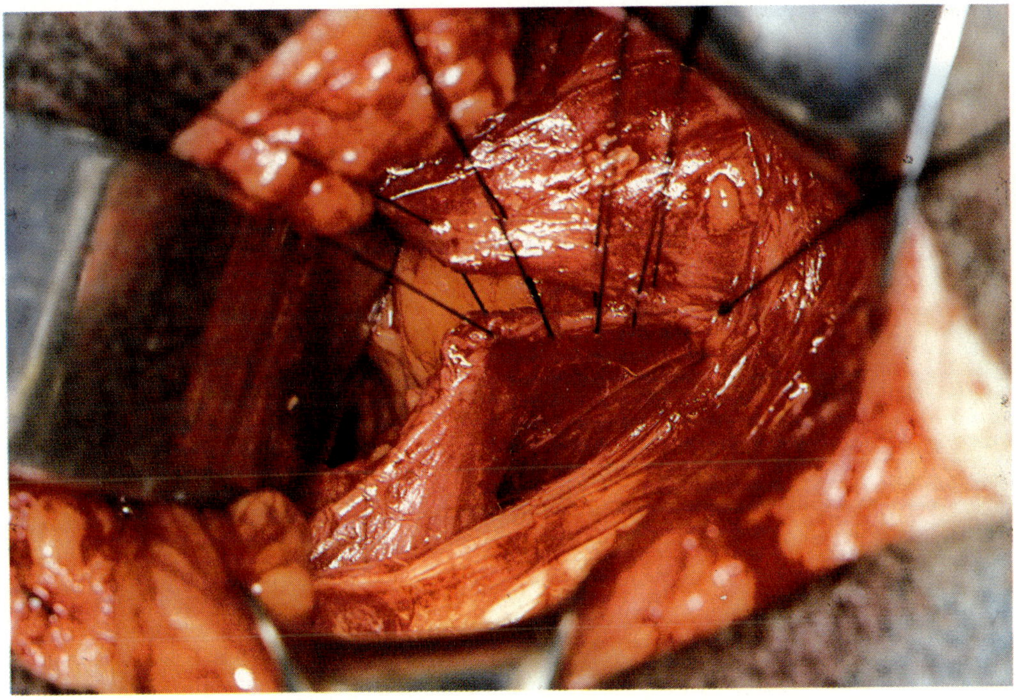

30

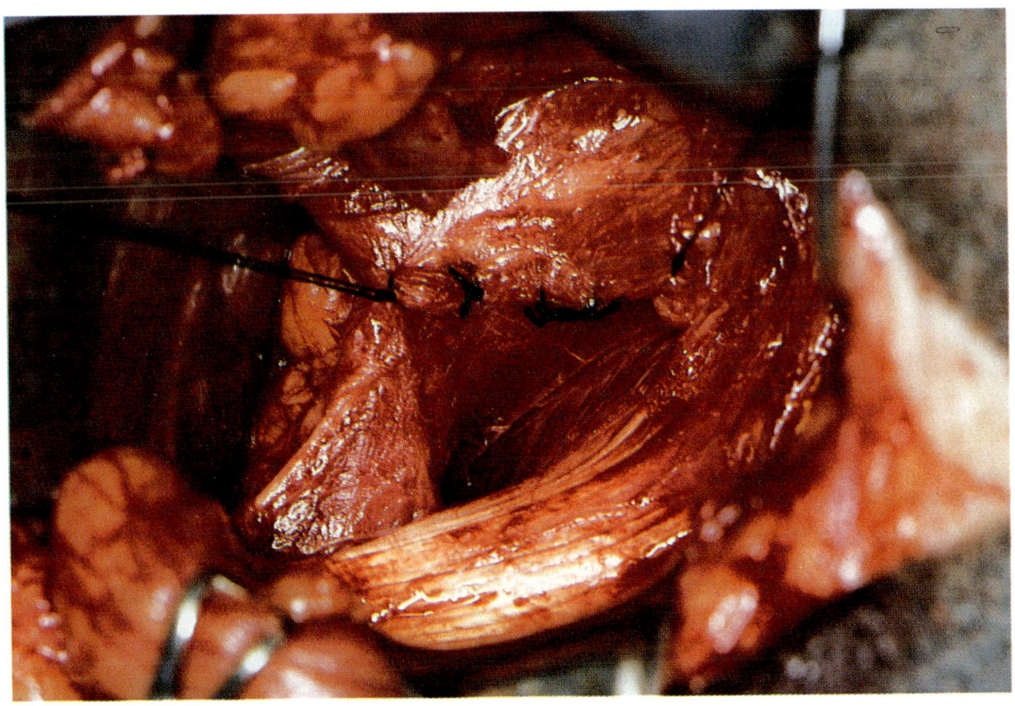

31

Figure 32 The normal anatomic in-continuity lateral closure of the fascia of the posterior inguinal wall, around the normal exit of the cremaster vessels, is illustrated. Accordingly, these vessels do not exit with the spermatic cord through the internal ring as is commonly thought.

Figures 33, 34 In this intraoperative photograph (Fig. 33) complementary to Figure 32, the suture for the closure of the fascial defect, lateral to the exit of the cremaster vessels (held in clamp), has been tied. The relationship of this closure to the small V-shaped fascial defect, in juxtaposition to the exit of the spermatic cord, is visible. The closure of this defect is completed with an additional suture of 3-0 silk, to obtain a snug closure of the internal ring around the exit of the cord (Fig. 34).

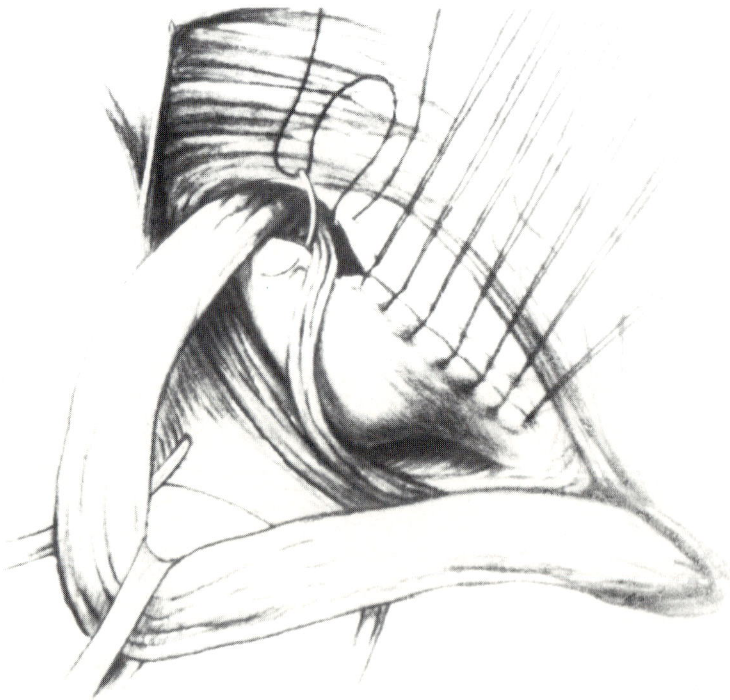

32

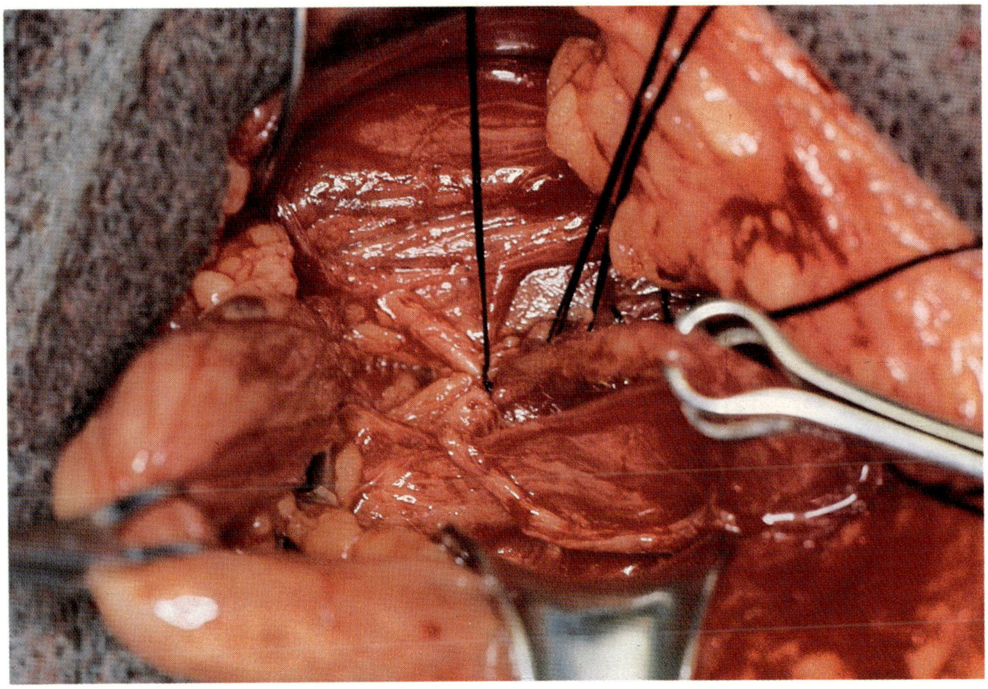

33

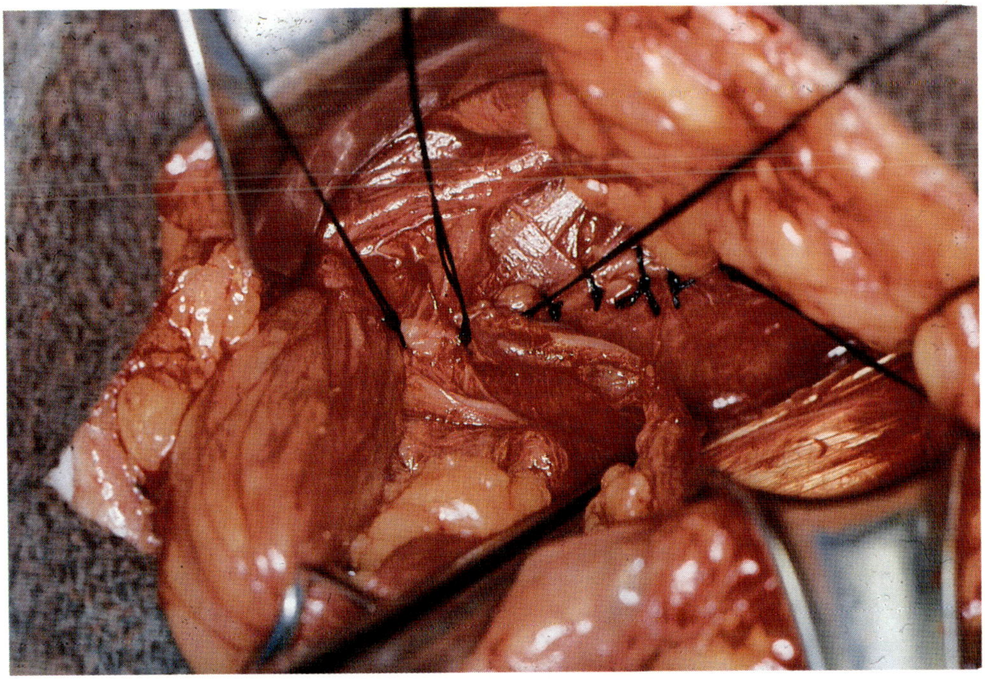

34

Figure 35 The reconstruction of the posterior inguinal wall is completed. Its relationships to the muscular and aponeurotic portions of the transversus abdominis superiorly, and to the anterior femoral sheath, inguinal ligament, and pyriform fossa inferiorly, are shown. Also, the conjoint lines of insertion into Cooper's ligament of the inferior segment of the fascia of the posterior inguinal wall superiorly, and of the fascial part of Gimbernat's ligament inferiorly, are visible as a slightly convex, curved line in the deep recess of the pyriform fossa.

Figure 36 This illustration of the completed reconstruction of the posterior inguinal wall conforms with the intraoperative photograph (Fig. 35), with the exception that in the photograph the internal oblique muscle is beneath the upper retractor and is not visible.

The normal arched configuration of the fasciculi of the internal oblique muscle, which commonly are interspersed with fatty areolar tissue, is shown. In the repair of an inguinal hernia, the poor holding power of this muscle for sutures and its distance from the inguinal ligament preclude their union. Such a union would fail to conform to the adage "Never suture red muscle to white fascia."

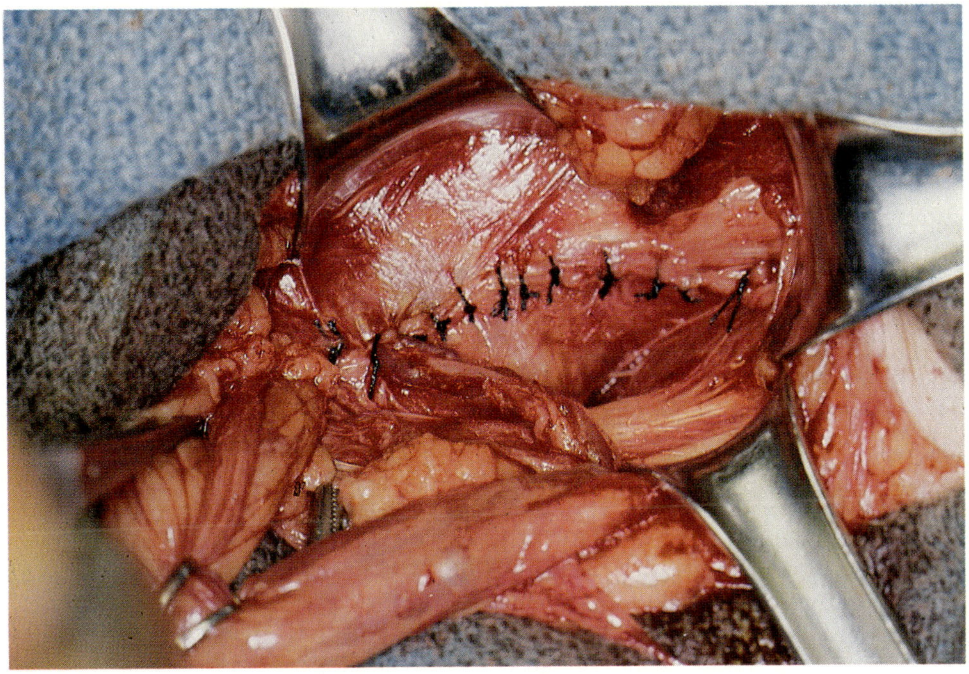

35

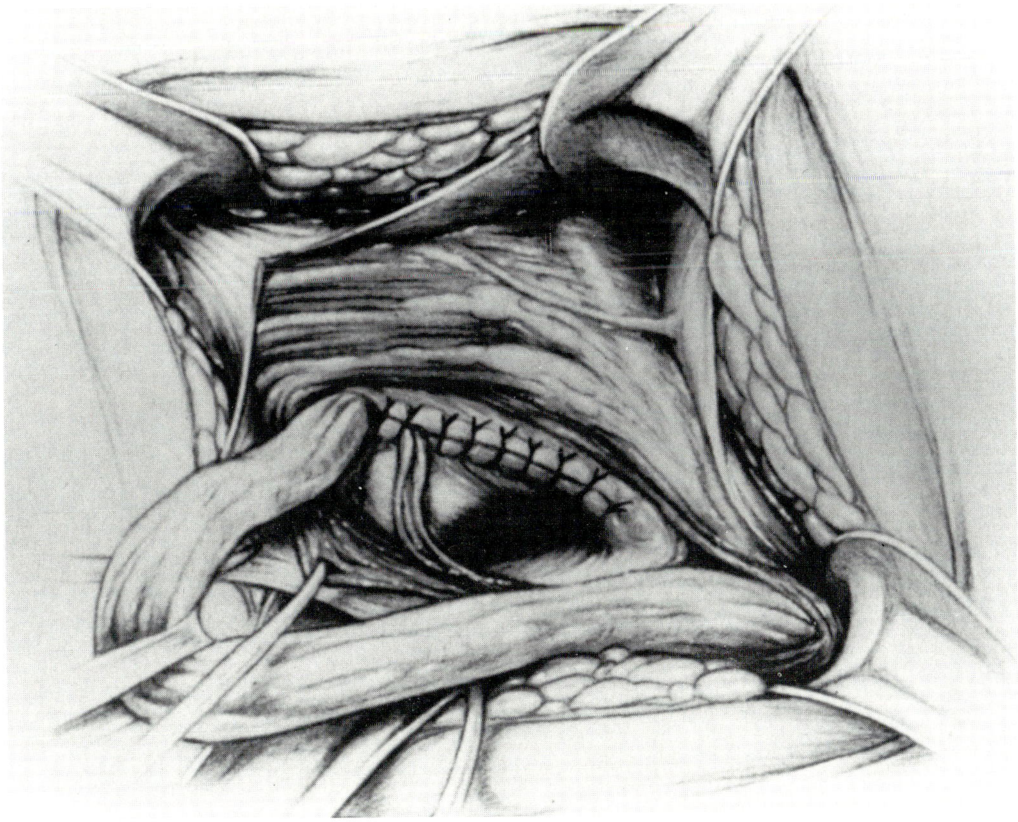

36

INTRAOPERATIVE ILLUSTRATIONS AND COMPLEMENTARY PHOTOGRAPHS
Continued

Figure 37 In this intraoperative photograph of the closure of the hernial defect, the cremaster vessels, held in forceps, are displaced downward and juxtaposed at approximately a 45-degree angle to the spermatic cord, with which they share a common but unanatomic exit from the internal ring. The relationship of the suture line medially to the subjacent inferior segment of the fascia of the posterior inguinal wall and its continuation laterally as the anterior femoral sheath are visible. Neither the internal oblique muscle superiorly nor the inguinal ligament inferiorly partakes in the reconstruction of the fascia of the posterior inguinal wall.

Figure 38 This illustration, which complements Figure 37, shows the cremaster vessels displaced laterally with the spermatic cord. The final suture in the reconstruction of the fascia of the posterior inguinal wall is being inserted.

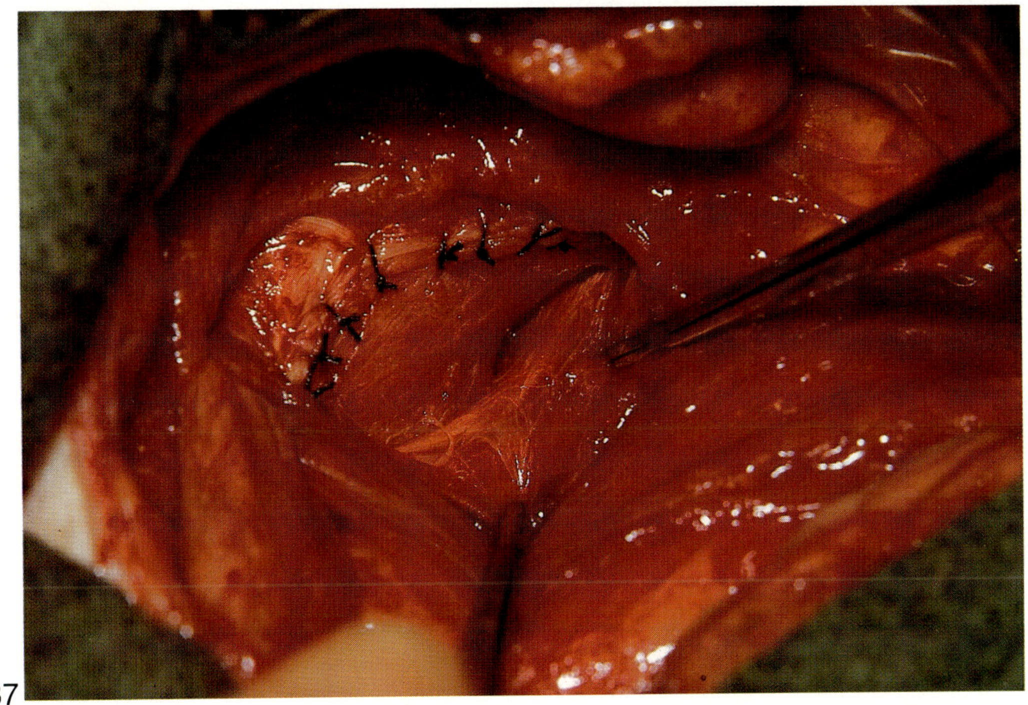

37

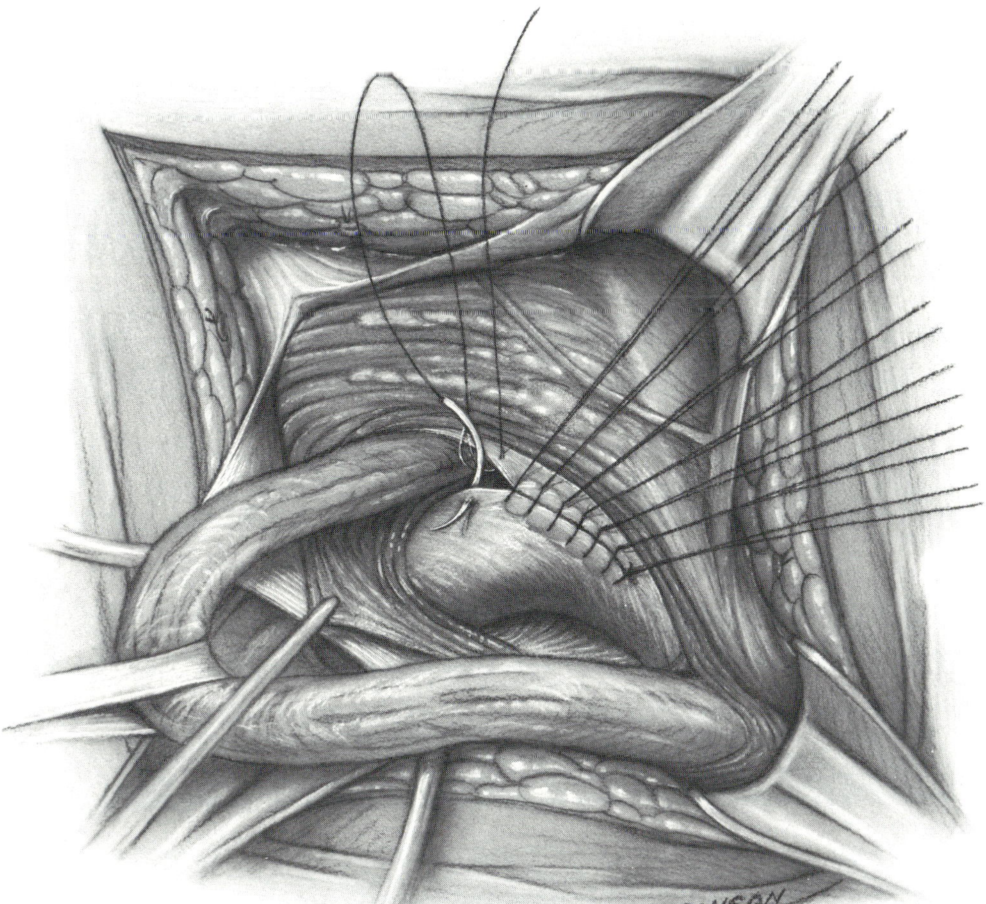

38

Figure 39 An intraoperative photograph of the pyriform fossa shows its relationship to the neighboring structures that form its boundaries. The inferior segment of the reconstructed fascia of the posterior inguinal wall, the superior boundary, is displaced upward and hidden from view.

The perpendicular suture strands in the center represent the site of the anatomic in-continuity restoration of the medial wall of the femoral sheath, which forms the lateral boundary. It is comparable to the site of the "transition" suture of McVay,[3] but differs in that it is more superficial and is in a normal, rather than distorted, anatomic plane of closure.

The inguinal ligament, as it arches over the reconstructed anterior femoral sheath (crural arch), continues medially to form the inferior boundary of the pyriform fossa. Ultimately it inserts, as the tendinous expansion of Gimbernat's ligament, into the

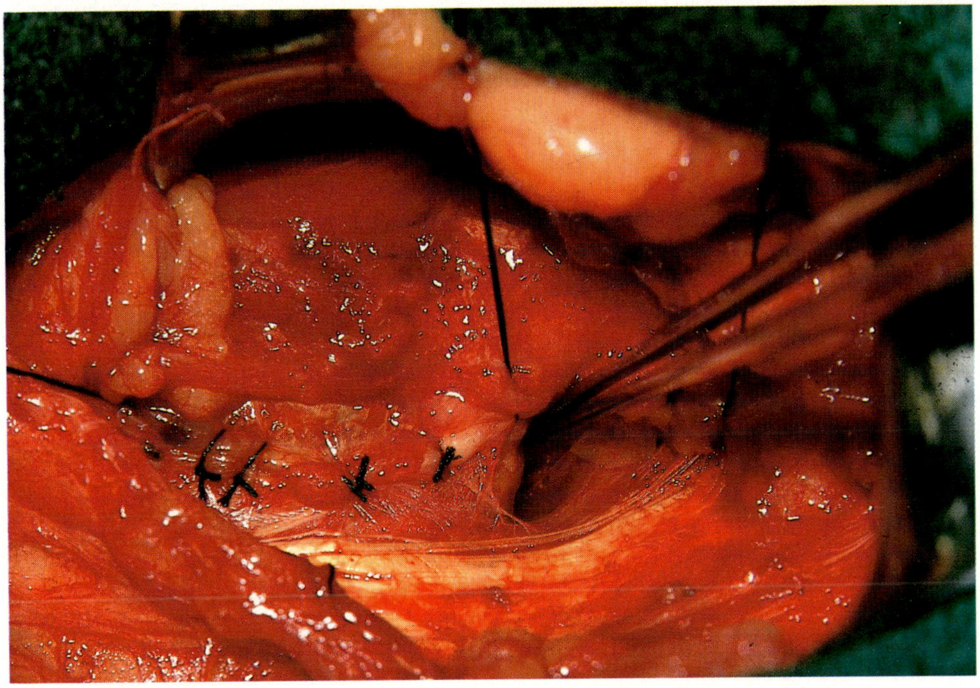

39

pubic tubercle, the juxtaposed medial angle of the fascia of the posterior inguinal wall, and the subjacent iliopectineal line (Cooper's ligament), to form the medial boundary of the fossa.

The floor of the pyriform fossa, which is clearly visible, is formed by the fascial (deep) part of Gimbernat's ligament. The lateral crescentic margin of this ligament is the medial boundary of the femoral sheath.

REFERENCES

1. De Gimbernat DA: *Nuevo Método De Operar En La Hernia Crural.* Madrid: Ibarra, 1793.
2. Lytle WJ: The inguinal and lacunar ligaments. J Anat *118*(2):241–251, 1974.
3. McVay CB: *Hernia.* Springfield: Charles C Thomas, 1954.

SECTION II

SURGICAL TECHNIQUES

OPERATION 1

REPAIR OF A DIRECT INGUINAL HERNIA AND SLIDING HERNIA OF THE BLADDER

A direct inguinal hernia is commonly referred to as a bulge of the fascia of the posterior inguinal wall. In its surgical repair, the generally accepted practice is neither to open the peritoneal sac nor to reduce the sliding hernia of the bladder that is invariably present. Frequently the bulge is simply inverted by suture approximation of the intact surfaces of the overlying attenuated fascia. However, this technique is considered surgically blind and is related to the higher incidence of recurrence following the repair of a direct hernia compared with that of an indirect hernia.

Inversion of the fascia of the posterior inguinal wall, or the incision and imbrication of its layers, is both unanatomic and unphysiologic. The experimental studies of Dunphy[1] have shown that suturing freshly cut margins of fascia evokes a greater fibroblastic response for wound healing than the inversion and suture approximation of their intact surfaces. Similarly, Farris, Smith, and Beattie[2] have demonstrated in rabbits that the distraction force required to disrupt the suture line of freshly cut margins of fascia is much greater than when an imbricated (Mayo) closure of the fascial layers is performed. Accordingly, even in the small direct hernial bulge the overlying attenuated fascia is excised rather than inverted, and the remaining cut margins of fascia, with their good "holding power," are sutured.

Ideally, the anatomy of repair in the surgical treatment of a direct inguinal hernia is based on the two specific findings that are peculiar to it—the large peritoneal sac and the sliding hernia of the bladder. When the overlying attenuated fascia of the posterior inguinal wall is excised, the peritoneal sac is always larger than anticipated and is comparable in size to that of a large indirect hernia. The major difference is the wider base or "neck" of the direct hernial sac.

Despite their comparable sizes the method of management of the two hernias differs. The sac of the indirect hernia, with few exceptions, is excised. In the direct hernia, isolation of the sac is infrequent and its excision is rare. The differences in treatment are difficult to understand, since the wider neck of the sac in the direct hernia permits the free ingress and egress of the omentum and small bowel. Therefore, when the intact sac of a direct hernia is simply and blindly inverted, an intermittent "battering ram" effect through this wide neck and against the overlying fascial closure is produced.

This hidden effect may be readily demonstrated when the peritoneal sac is isolated. Each time the sac is reduced by inversion into the peritoneal cavity, it herniates back, immediately and spontaneously, upon the release of the inversion force. In contrast, when the hernial sac is excised and its wide neck sutured, the anterior parietal peritoneal wall is restored to normal and the battering ram effect is eliminated.

The second characteristic component of a direct hernia is the sliding hernia of the bladder. When fully distended, it complements and reinforces the battering ram effect of the intact hernial sac. Ideally, therefore, the hernial sac should be excised and the sliding hernia of the bladder reduced.

The objections to surgical reduction of the sliding hernia have been the troublesome bleeding that may occur and the possibility of entering the bladder. Neither of these potential complications is a valid reason for not doing the proper anatomic repair that is required. The particular danger of entering the bladder is failing to recognize that it has occurred; once recognized, it is safely treated by suture closure of the site of entrance and insertion of an indwelling catheter, which is removed within seven to 10 days.

To avoid injury to the bladder in the repair of a direct inguinal hernia, Hoguet[3] stated, ". . .an indirect sac always can be found . . ., although very small." He continued, ". . .by traction outwards on the indirect sac. . .the direct sac may be pulled external to the vessels and the two sacs converted into one. By this proceeding, all possibility of injury to the bladder is eliminated. . . ."[3] This method, frequently referred to as Hoguet's maneuver, is considered more theoretical than practical and is certainly not a nicety of surgical technique. Furthermore, it produces a greater distortion of the anatomy of the bladder rather than restoring it to normal, and is not advocated.

The operation that is the ideal anatomic repair of a large direct inguinal hernia and sliding hernia of the bladder is described and illustrated here. This operation is purposely placed first because it includes detailed illustrations of the surgical anatomy of the posterior inguinal wall. Also, illustrations 1 through 13 are applicable to the comparable stages in the repair of the subsequent types of inguinal hernias that will be discussed and will serve as an immediate reference guide.

REPAIR OF A DIRECT INGUINAL HERNIA AND SLIDING HERNIA OF THE BLADDER

Continued

1 An oblique inguinal incision 7 to 8 cm in length is outlined and cross-hatched to facilitate its later closure. It begins approximately 2 cm above the midportion of the inguinal ligament and extends obliquely down to the level of the pubic tubercle.

2 Digital pressure for hemostasis is maintained as the skin incision is deepened into the subcutaneous fatty tissue layer.

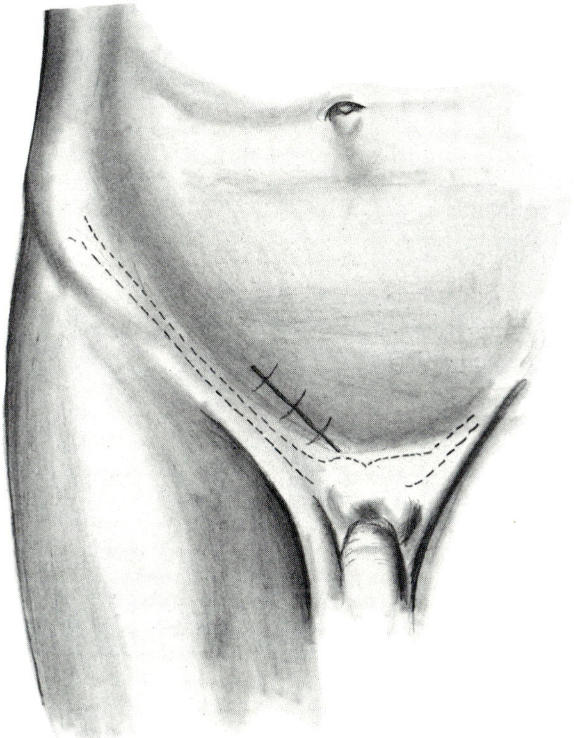

1

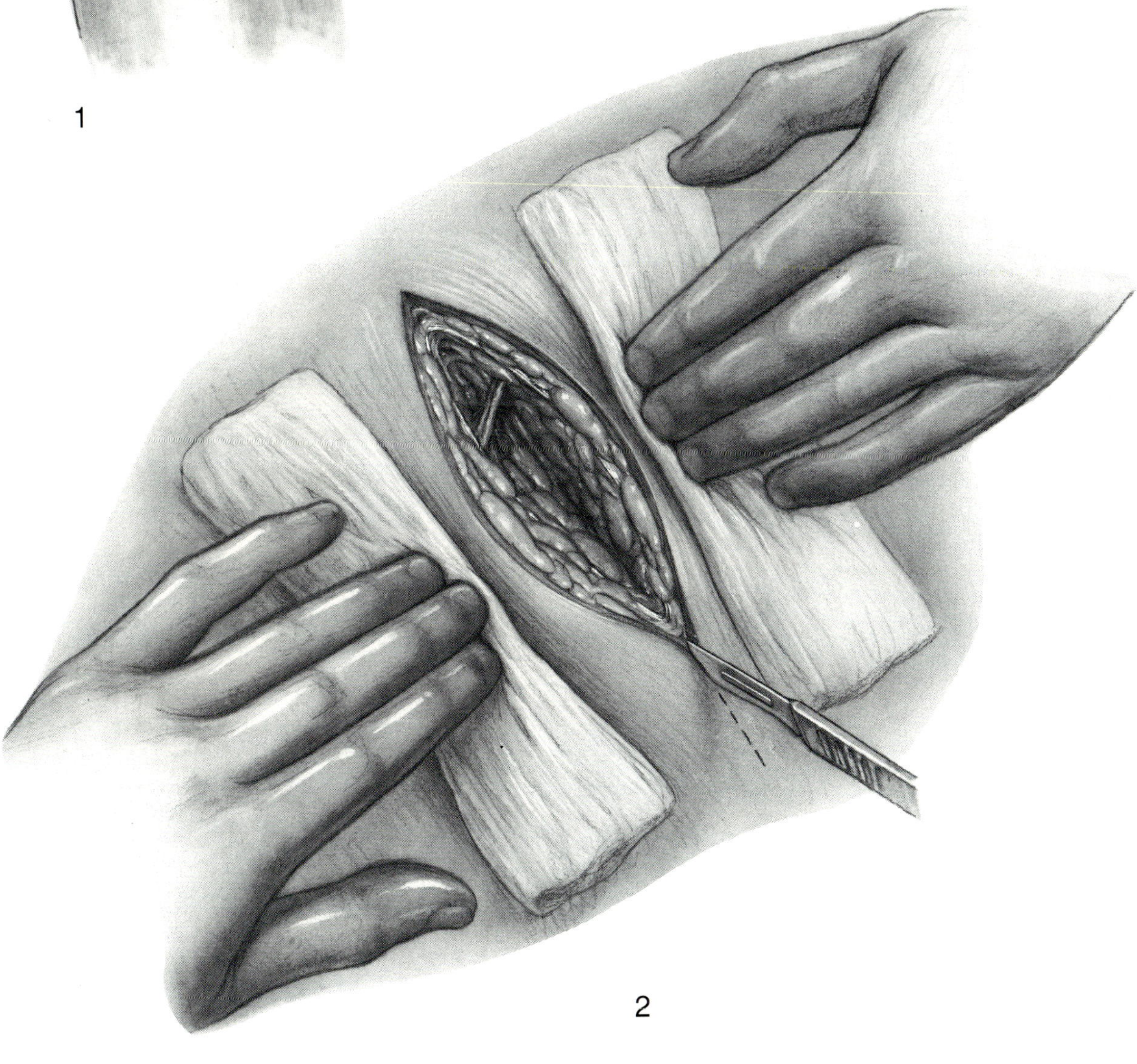

2

3 The external superficial pudendal vein is transected between clamps. The ligated ends of the previously severed external superficial epigastric vein are visible.

4 An incision is made through the preaponeurotic fibroareolar tissue layer, and a portion of the underlying fatty areolar tissue is herniated through the opening.

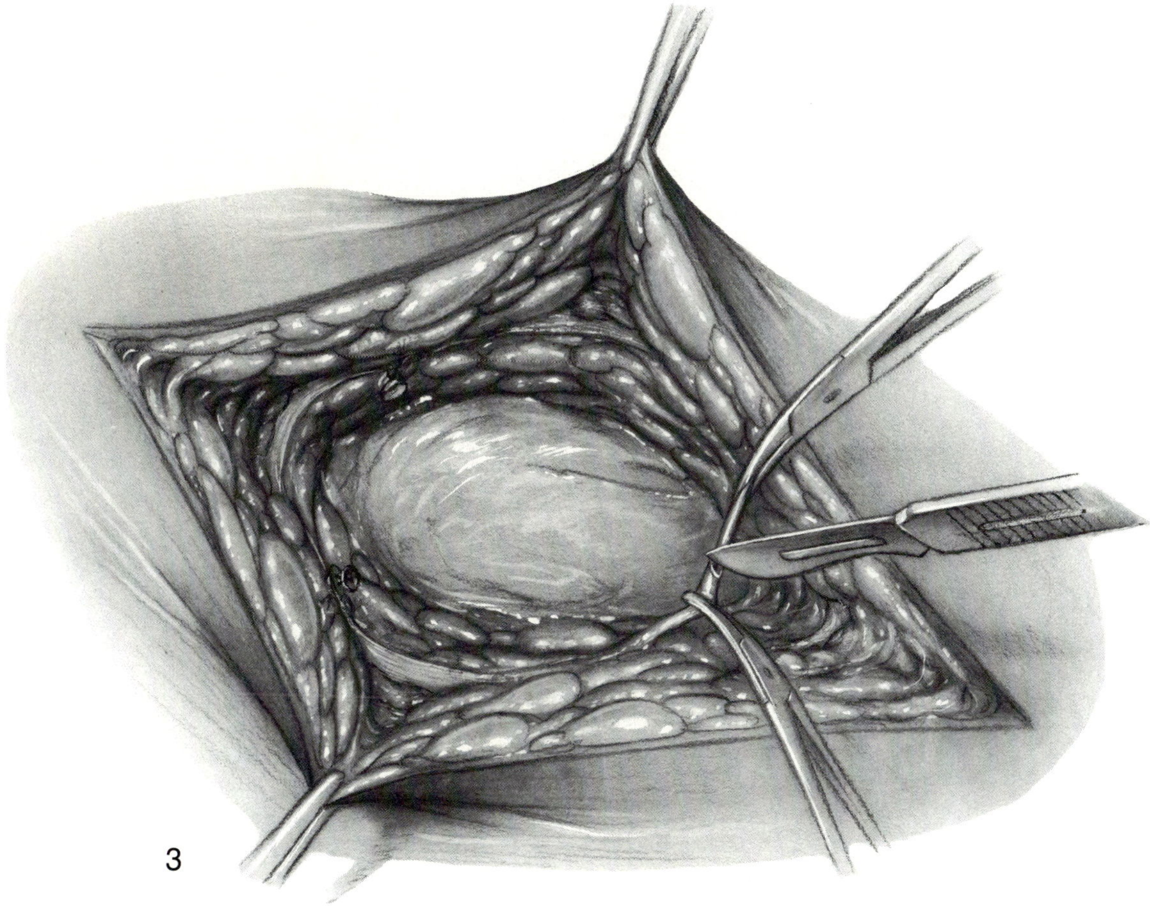

3

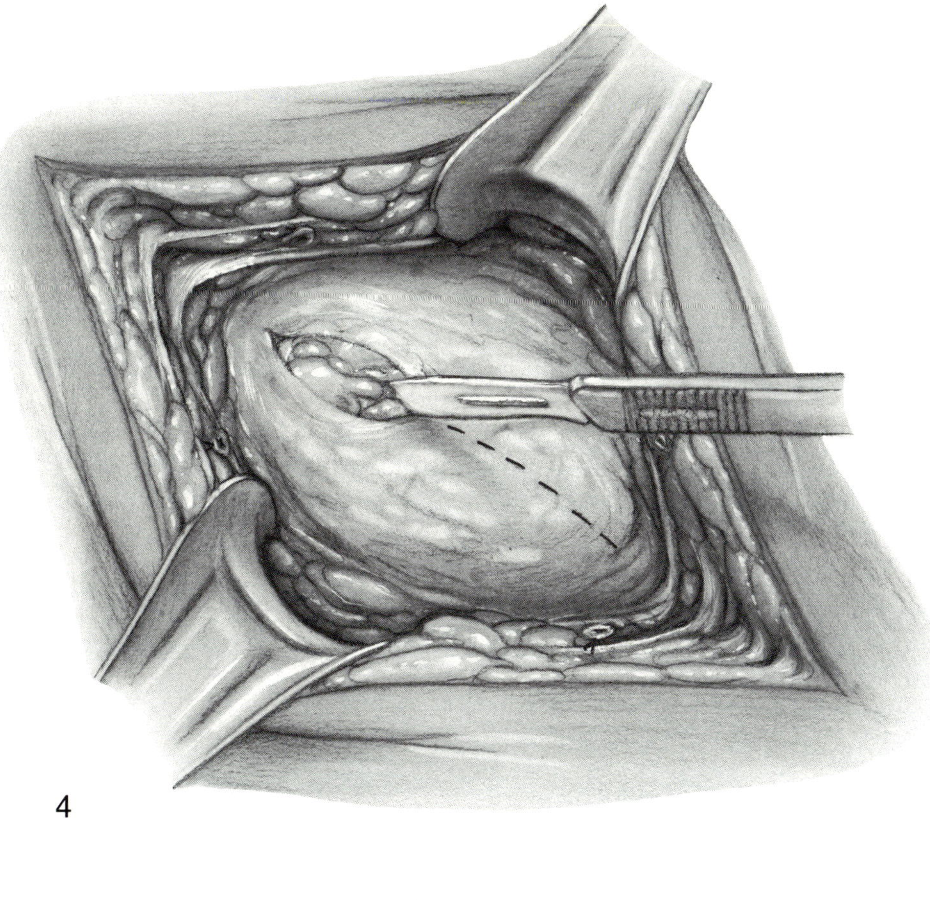

4

REPAIR OF A DIRECT INGUINAL HERNIA AND SLIDING HERNIA OF THE BLADDER

Continued

5 Using a gauze-covered index finger, the aponeurosis of the external oblique muscle and its intercrural fibers are exposed by blunt dissection of the overlying fatty areolar tissue.

6 A "stab" incision in the external oblique aponeurosis, made laterally, is extended medially by scissor dissection through the external (subcutaneous) inguinal ring (*dashed line*). Its relationship to the cremaster "veil" and ilioinguinal nerve, which overlie the spermatic cord, is evident.

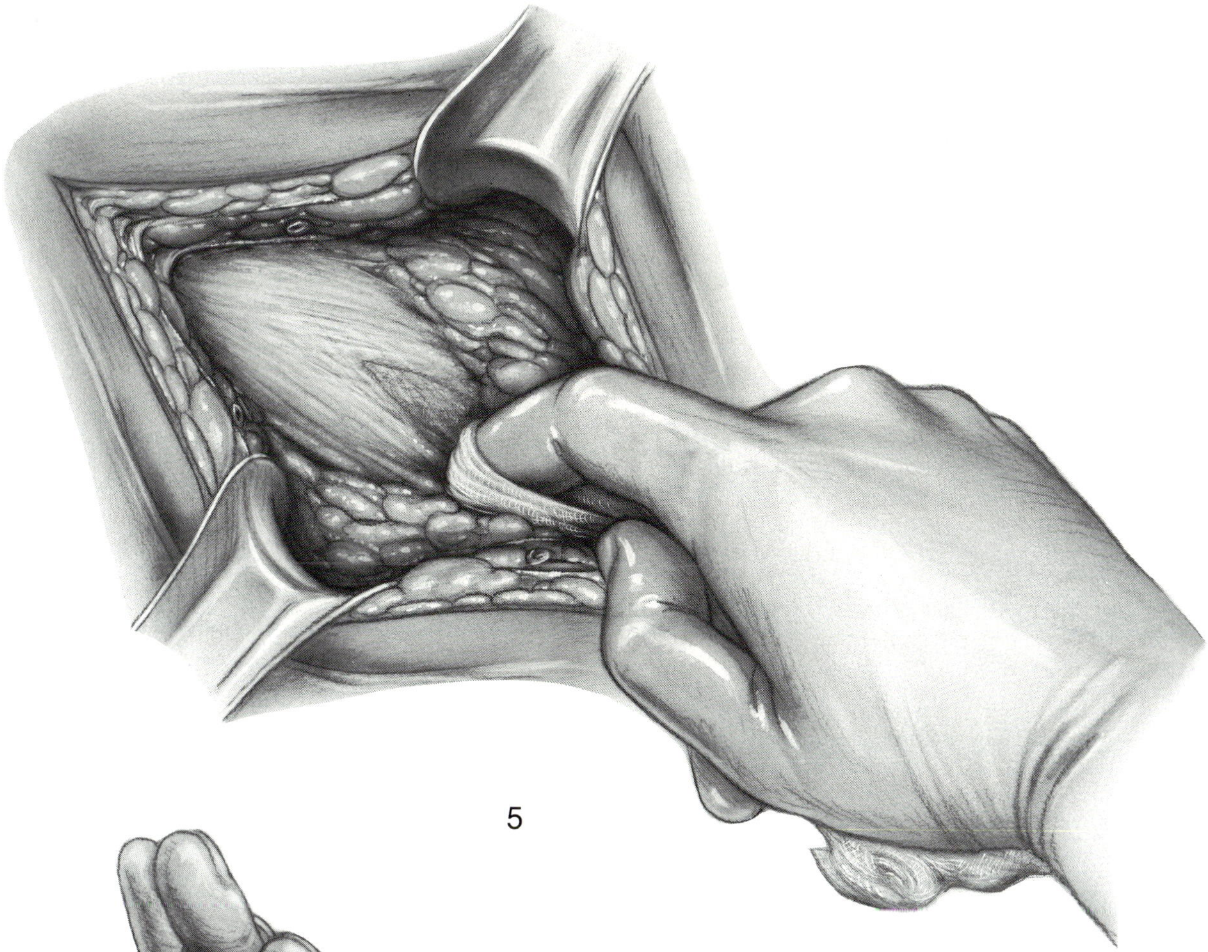

5

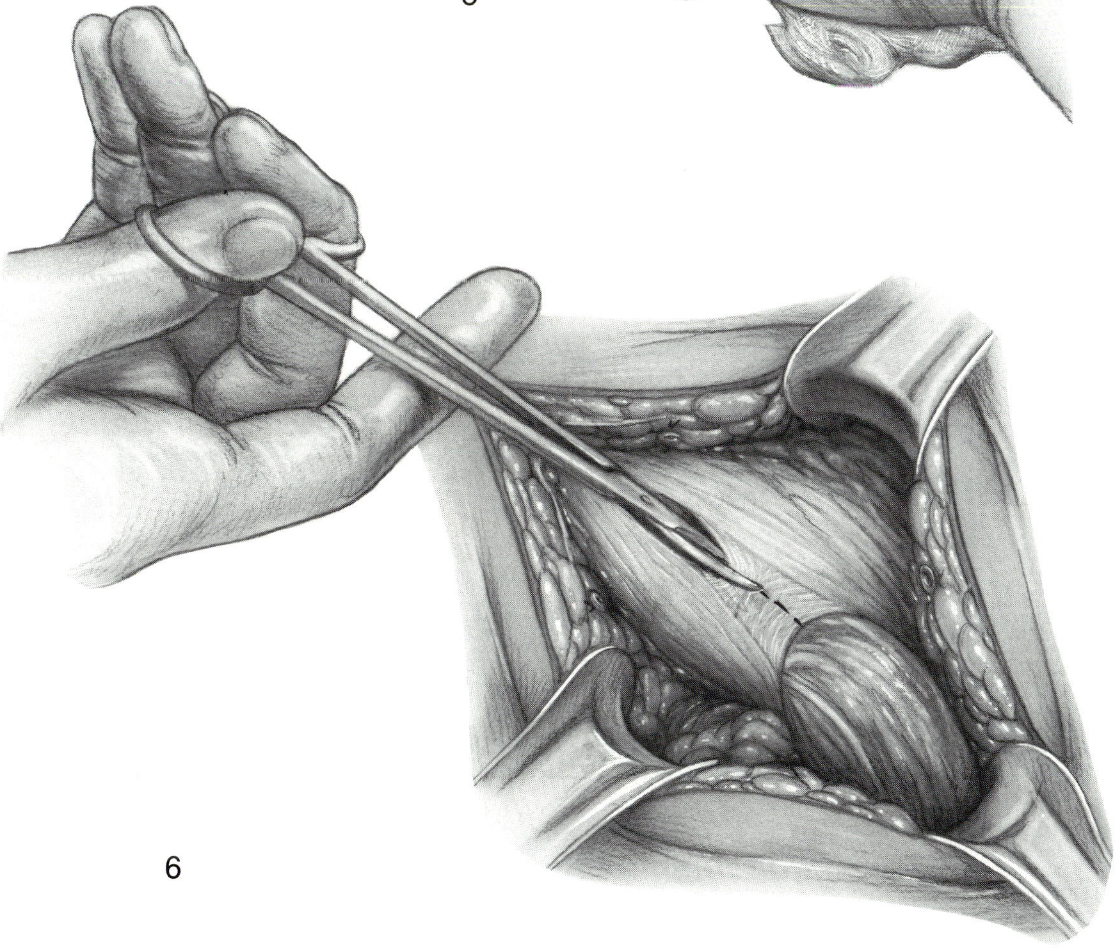

6

REPAIR OF A DIRECT INGUINAL HERNIA AND SLIDING HERNIA OF THE BLADDER
Continued

7 The superior (medial) and inferior (lateral) leaflets of the incised external oblique aponeurosis are retracted to expose the iliohypogastric nerve superiorly and ilioinguinal nerve inferiorly. Loose fatty areolar tissue, which has poor holding power, is interposed between the fasciculi of the internal oblique muscle and precludes the use of this muscle in the repair of inguinal hernias.

8 The cremaster muscle, which originates from the internal oblique muscle, is incised. The thick texture of its fibers is more commonly seen in the indirect rather than the direct inguinal hernia.

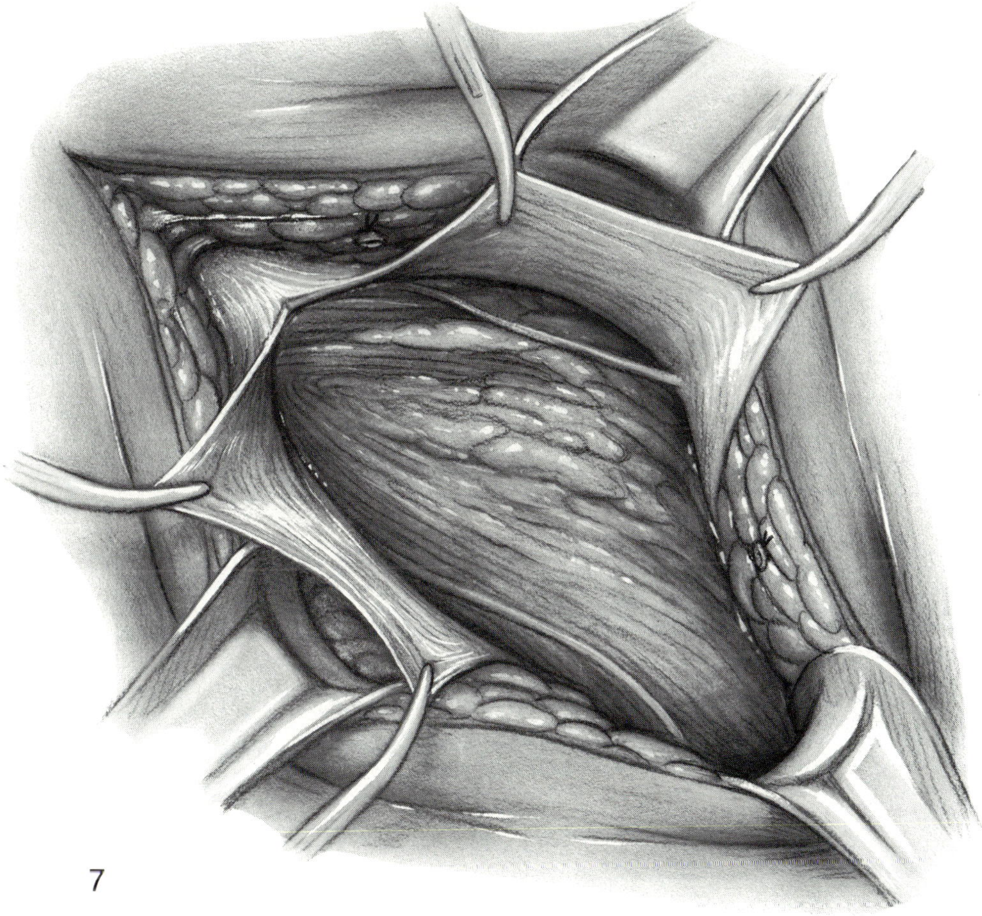

7

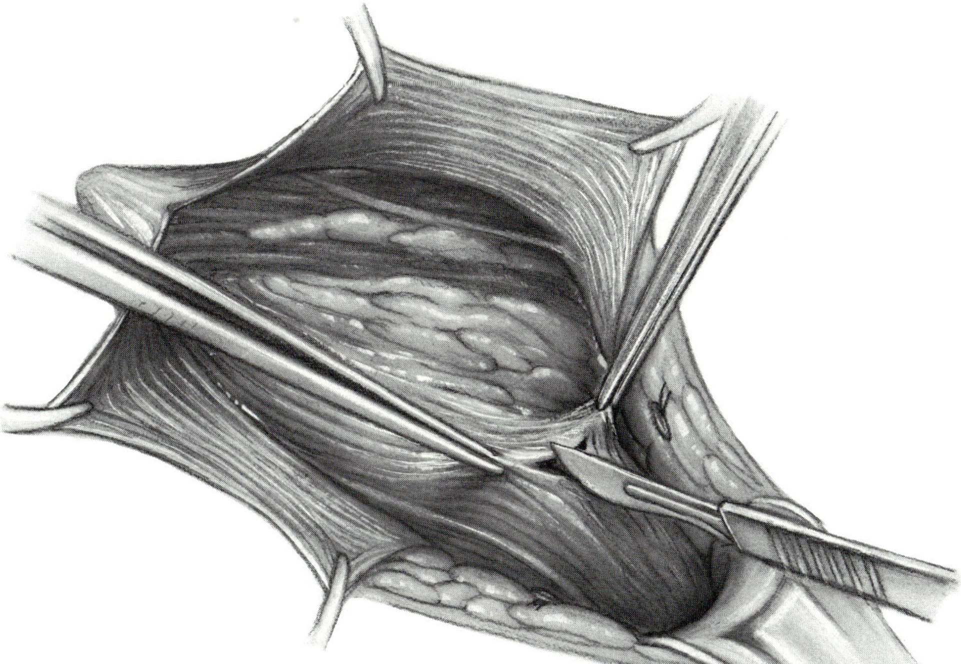

8

REPAIR OF A DIRECT INGUINAL HERNIA AND SLIDING HERNIA OF THE BLADDER

Continued

9, 10 The opening in the cremaster veil is extended laterally with scissors (**9**) and medially by scalpel (**10**).

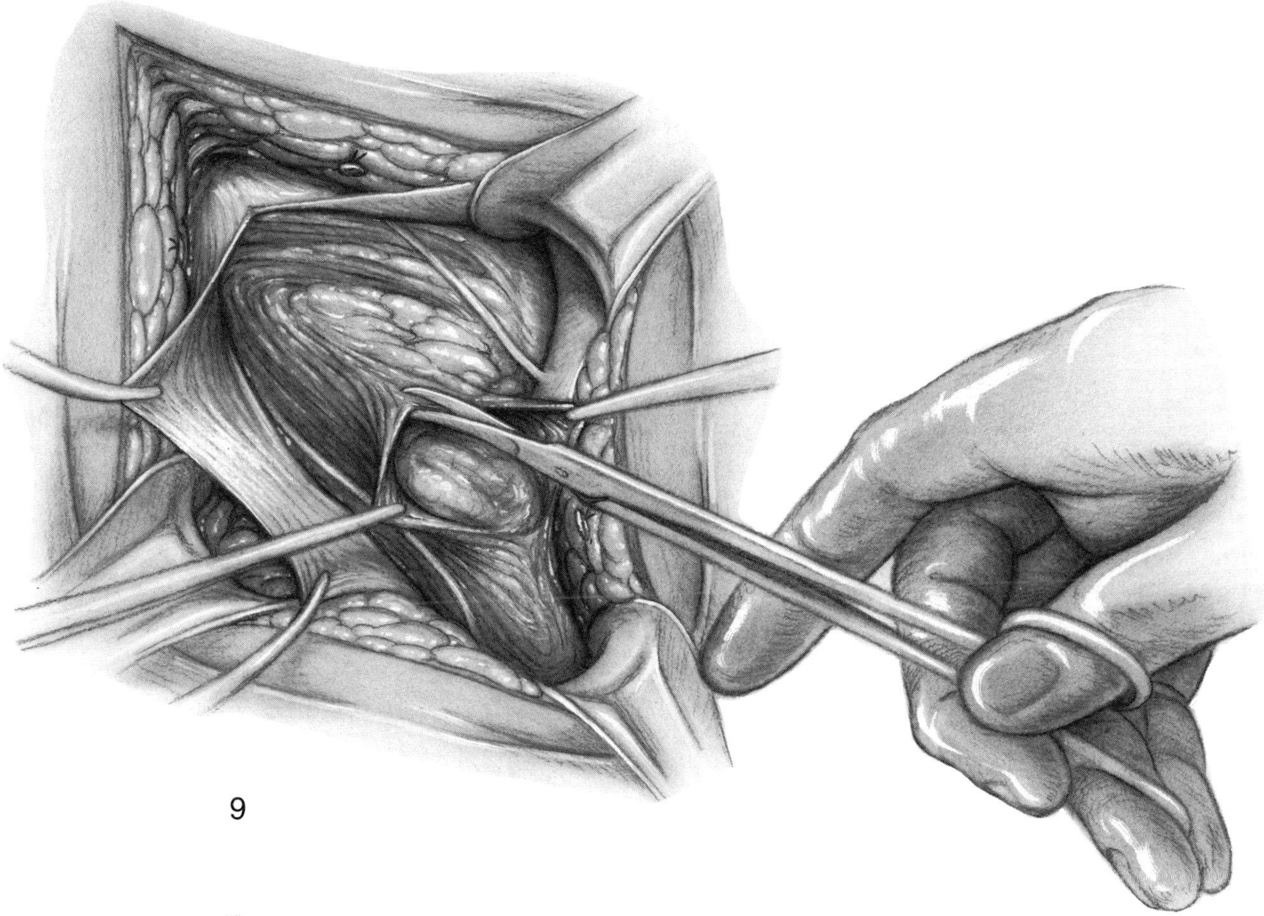

9

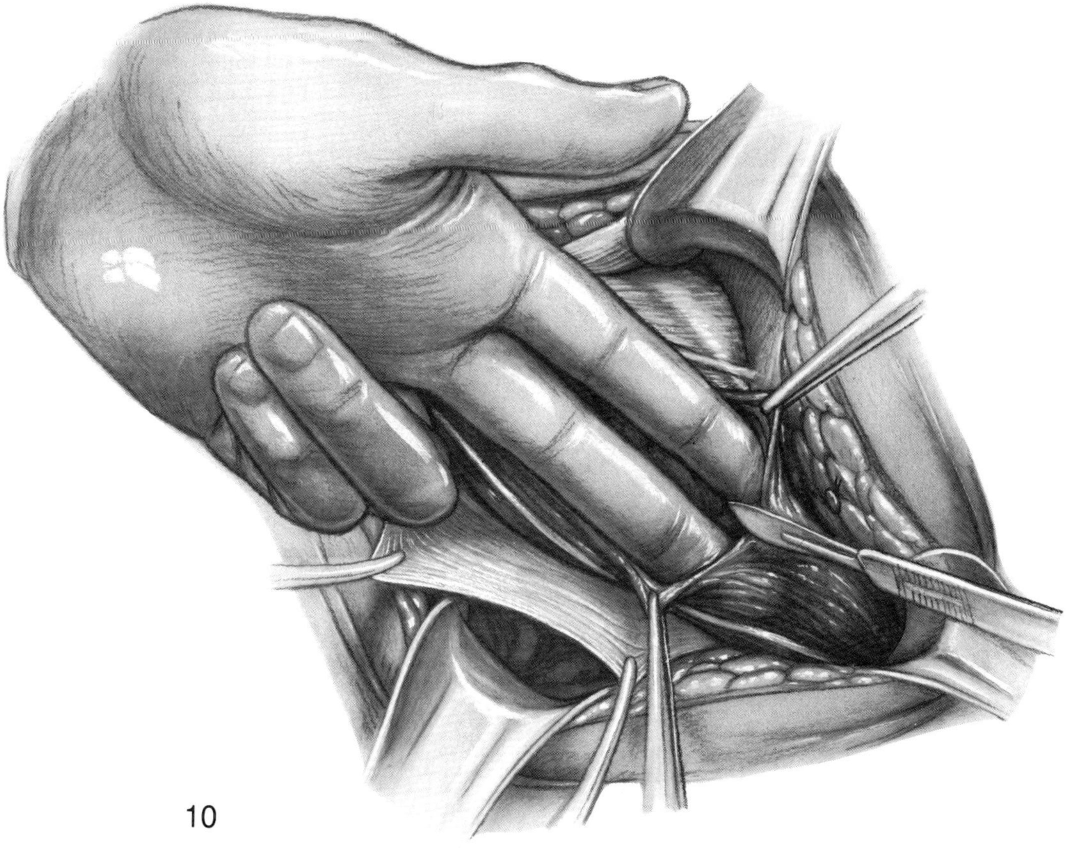

10

REPAIR OF A DIRECT INGUINAL HERNIA AND SLIDING HERNIA OF THE BLADDER
Continued

11 The cut margins of the cremaster muscle are elevated by tissue forceps to show the contiguous attachment of its fibers, laterally, to the inguinal ligament. Frequently, the cremaster veil is poorly defined. Once it is incised, however, the resulting increase in tissue turgor clearly defines its muscle fibers.

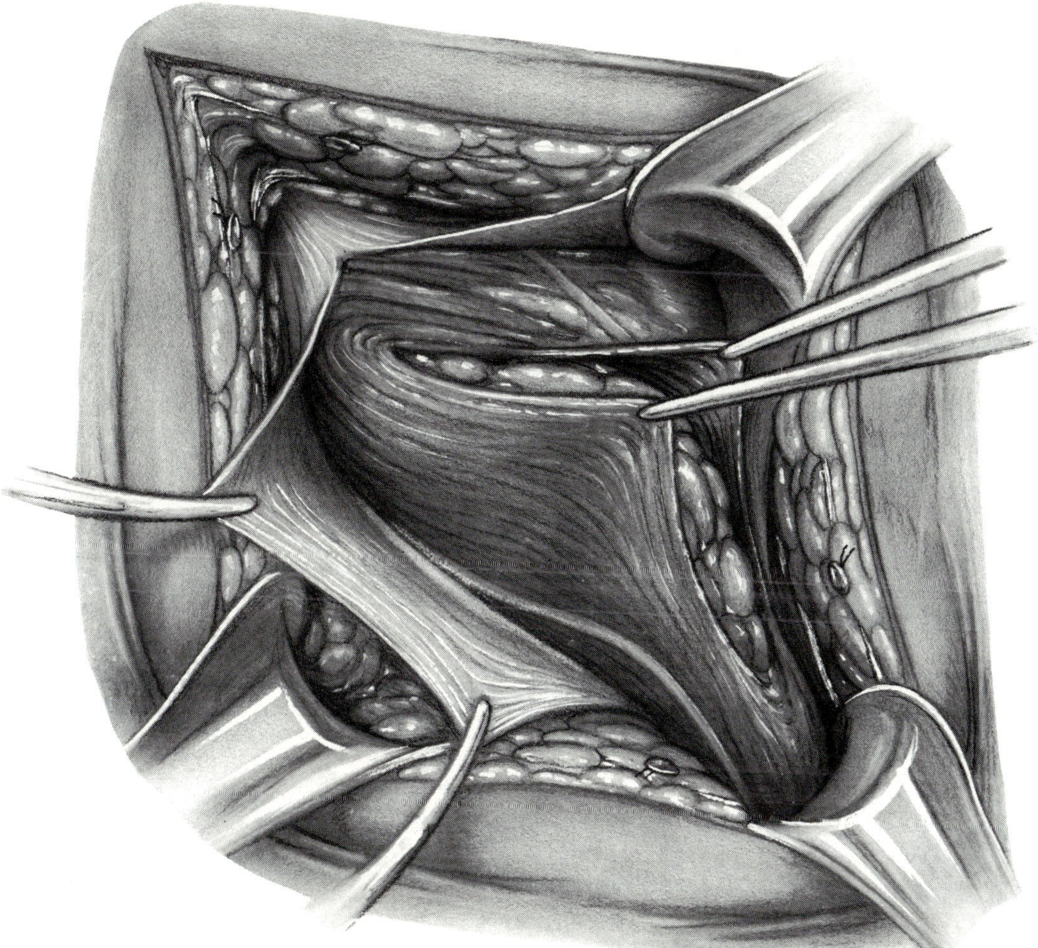

11

12 The spermatic cord structures are picked up between the thumb and index finger, and the "mesentery of the cord" (MacLeod), between the vas deferens and the external spermatic (cremaster) vessels, is tented on the finger. The genital branch of the genitofemoral nerve, between the cremaster vessels and retracted fibers of the cremaster muscle, is visible.

13 The tip of the index finger is herniated through the mesentery, and the subjacent medial protrusion of the direct inguinal hernia, distinct from the cord, is visible.

In the direct inguinal hernia of moderate or large size, the thinned-out fibers of the cremaster muscle frequently are splayed onto its outer surface, which facilitates the digital dissection of both the muscle and cord from the hernia.

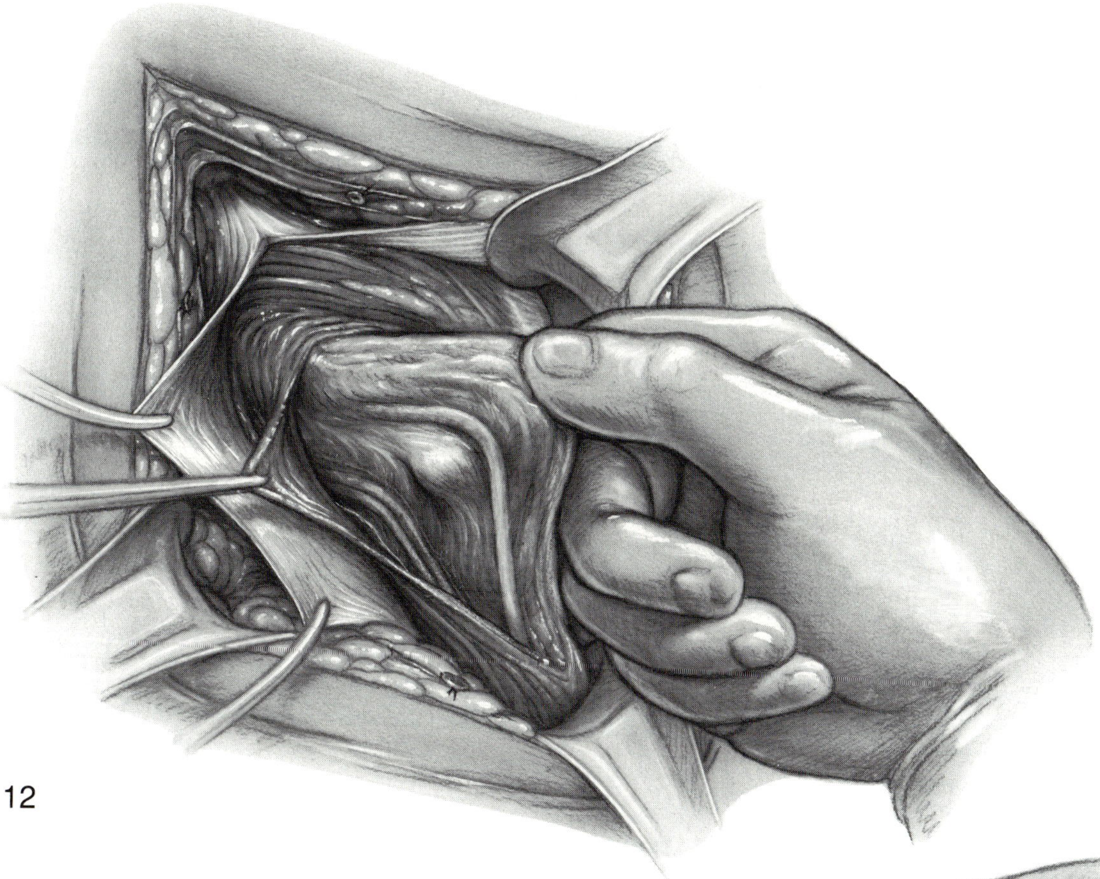

12

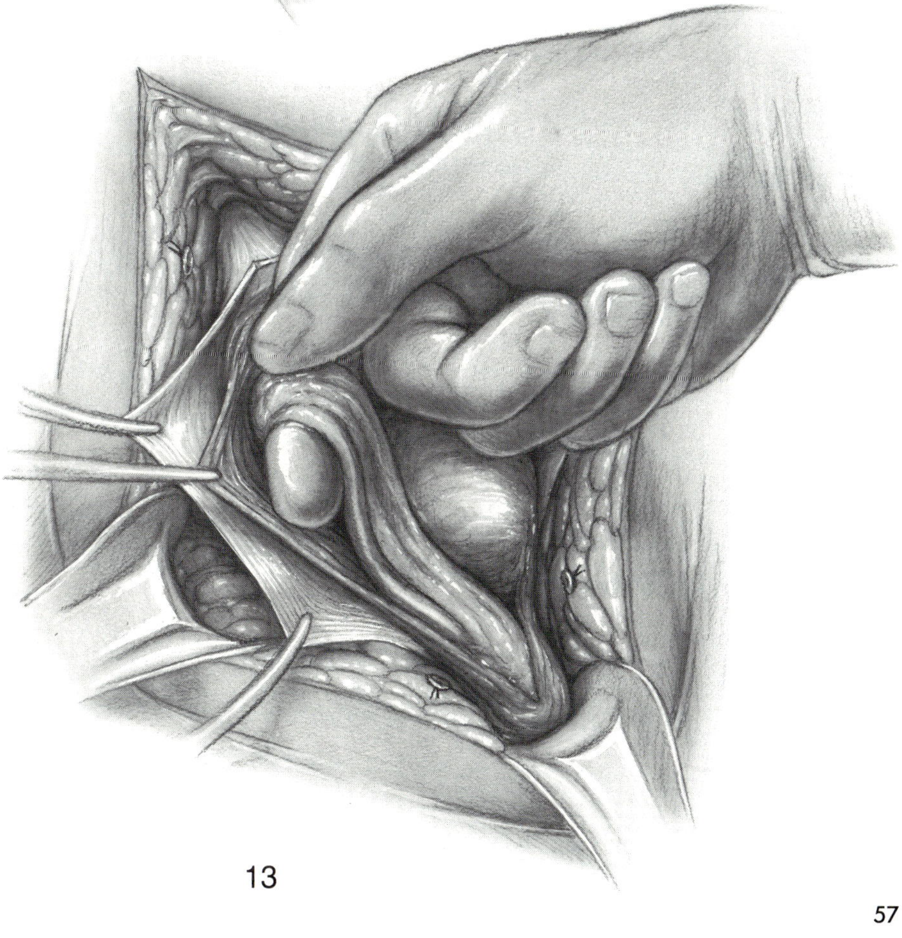

13

REPAIR OF A DIRECT INGUINAL HERNIA AND SLIDING HERNIA OF THE BLADDER

Continued

14 The spermatic cord, encircled by a tape, is retracted out and up to show its independence from the large direct inguinal hernia that protrudes through Hesselbach's triangle. This triangle is bounded laterally and superiorly by the deep epigastric vessels that form its base; medially by the lateral border of the lower third of the rectus sheath; and inferiorly by the inner third of the inguinal ligament.

14A In this direct inguinal hernia, the fascia of the posterior inguinal wall is so attenuated that it gives a transparency to the underlying tissues.

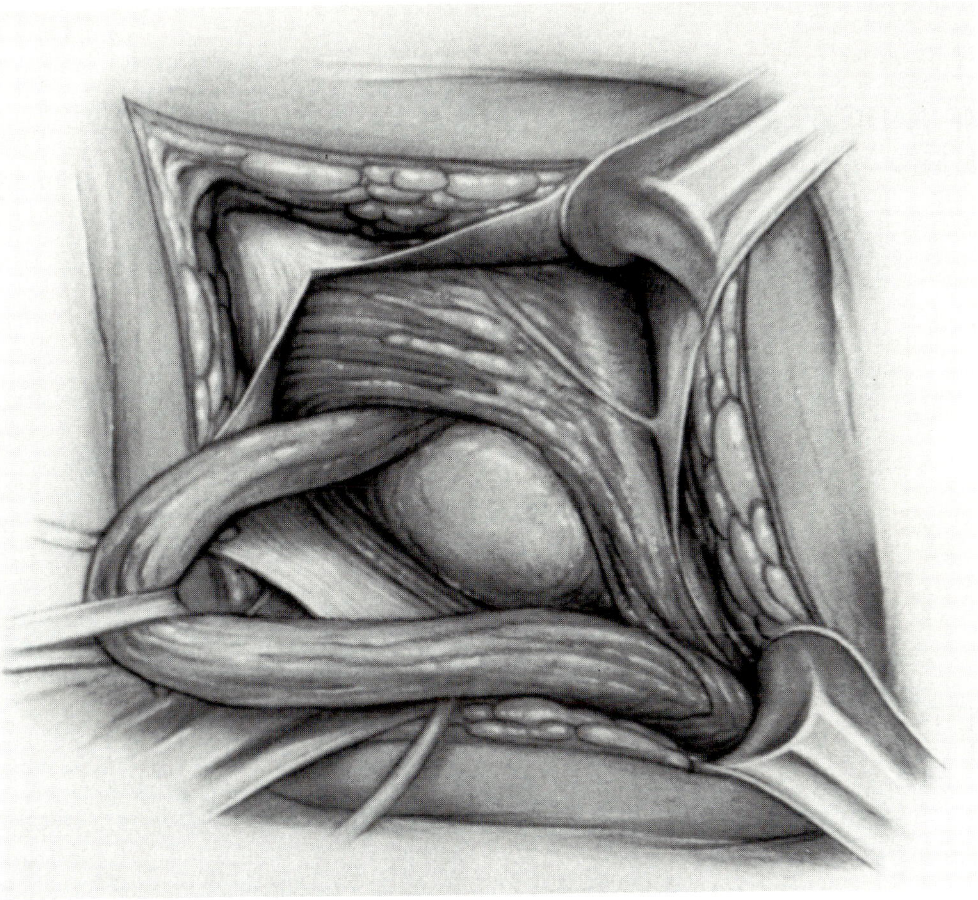

14

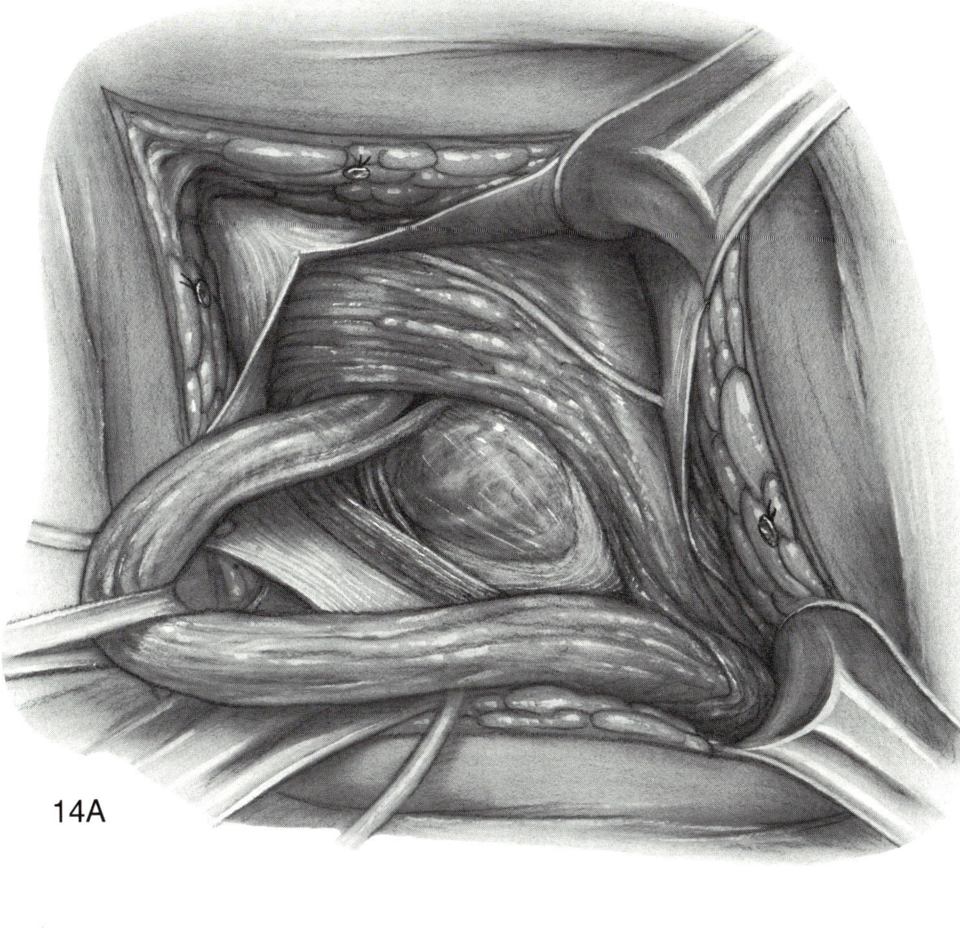

14A

REPAIR OF A DIRECT INGUINAL HERNIA AND SLIDING HERNIA OF THE BLADDER

Continued

15 The summit of the attenuated fascia of the posterior inguinal wall, grasped in a clamp, is tented by traction as an incision is made and continued circumferentially (*dashed line*) through the intact fascia of the posterior inguinal wall at the base of the direct hernia. The protrusion of preperitoneal fat through the site of the partially completed incision is visible.

16 The circumferential incision in the fascia of the posterior inguinal wall is completed, and the attenuated fascia over the summit of the direct hernia is inverted by upward traction with clamps.

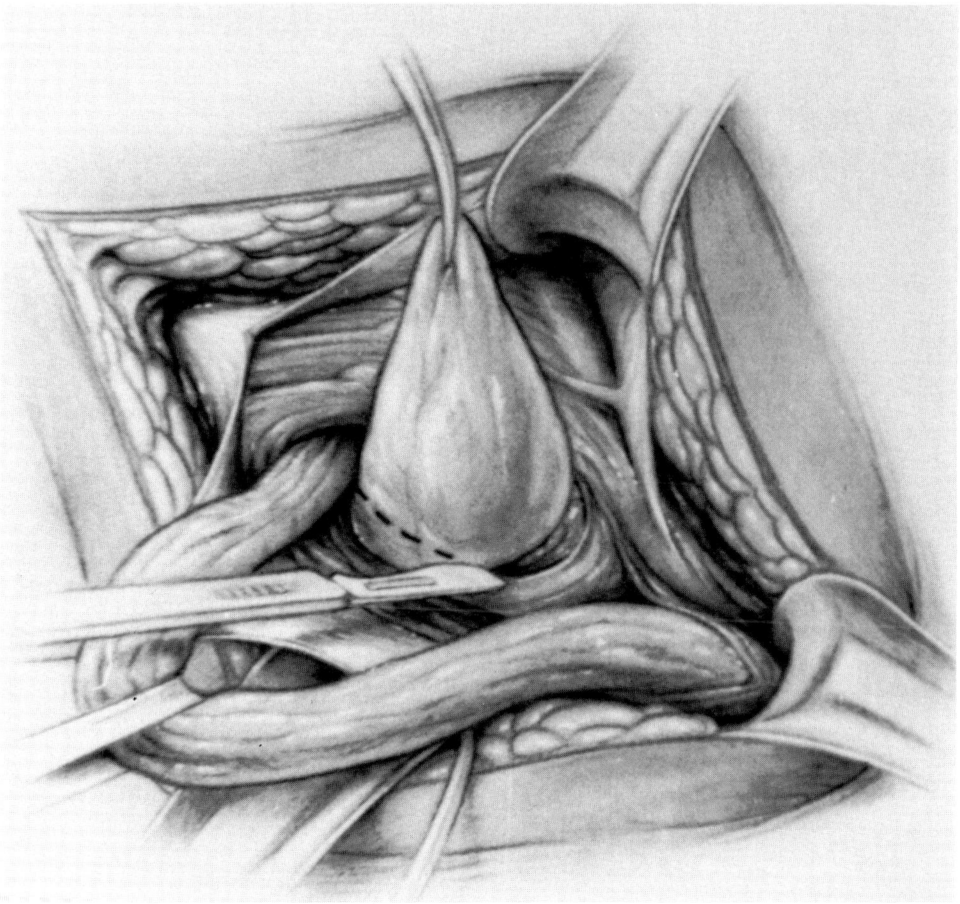

15

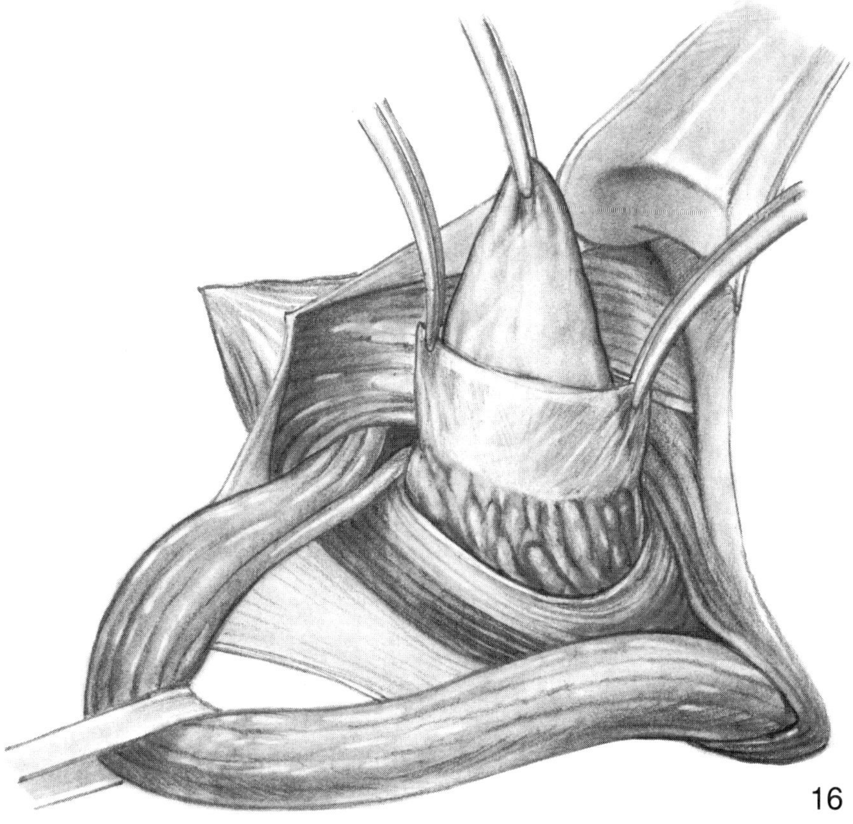

16

REPAIR OF A DIRECT INGUINAL HERNIA AND SLIDING HERNIA OF THE BLADDER
Continued

17 The inverted cone of attenuated fascia is seen immediately before its removal. The normal thickness of the cut margin of the intact fascia of the posterior inguinal wall is clearly shown.

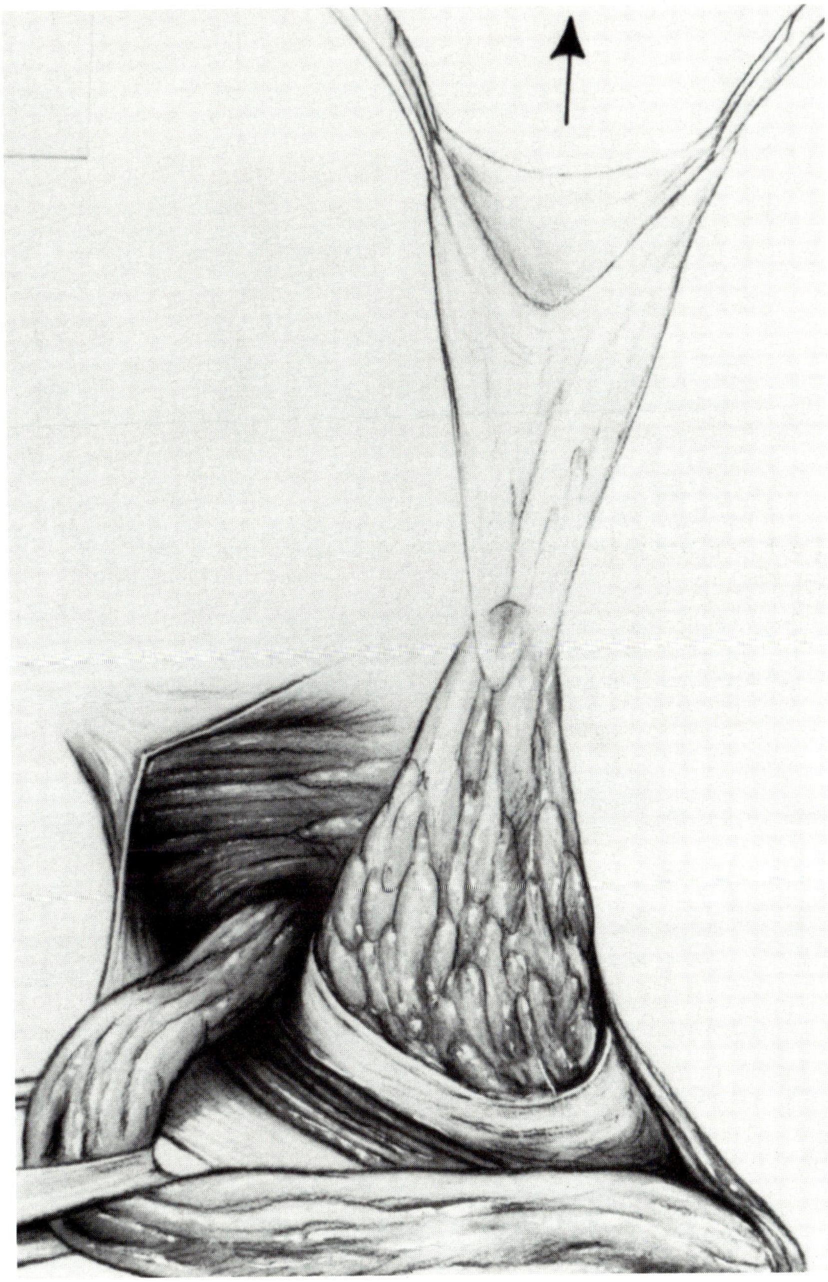

17

REPAIR OF A DIRECT INGUINAL HERNIA AND SLIDING HERNIA OF THE BLADDER
Continued

18 The sac of the direct hernia is opened, preparatory to reduction of the sliding hernia of the bladder that is invariably present in a large direct inguinal hernia.

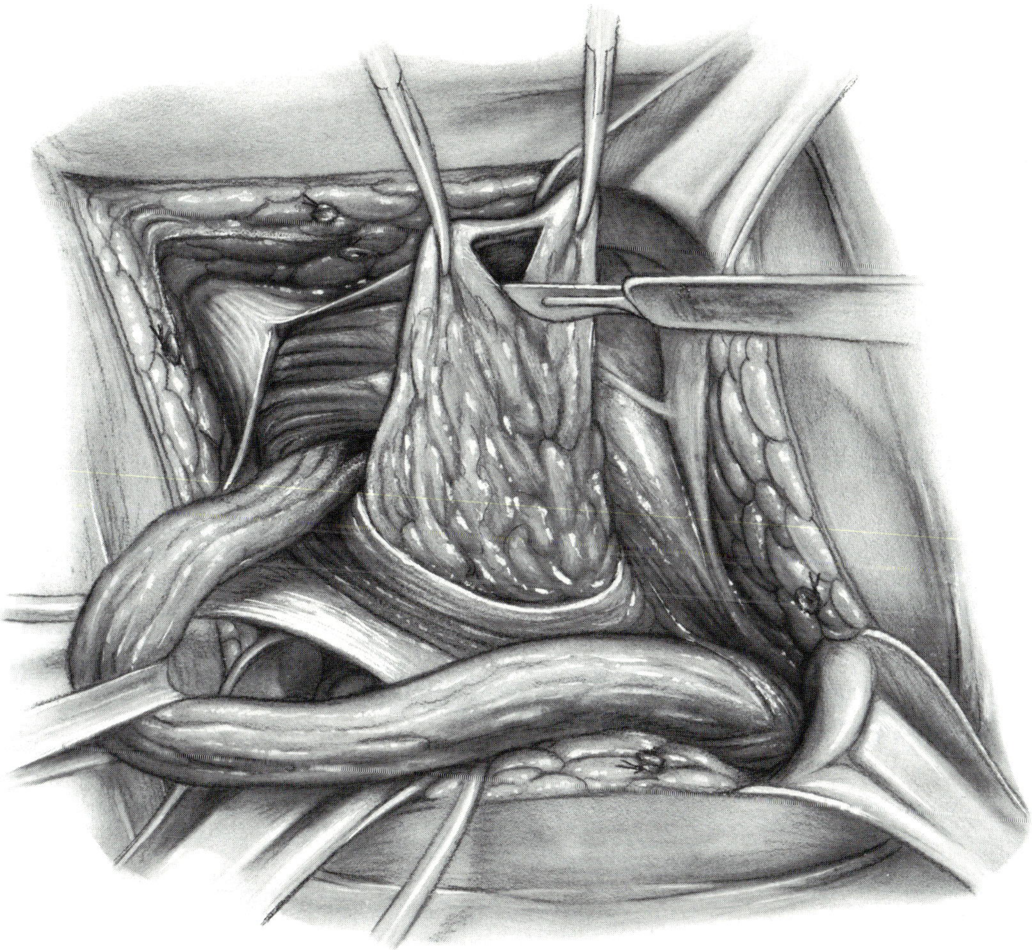

18

REPAIR OF A DIRECT INGUINAL HERNIA AND SLIDING HERNIA OF THE BLADDER

Continued

19, 19A The left index finger is inserted into the lumen of the direct hernial sac, and outward traction is maintained with clamps as the sliding hernia of the bladder is mobilized from its medial wall by scissors dissection (**19**). The dissection of the sliding hernia of the bladder is completed as indicated by the exposure of the obliterated hypogastric artery, elevated on the scissors (**19A**).

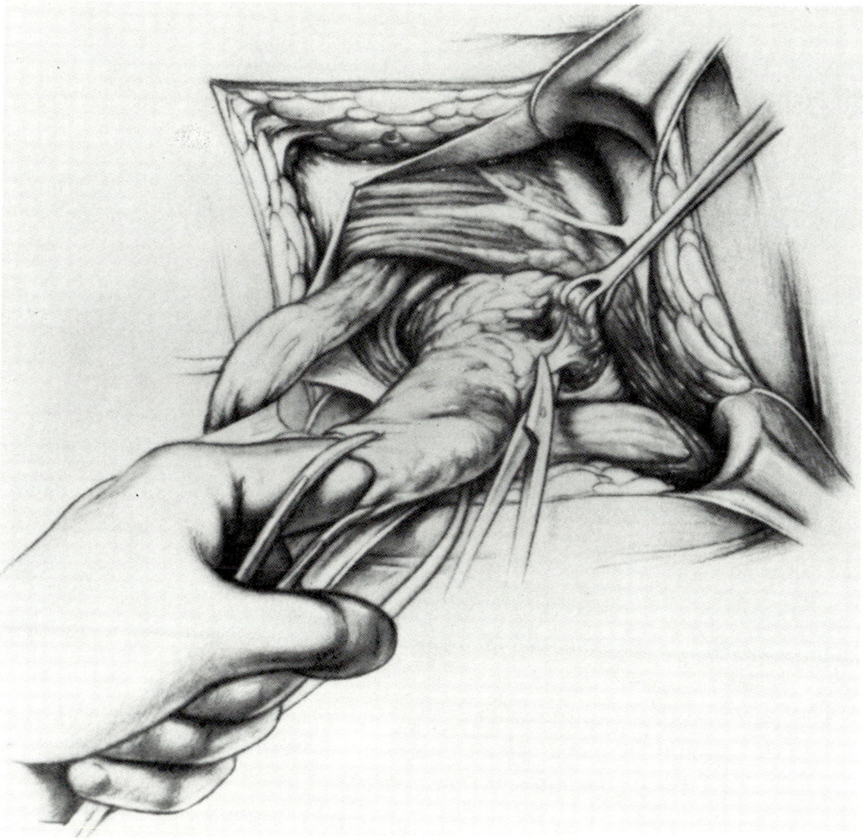

19

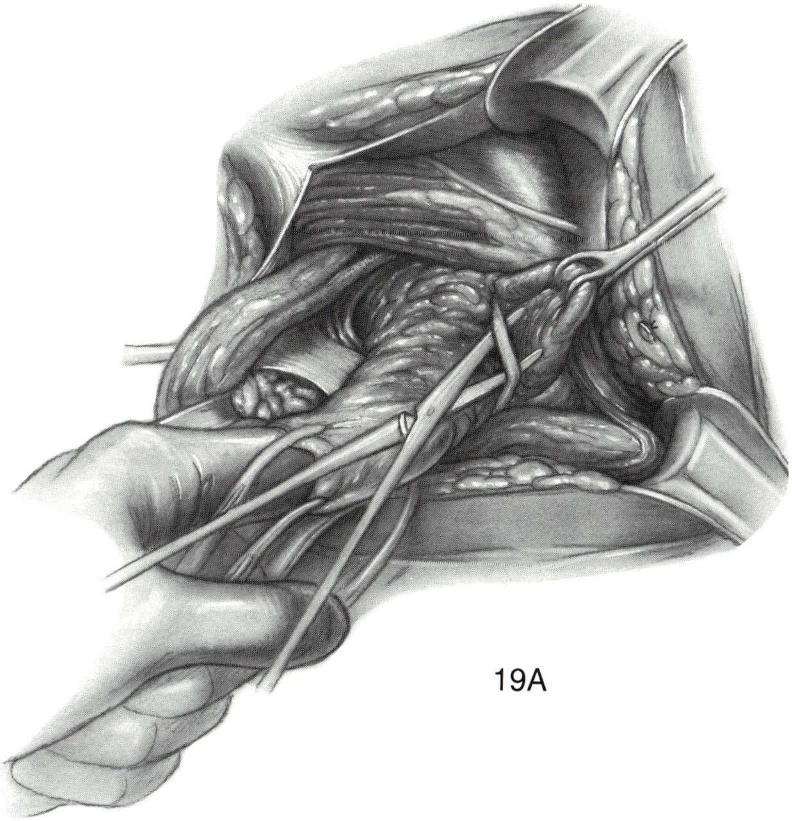

19A

REPAIR OF A DIRECT INGUINAL HERNIA AND SLIDING HERNIA OF THE BLADDER
Continued

20 The outer wall of the hernial sac is bisected with scissors to the level of the neck of the sac (*circular dashed line*). The inner wall is similarly bisected and the redundant leaflets of the hernial sac are excised.

21 The wide neck of the previously excised peritoneal sac is closed by the insertion of interrupted horizontal everting mattress sutures of 3-0 silk. If preferred, a continuous suture of 3-0 chromic catgut may be used. The suture is started at either angle of the neck of the sac, and, on reaching its opposite angle, is returned as an over-and-over suture (baseball stitch) to the starting angle, where it is tied to the opposing suture strand.

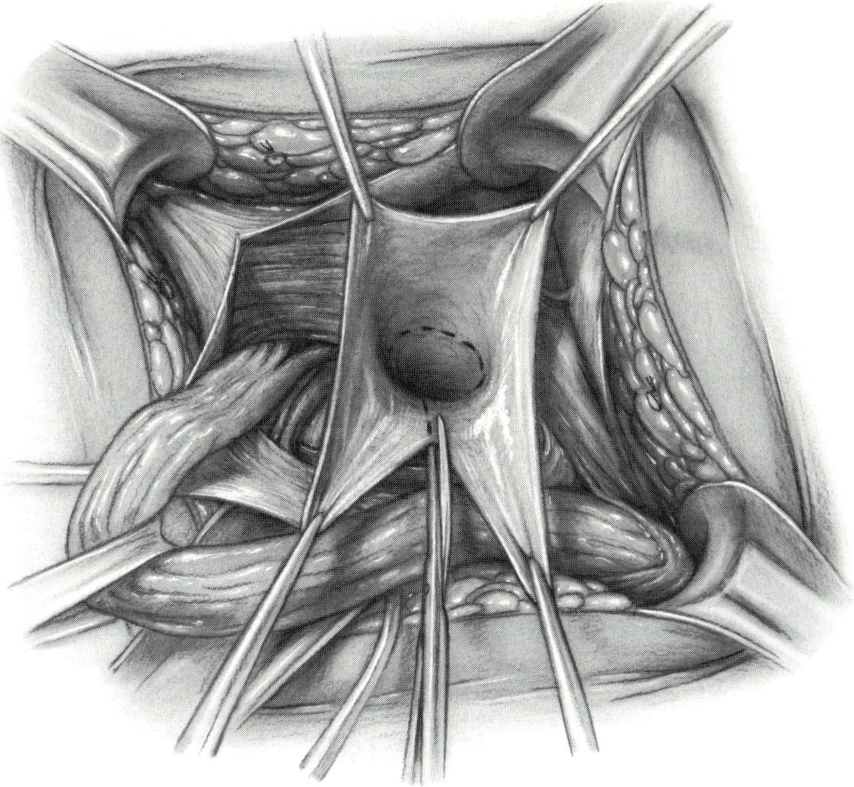

20

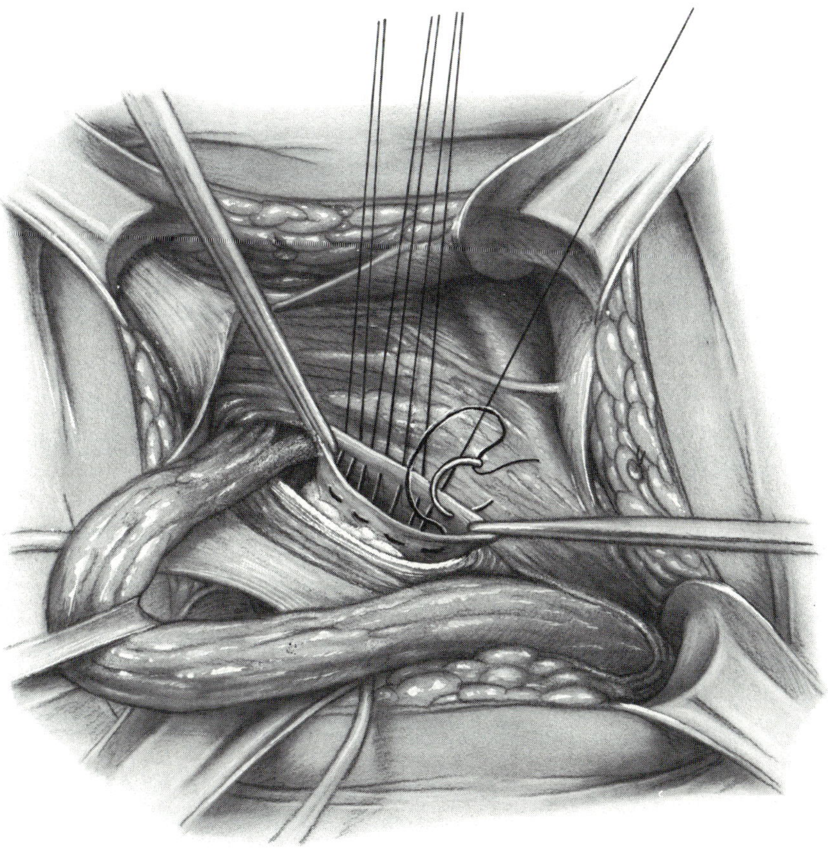

21

REPAIR OF A DIRECT INGUINAL HERNIA AND SLIDING HERNIA OF THE BLADDER

Continued

22 The mattress sutures are tied and the everted cut margins of the peritoneum are approximated with interrupted sutures of 3-0 silk.

23 The tip of a Mixter clamp is readily inserted between the overlying inguinal ligament and the underlying anterior femoral sheath to demonstrate that the ligament has only a contiguous anatomic relationship to the sheath in the surgical reconstruction of the fascia of the posterior inguinal wall.

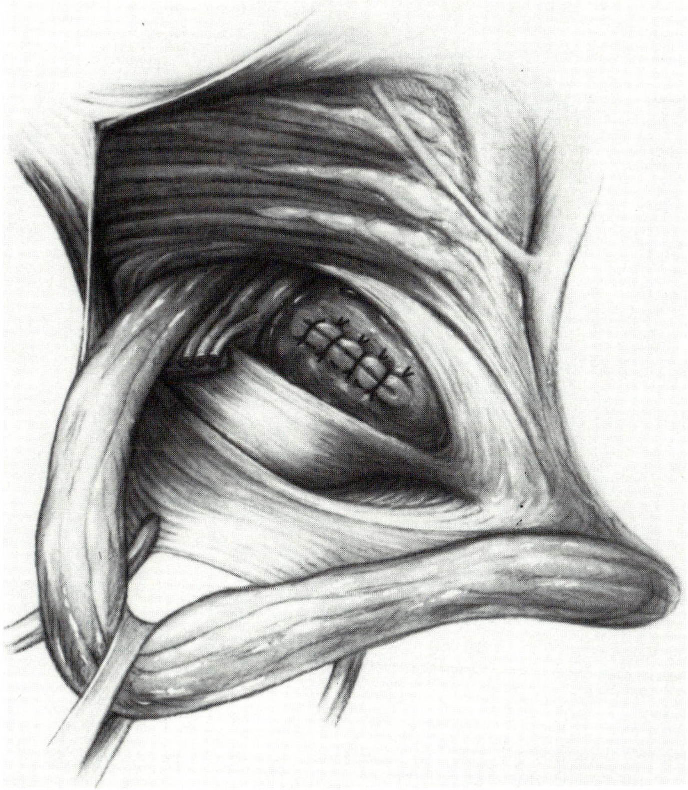

22

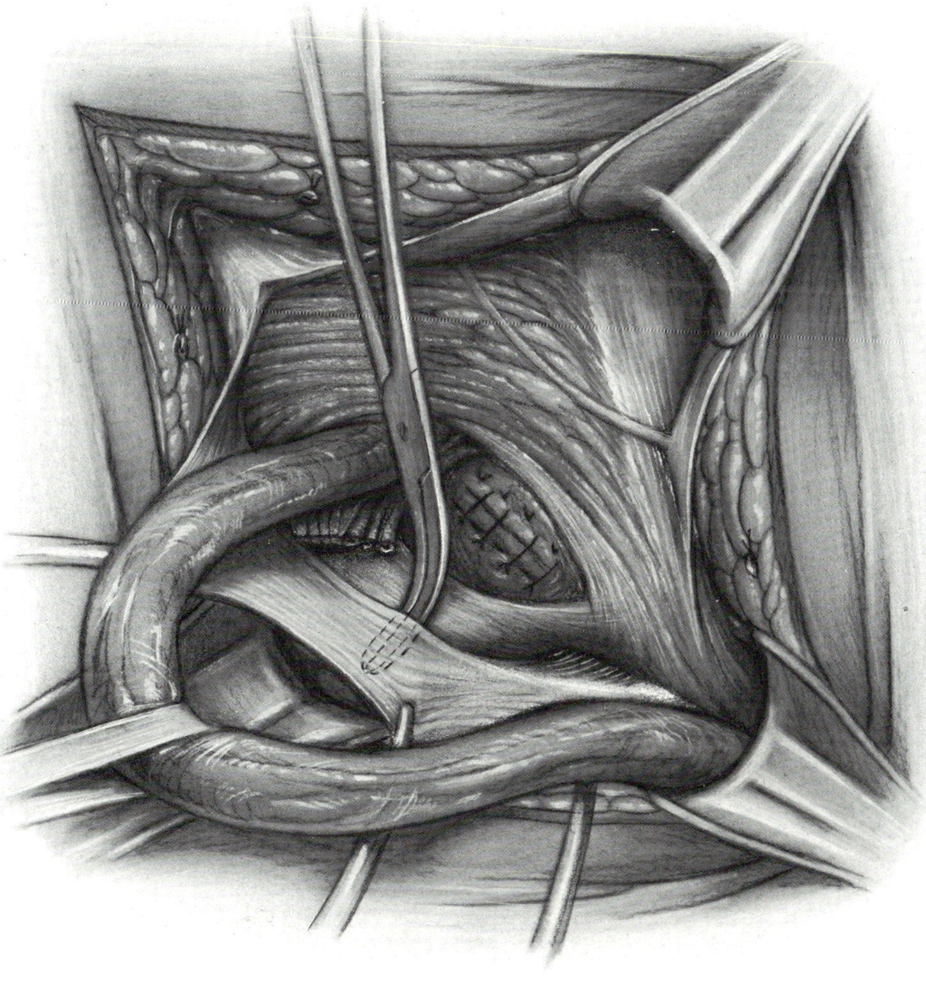

23

REPAIR OF A DIRECT INGUINAL HERNIA AND SLIDING HERNIA OF THE BLADDER

Continued

24 The inferior segment of the fascia of the posterior inguinal wall is pulled up and medially to demonstrate its insertion along Cooper's ligament, in common with the fascial (lacunar) component of Gimbernat's ligament.

25 The inferior segment of the fascia of the posterior inguinal wall, at the site of its continuation as the anterior femoral sheath, is pulled down, and the peritoneal wall and subjacent intraperitoneal viscera are retracted superiorly to expose Cooper's ligament. The relationship of this ligament to the surrounding structures is clearly depicted. Also shown is the inserted but untied "crown" suture for closure of the medial angle of the fascia of the posterior inguinal wall.

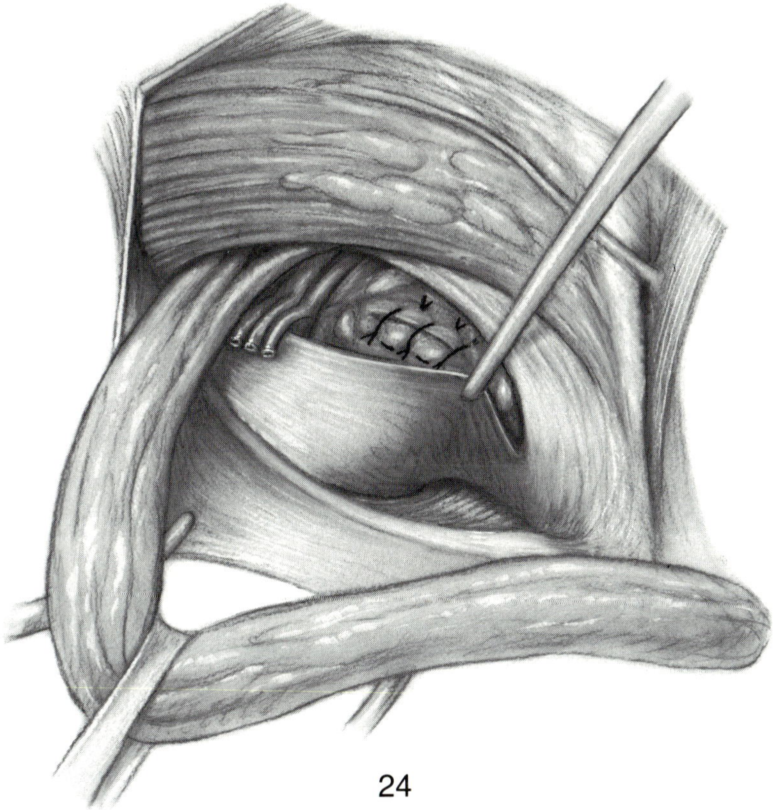

24

25

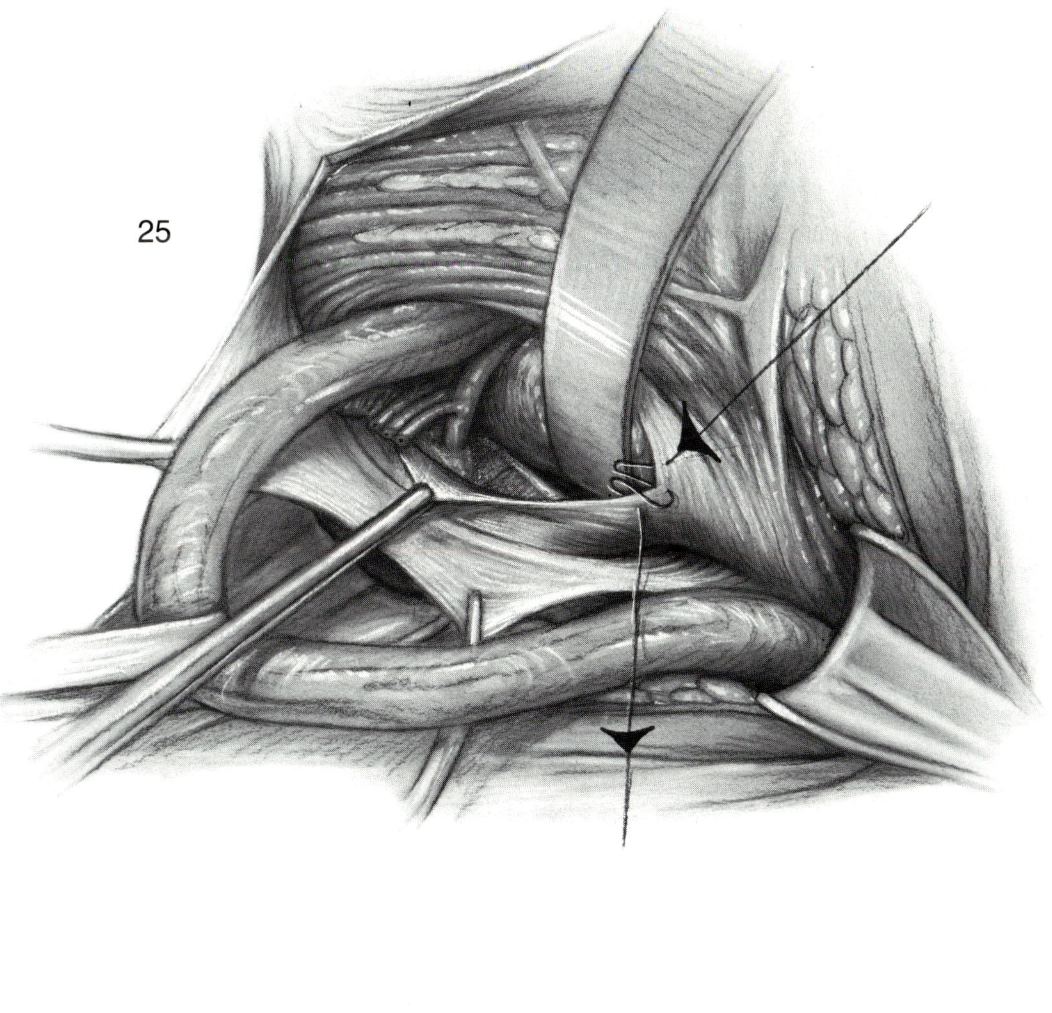

REPAIR OF A DIRECT INGUINAL HERNIA AND SLIDING HERNIA OF THE BLADDER

Continued

26, 27 For purposes of illustration, the inferior segment of the fascia of the posterior inguinal wall, its lateral extension as the anterior femoral sheath, and the underlying transversalis fascia (true femoral sheath) have been excised. Medially, the origin of Cooper's ligament, the juxtaposed insertion of the paddle-shaped expansion of the inguinal liagment (tendinous portion of Gimbernat's ligament), and the medial angle of expansion of the superior segment of the fascia of the posterior inguinal wall may be seen.

Extending laterally from the medial angle, between the inguinal ligament and Cooper's ligament, is the triangular fascial expansion of Gimbernat's ligament, the base of which terminates in a crescentic fascial margin that forms the unyielding medial boundary of the femoral sheath (**26**). The femoral vessels are retracted, rendering visible the intimate apposition of the fibers of the concave crescentic fascial margin of Gimbernat's ligament and the underlying pectineus fascia, at their insertion and origin, respectively, in relation to Cooper's ligament (**27**).

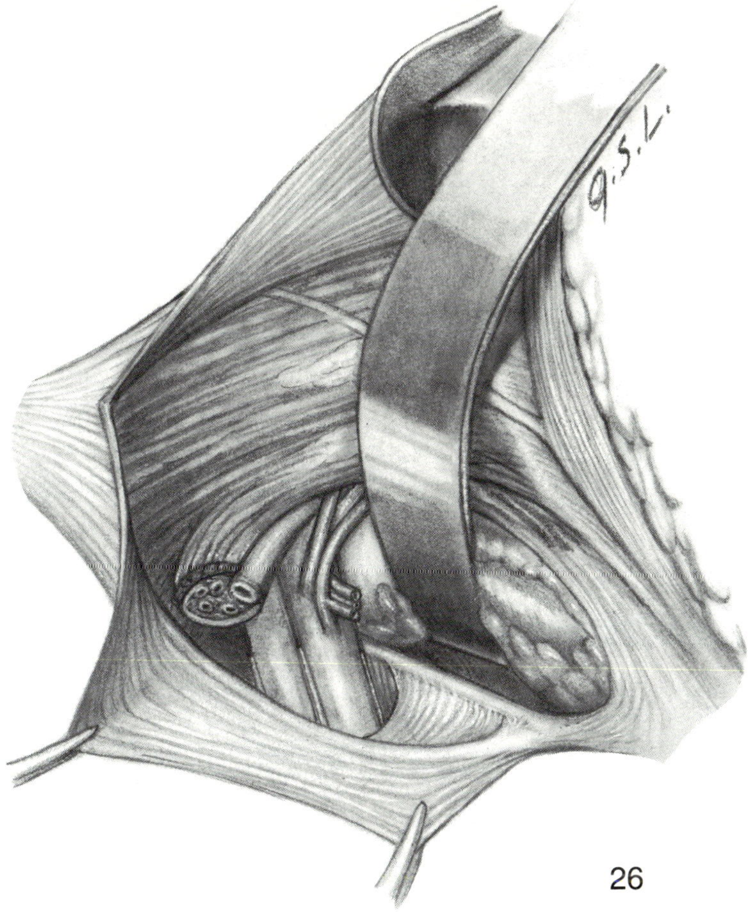

26

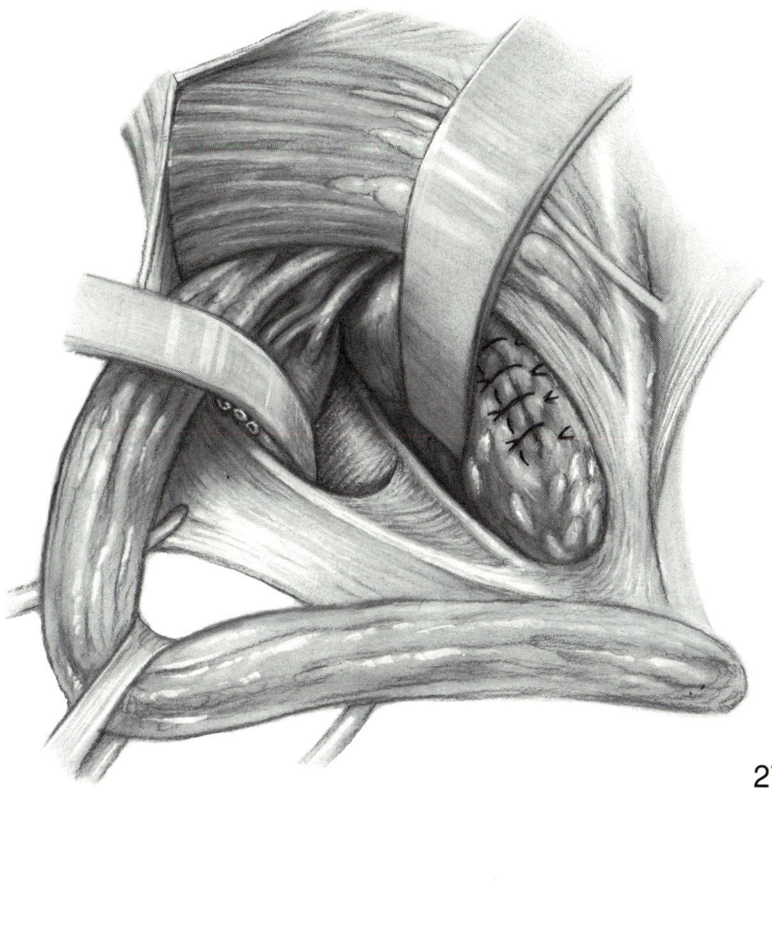

27

REPAIR OF A DIRECT INGUINAL HERNIA AND SLIDING HERNIA OF THE BLADDER

Continued

28, 29, 30 The closure of the defect in the fascia of the posterior inguinal wall (the "floor") is begun by the insertion of the crown suture to close its medial angle. The interrupted suture of 3-0 silk is first inserted through the superior segment of fascia and then, from the inside out, through the intact fascial wall at its medial angle (**28**). A good "bite" of this fascial wall is required to prevent the recurrence of a hernia at this site. The suture is then inserted through the inferior segment of the fascia of the posterior inguinal wall (**29**); when tied, it completes the closure of the medial angle of the fascial defect. A diagrammatic representation of the completed insertion of the untied crown suture is shown (**30**).

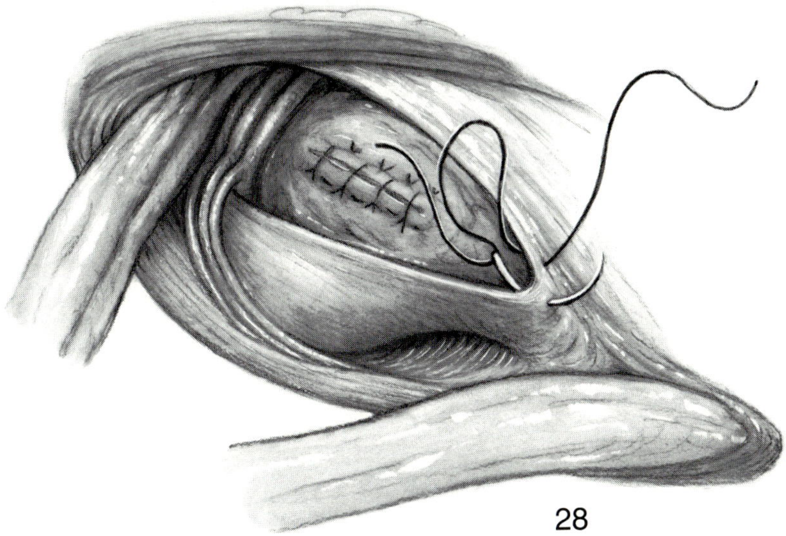

28

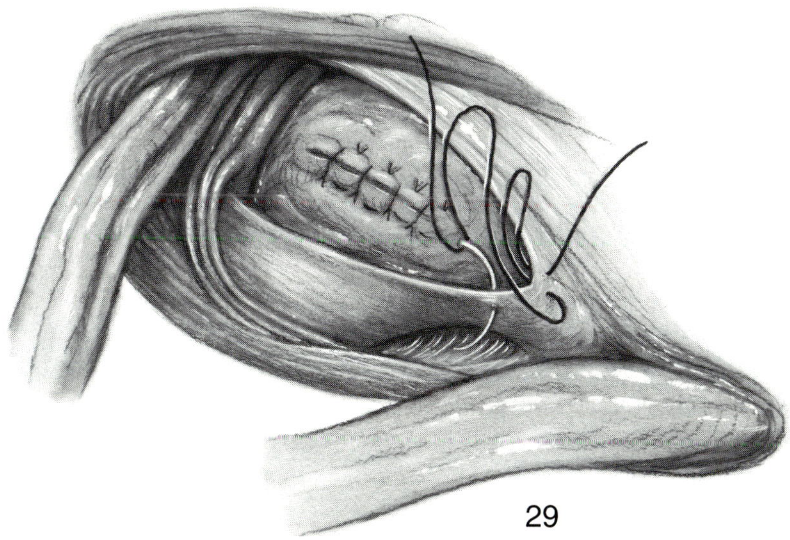

29

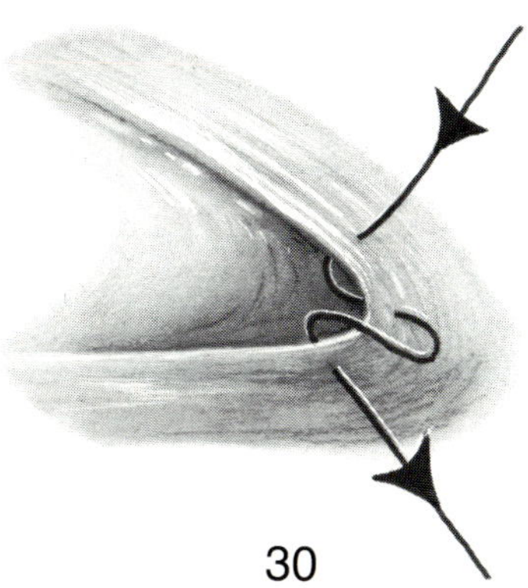

30

REPAIR OF A DIRECT INGUINAL HERNIA AND SLIDING HERNIA OF THE BLADDER

Continued

31 The reconstruction of the posterior inguinal wall (floor) is continued laterally, using interrupted sutures of 3-0 silk. A portion of the needle of one of these sutures is inserted through the inferior (lateral) segment of the posterior inguinal wall, which at this level is commonly referred to as the anterior femoral sheath. This suture corresponds to the approximate location of the transition suture of McVay for the closure of the defect in the medial wall of the femoral sheath. It differs, however, in that the normal anatomic plane for the in-continuity closure of the fascia of the posterior inguinal wall is maintained. Furthermore, since there is no defect in the medial wall of the femoral sheath to close, the trough deformity inherent in the use of the transition suture is avoided.

32 The fascial reconstruction is continued in its normal plane around the exit of the cremaster vessels, which may be sacrificed if desired. Maintenance of these vessels, however, does not produce a weakness in the repair of the fascia of the posterior inguinal wall but is simply a restoration of their normal anatomic site of exit.

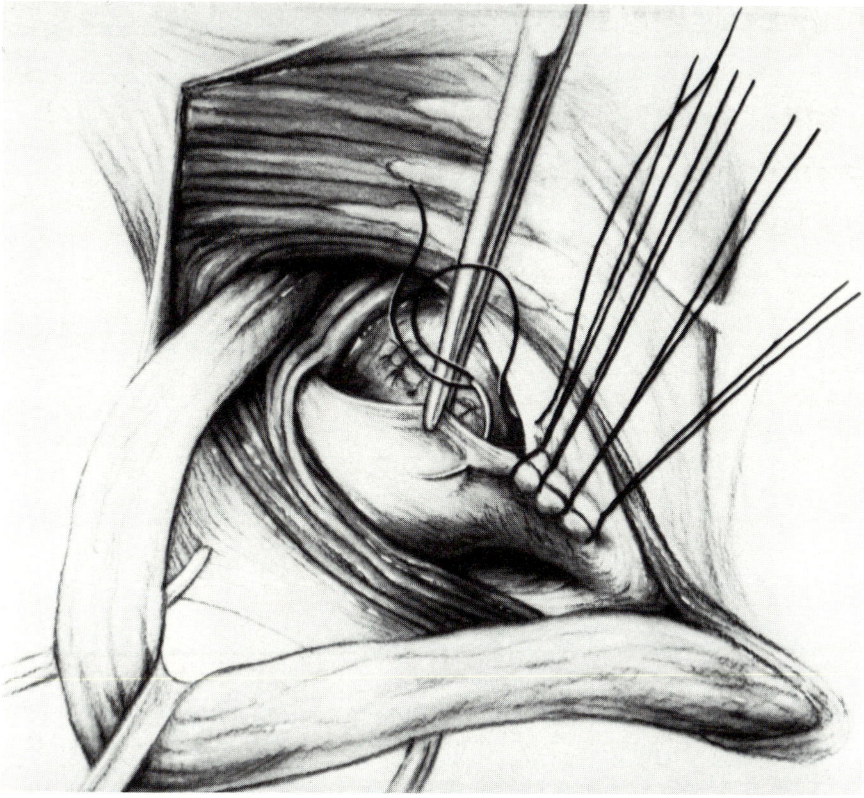

31

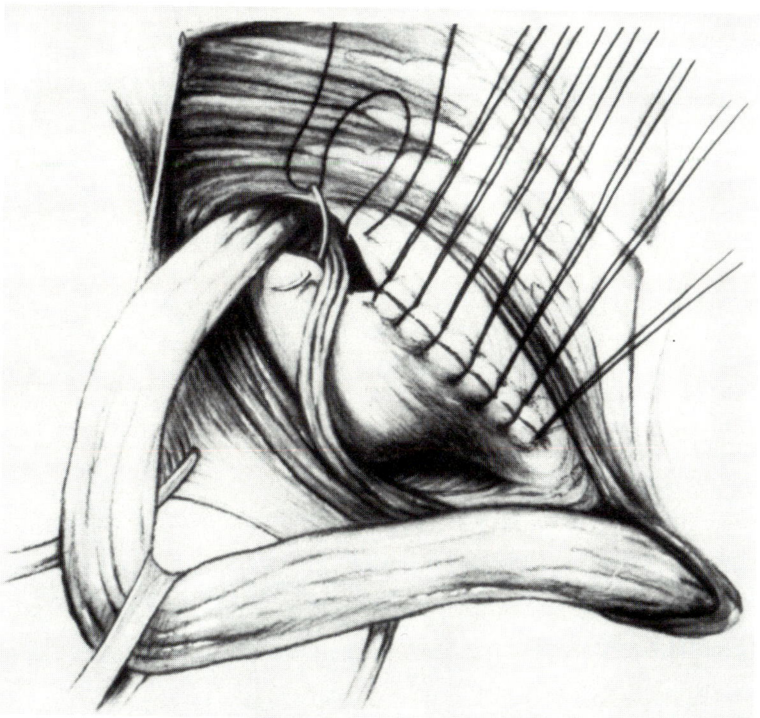

32

REPAIR OF A DIRECT INGUINAL HERNIA AND SLIDING HERNIA OF THE BLADDER

Continued

33 In this alternate technique, the cremaster vessels are displaced laterally beneath the cord, instead of having their normal exit through the reconstructed fascia of the posterior inguinal wall.

34 The one-layer reconstruction of the fascia of the posterior inguinal wall is completed, and its relationship to the pyriform fossa may be seen. This fossa is bounded superiorly by the inferior segment of the fascia of the posterior inguinal wall; inferiorly by the shelving border of the inguinal ligament; medially by the tendinous paddle-shaped portion of Gimbernat's ligament and its expansion onto the adjacent fascia of the posterior inguinal wall; and laterally by the medial wall of the anterior femoral sheath. The floor of the fossa is formed by the fascial or lacunar portion of Gimbernat's ligament.

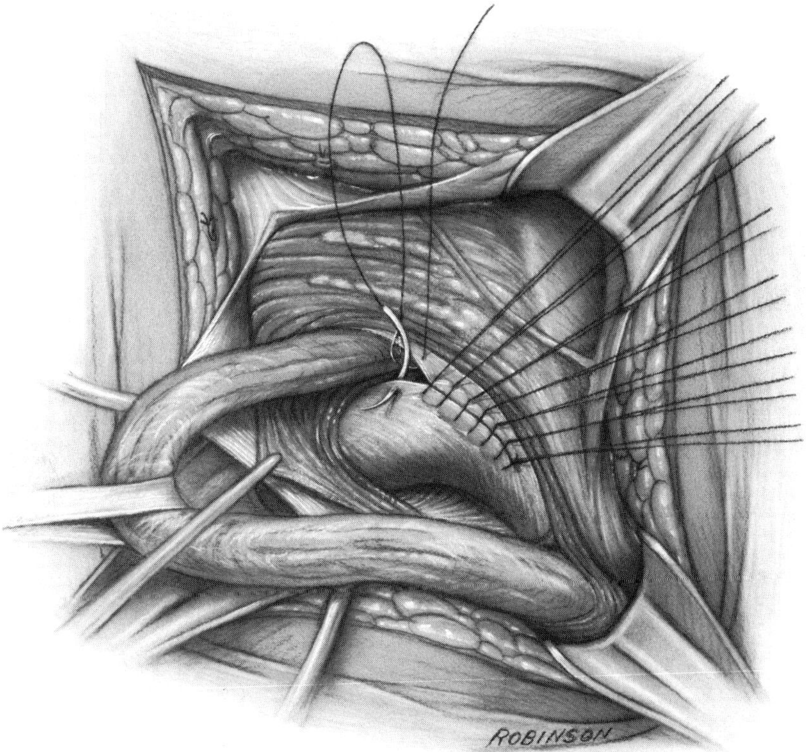

33

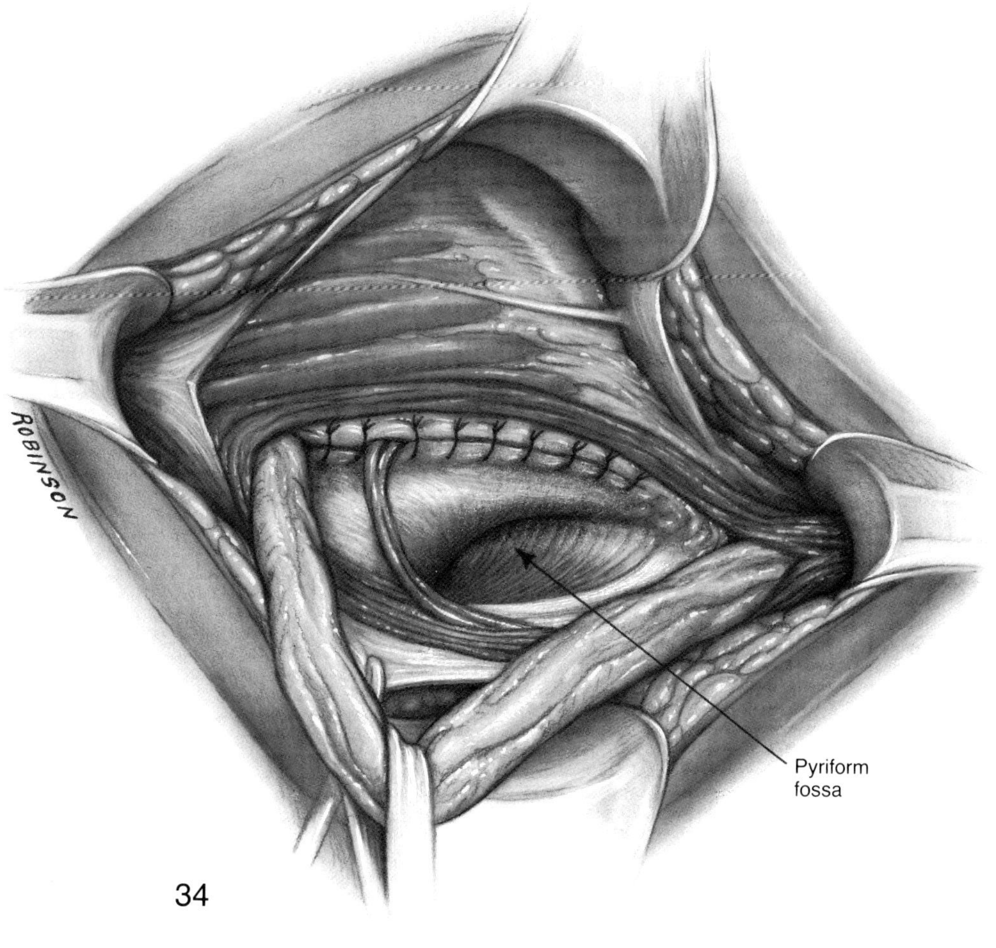

34

REPAIR OF A DIRECT INGUINAL HERNIA AND SLIDING HERNIA OF THE BLADDER

Continued

35 The spermatic cord is placed on the reconstructed posterior inguinal wall, and the separated margins of the cremaster muscle are approximated with interrupted sutures of 4-0 silk. This closure of the cremaster muscle is more applicable to the repair of the indirect rather than the direct inguinal hernia, because of the frequent anatomic variations inherent in the latter.

36 The superior (medial) and inferior (lateral) leaflets of the aponeurosis of the external oblique muscle are approximated with interrupted sutures of 3-0 silk.

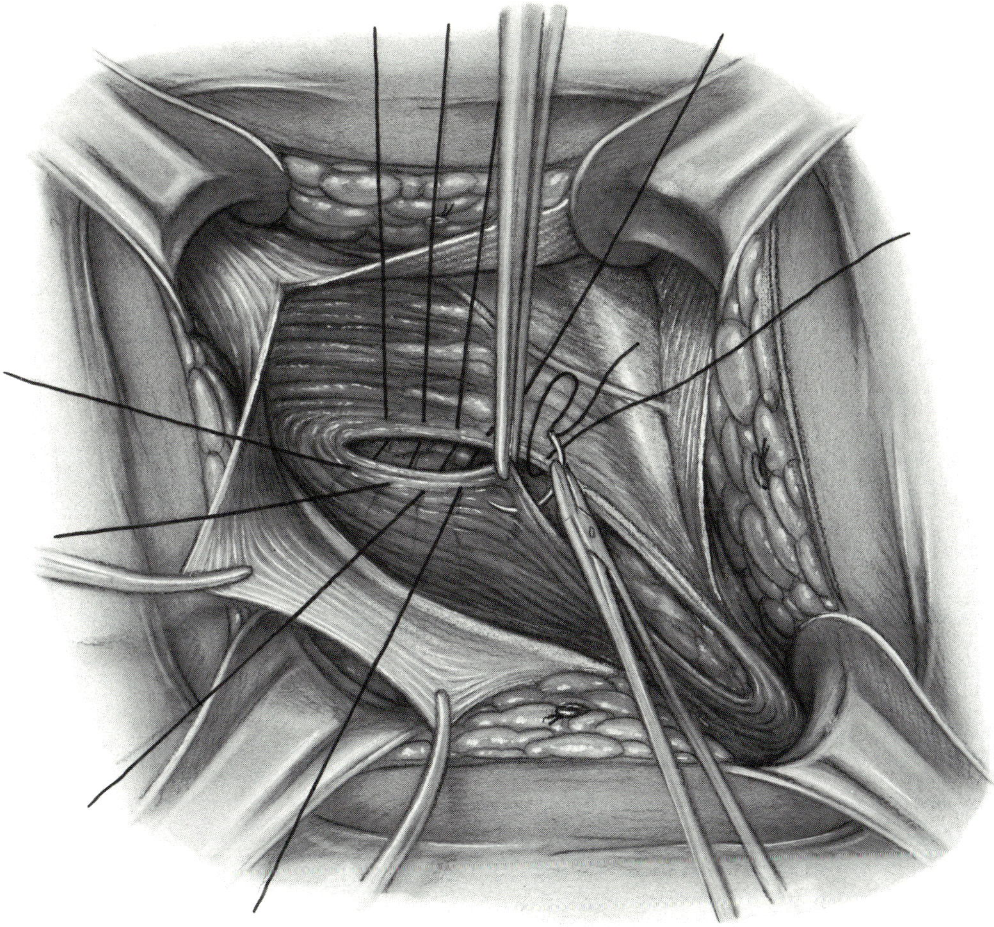

35

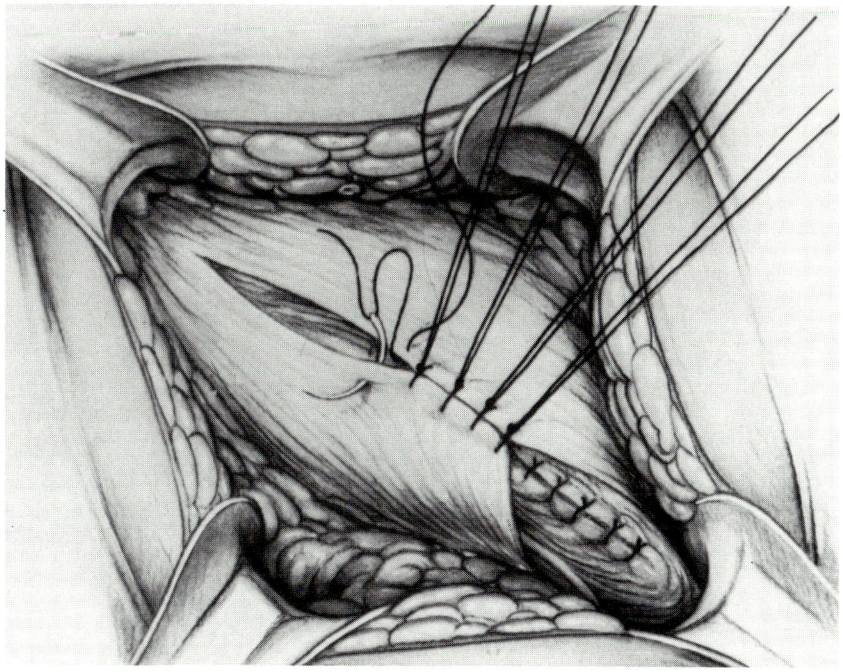

36

REPAIR OF A DIRECT INGUINAL HERNIA AND SLIDING HERNIA OF THE BLADDER

Continued

37, 38 The subcutaneous (deep) fascial layer (Scarpa's fascia) is closed with interrupted sutures of 4-0 silk (**37**). The skin is closed with interrupted sutures of 4-0 silk, threaded on straight needles that are inserted separately, then individually withdrawn, and the suture is tied (**38**). A wound dressing is not applied.

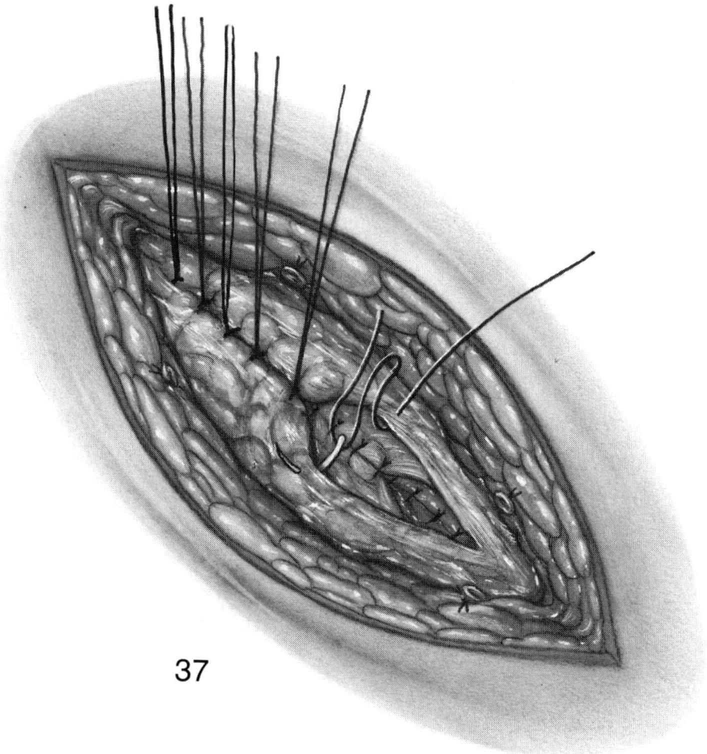

37

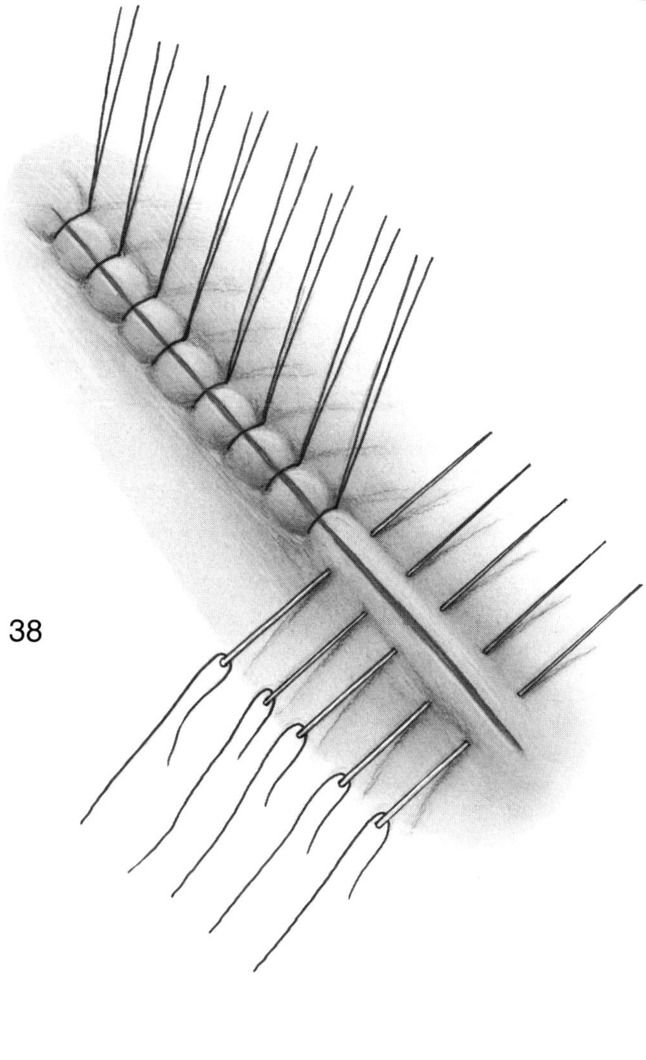

38

REPAIR OF A DIRECT INGUINAL HERNIA AND SLIDING HERNIA OF THE BLADDER
Continued

REFERENCES

1. Dunphy, JE: On the nature and care of wounds (Moynihan Lecture). Ann R Coll Surg Engl *26*:69–87, 1960.
2. Farris, JM, Smith, GK, and Beattie, AS: Umbilical hernia: An inquiry into principles of imbrication and a note on the preservation of the umbilical dimple. Am J Surg *98*:236–242, 1959.
3. Hoguet, JP: Direct inguinal hernia. Ann Surg *72*:671–674, 1920.

DISCUSSION

Chester B. McVay, M.D.

I prefer a transverse incision that follows the lines of skin cleavage. It crosses the position of the abdominal inguinal ring, which is determined as half the distance between the pubic tubercle and the anterosuperior iliac spine. The length of the incision depends upon the size of the hernia, and its transverse or oblique direction depends upon the habitus of the patient. It does, however, follow the lines of skin cleavage. The exposure with the "groin crease" incision is just as good as with the oblique incision: cosmetically, the scar is much more acceptable.

I begin the incision of the intercrural fascia at the subcutaneous inguinal ring and progress laterally, as I think it is easier in this way to identify the ilioinguinal nerve.

In a direct hernia I do not open the cremaster muscle as depicted. I am, however, in perfect agreement with Madden regarding the excision of the attenuated fascia of the posterior inguinal wall, since it is worthless as a constituent in the operative repair. I notice, however, that Madden leaves a remnant of the fascia of the posterior inguinal wall inferiorly or caudally, to be used in the closure of the hernial defect. I believe that this segment of fascia is of insufficient holding power for the reconstruction of the posterior inguinal wall. Therefore, I excise it completely, down to Cooper's ligament.

The hernial defect should be closed with a fascial layer of good holding power and without tension on the suture line. Accordingly, I prefer to suture the rectus sheath to Cooper's ligament, which represents the normal insertion of the posterior inguinal wall. To do so, however, a relaxing incision in the rectus sheath is mandatory, in order to permit its "slide" for approximation without tension to Cooper's ligament.

In the treatment of the large direct inguinal hernia, Madden's method is to open the sac, reduce the sliding hernia of the urinary bladder that is invariably present, and excise the redundant sac. My own preference is simply to reduce the peritoneal bulge without entering the peritoneal cavity. Therefore, I am not concerned about injuring the urinary bladder, nor am I interested in seeing the anatomic remnant of the obliterated hypogastric artery following the mobilization of the bladder from the hernial sac, as depicted by Madden.

OPERATION 2

ANATOMIC REPAIR OF A COMBINED INDIRECT-DIRECT INGUINAL HERNIA

Plate VIII
Plate IX
Plate X

This repair of an indirect-direct inguinal hernia is called anatomic because the tissues of the groin are opened in layers and, after excision of the indirect hernial sac and reconstruction of the direct hernial defect in the posterior inguinal wall, they are simply closed in layers in a reverse fashion. None of the normal anatomic structures are removed. Furthermore, no synthetic prosthesis, as a tissue support, is used.

1 An oblique inguinal incision is made about 2 cm superior to and paralleling the medial half of the inguinal ligament (*dashed outline*). It starts at the level of the internal ring (*lateral X*) and extends medially for a distance of approximately 7 cm, terminating in close proximity to the pubic tubercle (*medial X*).

Although this incision is preferred by the author, many surgeons—perhaps even the majority—would use the more anatomic transverse groin crease incision.

2 The thin preperitoneal areolar tissue layer is held taut in tissue forceps to demonstrate the relationship of the preperitoneal fatty tissue layer ("lipoma") to the spermatic cord structures (spermatic vessels and vas deferens). The fibroareolar tissue between the vas deferens and the subjacent genital branch of the genitofemoral nerve and cremaster vessels was termed by MacLeod the "mesentery of the cord." Through an opening in this relatively avascular mesentery, the cord will be mobilized on the index finger.

3, 3A By scissors dissection, the preperitoneal fatty tissue is severed from its loose attachment to the hernial sac (**3**). It is then ligated cephalad with a transfixion suture ligature of 3-0 silk, and the redundant segment is excised with scissors (**3A**).

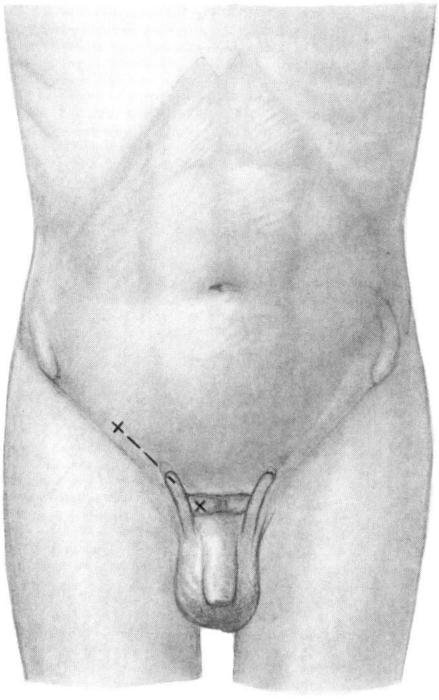

1

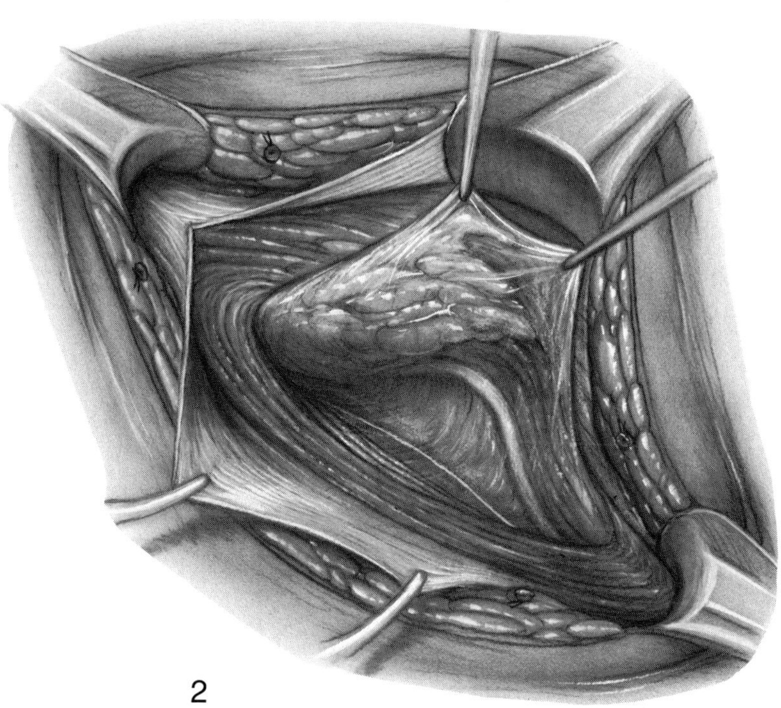

2

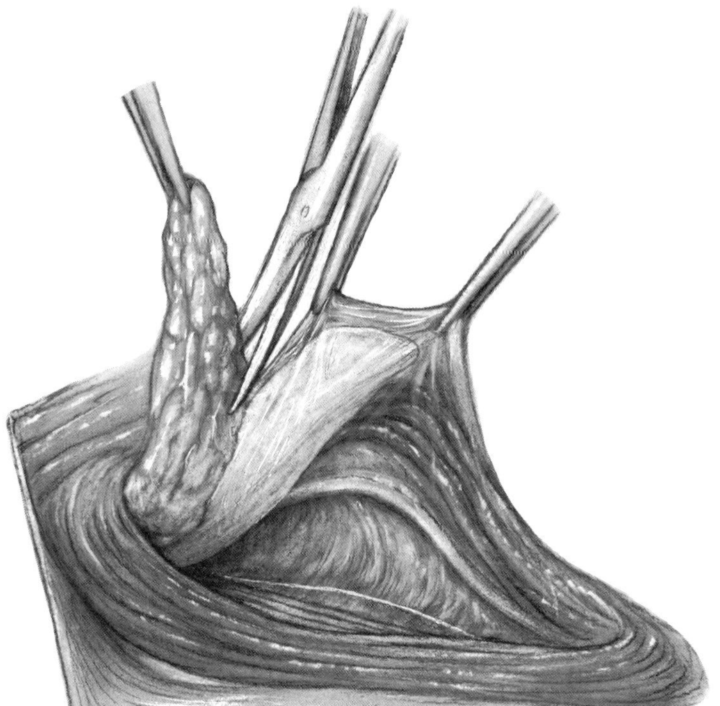

3

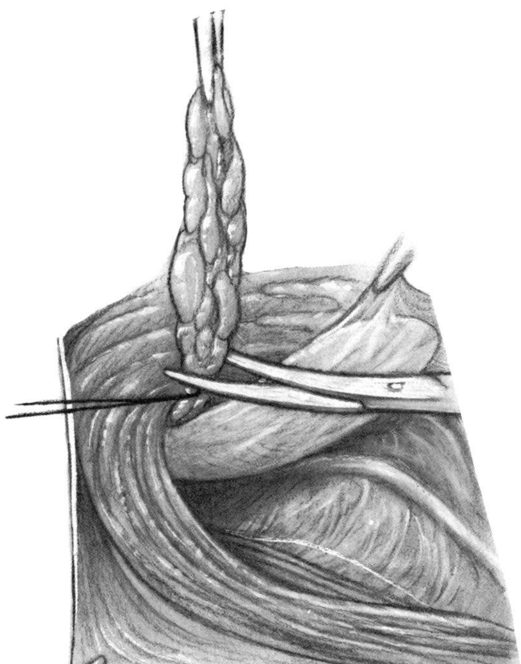

3A

ANATOMIC REPAIR OF A COMBINED INDIRECT-DIRECT INGUINAL HERNIA
Continued

4 Tissue countertraction is maintained as scissors dissection of the fibroareolar tissue from its attachment to the hernial sac is commenced (*dashed line*).

5 The hernial sac is opened after being mobilized laterally to expose the angle of convergence of the spermatic vessels and the vas deferens. This angle is the anatomic landmark for the level of high ligation and excision of the sac.

A commonly practiced alternate technique of mobilizing the sac is to insert the index finger into the opened sac; by a combination of digital countertraction and scissors dissection, the sac is separated from the cord. Dissection of the unopened sac is preferred because the double thickness of its intact wall decreases the incidence of inadvertent tears. Furthermore, it provides a distinctive "white border" that facilitates both its identification and mobilization.

The bulge of preperitoneal fat beneath the oval attenuated fascia of the posterior inguinal wall (the accompanying direct hernia) is visible.

6, 6A The left index finger is inserted into the lumen of the sac, then beneath the deep epigastric vessels, to elevate the anterior parietal peritoneum and overlying layer of preperitoneal fat through the fascial defect in the posterior inguinal wall (**6**). This direct hernial component is treated by an elliptical excision of the overlying attenuated fascia and suture closure of the fascial defect in the posterior inguinal wall. Should the deep epigastric vessels pose a technical problem, they are doubly clamped, transected (**6A**), and ligated.

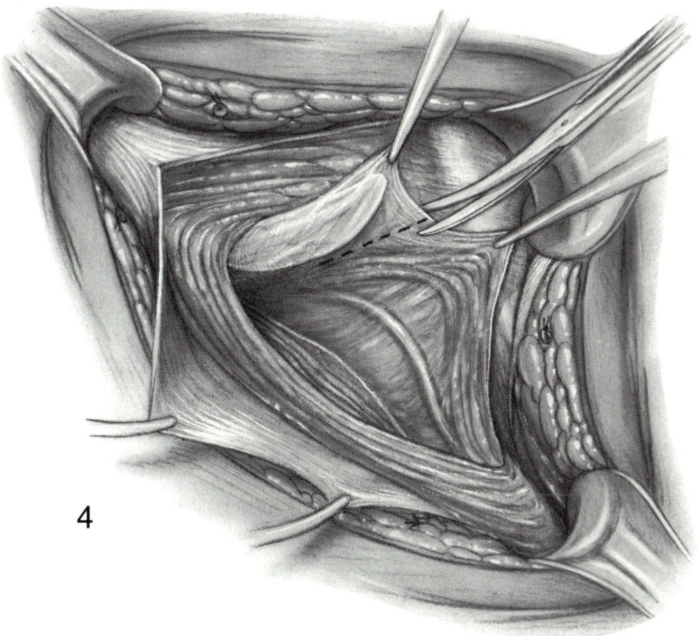

4

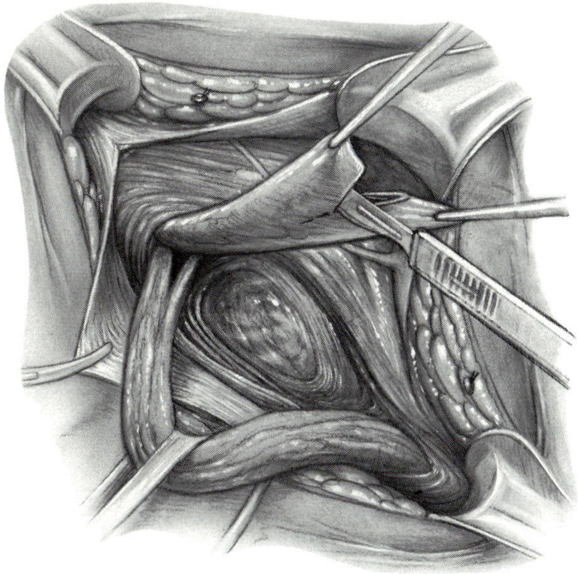

5

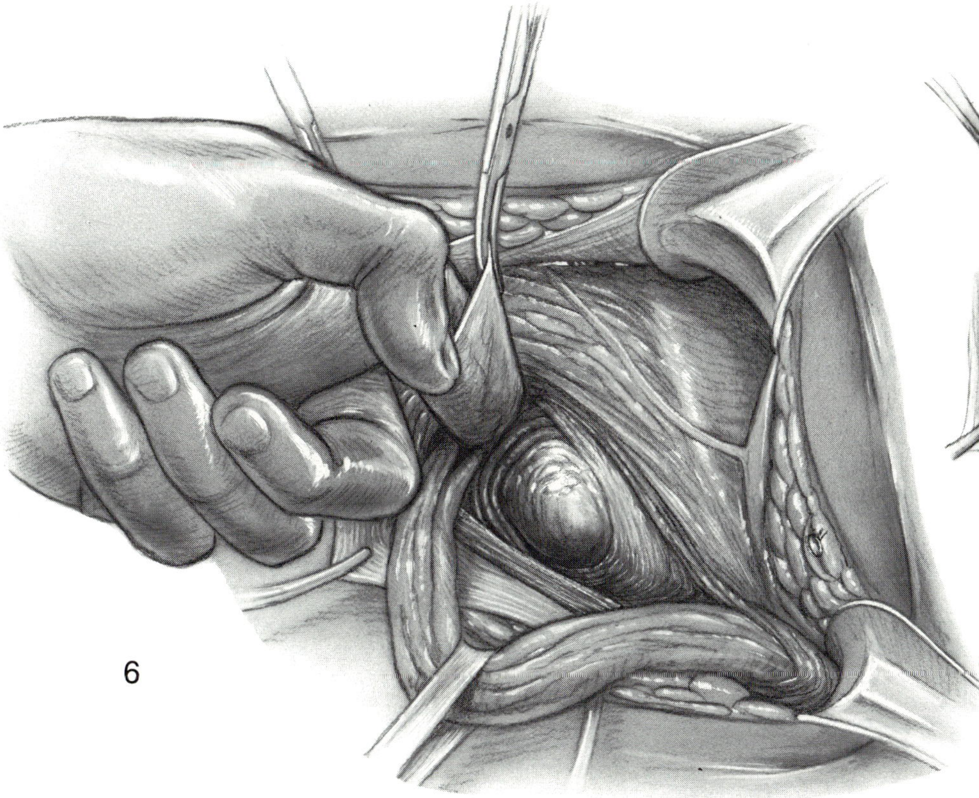

6

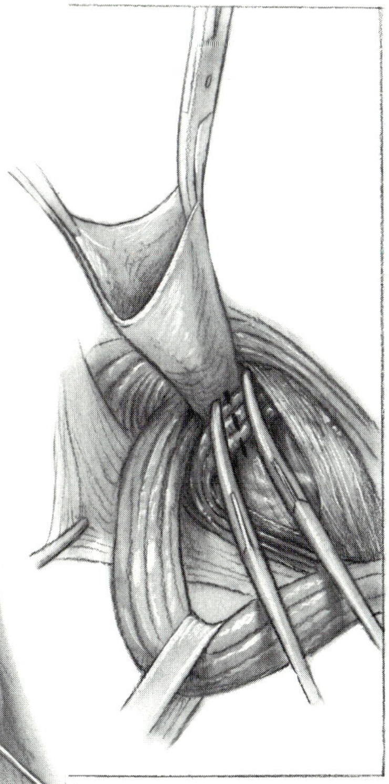

6A

ANATOMIC REPAIR OF A COMBINED INDIRECT-DIRECT INGUINAL HERNIA
Continued

7, 8 For intraoperative detection of a potential or existing direct inguinal hernia, the left index finger is inserted into the open sac of the indirect inguinal hernia and beneath the deep epigastric vessels to elevate the posterior inguinal wall and test its fascial integrity (**7**). In like manner, the tip of the finger can be directed down and the femoral "ring" explored to rule out the presence of a concomitant femoral hernia (**8**).

In both of these illustrations, the deep epigastric vessels—the artery in the middle and an accompanying vein on each side—are clearly shown. Also visible are the transected open end of the cremaster artery at its origin from the deep epigastric artery and the open ends of the cremaster tributary veins on each side. The pyriform fossa and its anatomic relationship to the fascia of the posterior inguinal wall also may be seen.

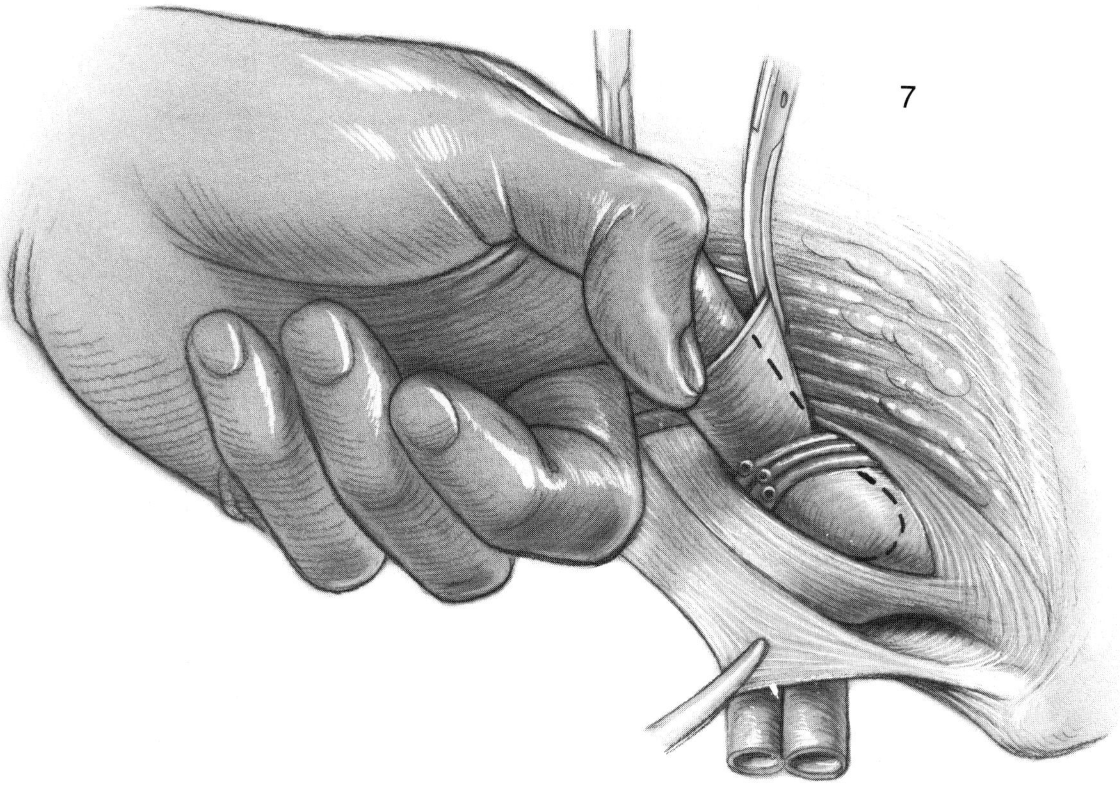

7

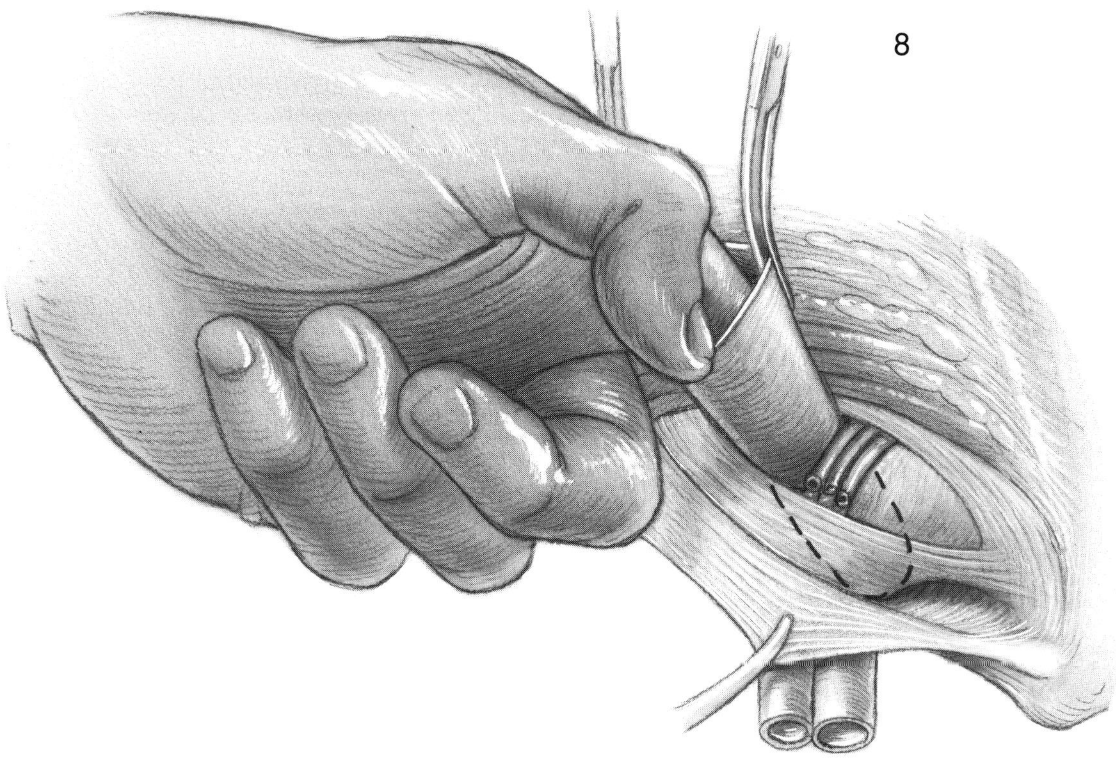

8

ANATOMIC REPAIR OF A COMBINED INDIRECT-DIRECT INGUINAL HERNIA
Continued

9, 9A, 9B The open and empty hernial sac is triangulated with clamps (**9**), and its neck is transfixed with the needle of a swaged suture of 3-0 silk (**9A**). After being inserted, the suture is tied on one side of the neck of the sac, and its strands are then tied on the opposite side (**9B**).

9C The insertion of the transfixion suture is completed, and its relationship to the angle of convergence of the spermatic vessels and vas deferens is visible. The redundant portion of the sac is resected with scissors (*dashed line*).

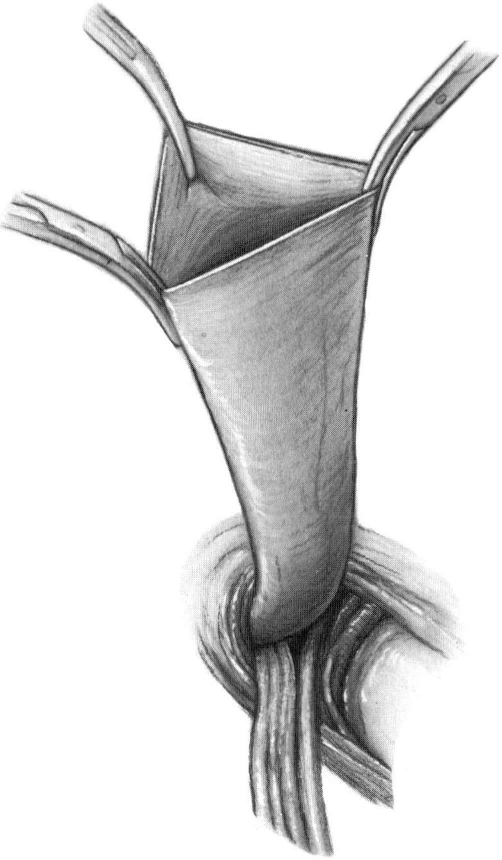

9

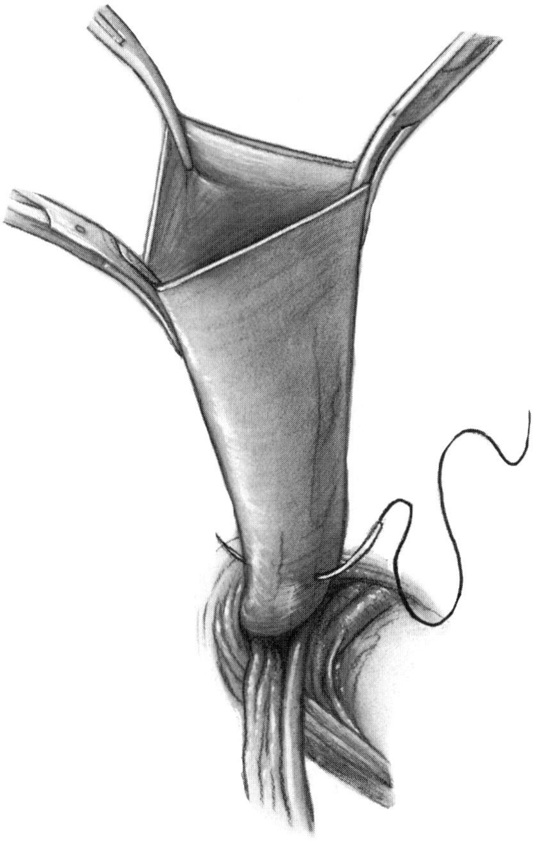

9A

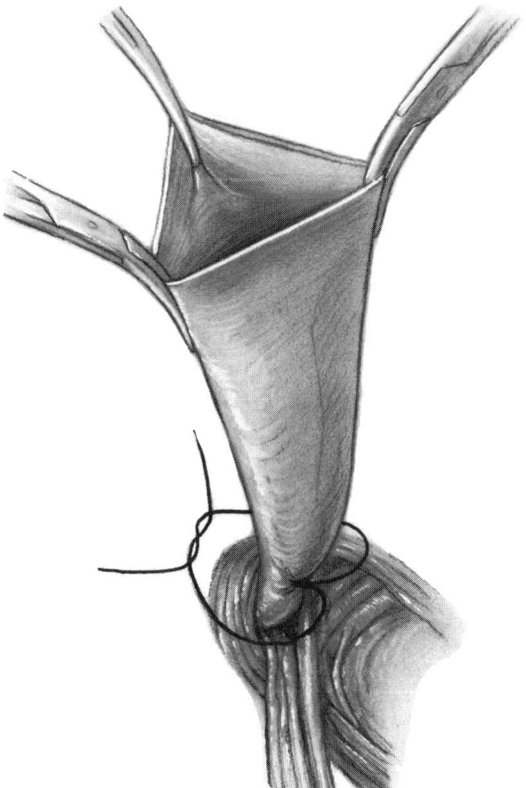

9B

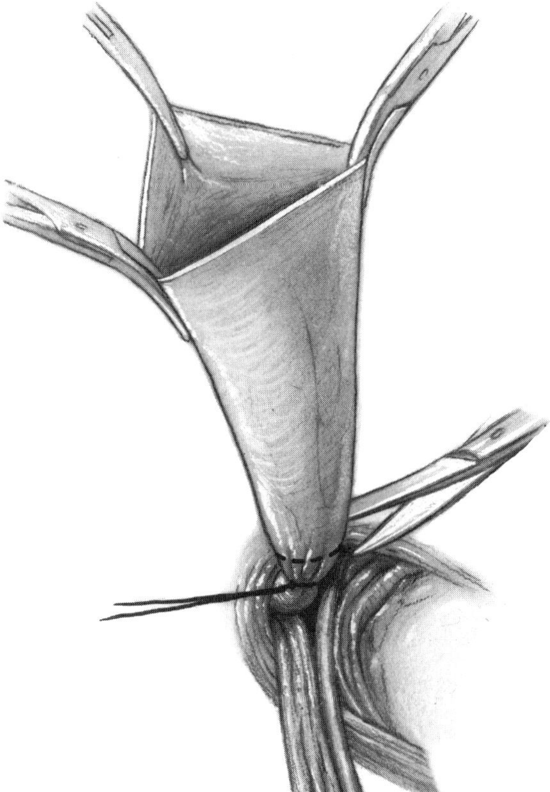

9C

ANATOMIC REPAIR OF A COMBINED INDIRECT-DIRECT INGUINAL HERNIA

Continued

10, 10A The retracted cuff of the ligated neck of the sac of the indirect inguinal hernia is indicated by the *circular dashes.* The attenuated fascia of the posterior inguinal wall has been excised, and the medial angle crown suture of 3-0 silk is tied. For technical expediency, the remaining sutures (3-0 silk) are first inserted (**10**) and subsequently tied in sequence to complete the single-layer closure of the direct hernial defect in the fascia of the posterior inguinal wall (**10A**). The cremaster vessels have their exit through the line of fascial reconstruction, medial to the snug closure of the internal ring about the exit of the spermatic cord. This is their normal site of exit, and its maintenance does not weaken the surgical repair.

Neither the internal oblique muscle nor the inguinal ligament participates in the surgical repair of the combined indirect-direct inguinal hernia. The cord is placed on the single-layer fascial reconstruction of the posterior inguinal wall, and the overlying cremaster veil, external oblique aponeurosis, subcutaneous fascia, and skin are closed serially in layers to complete the operation.

In the indirect (congenital) inguinal hernia, even if it is small, exposure of the internal ring almost invariably shows a V-shaped fascial defect that requires two or three sutures (3-0 silk) to obtain a snug closure of the internal ring around the exit of the cord. This is true in children as well as in adults. Failure to close this defect in the fascia is believed to be the anatomic basis for the subsequent "recurrence" of the hernia. This belief is supported by the oft-repeated statement, "The recurrence of an indirect inguinal hernia is usually at the internal ring." Rather than a recurrence, however, it is thought to be a primary hernia through the uncorrected pre-existing fascial defect around the internal ring.

In the treatment of inguinal hernias in infants aged six to 12 months, the "Scottish technique" has proved popular. This consists of making a small incision in the external oblique aponeurosis lateral to the external ring, which is not opened, and "teasing" the sac from the cord to expose its neck. The unopened sac is twisted on itself and occluded at its base with a transfixion suture of 4-0 silk. The redundant portion of the twisted sac is excised, and the incision in the aponeurosis is closed.

Undoubtedly, completely satisfactory results have been obtained with this technique. Unfortunately, however, they are difficult to substantiate in scientific fact. To do so would require the follow-up of a large number of these infants through adolescence into adult life. Such a necessary and admittedly most difficult study, to the author's knowledge, has not been reported.

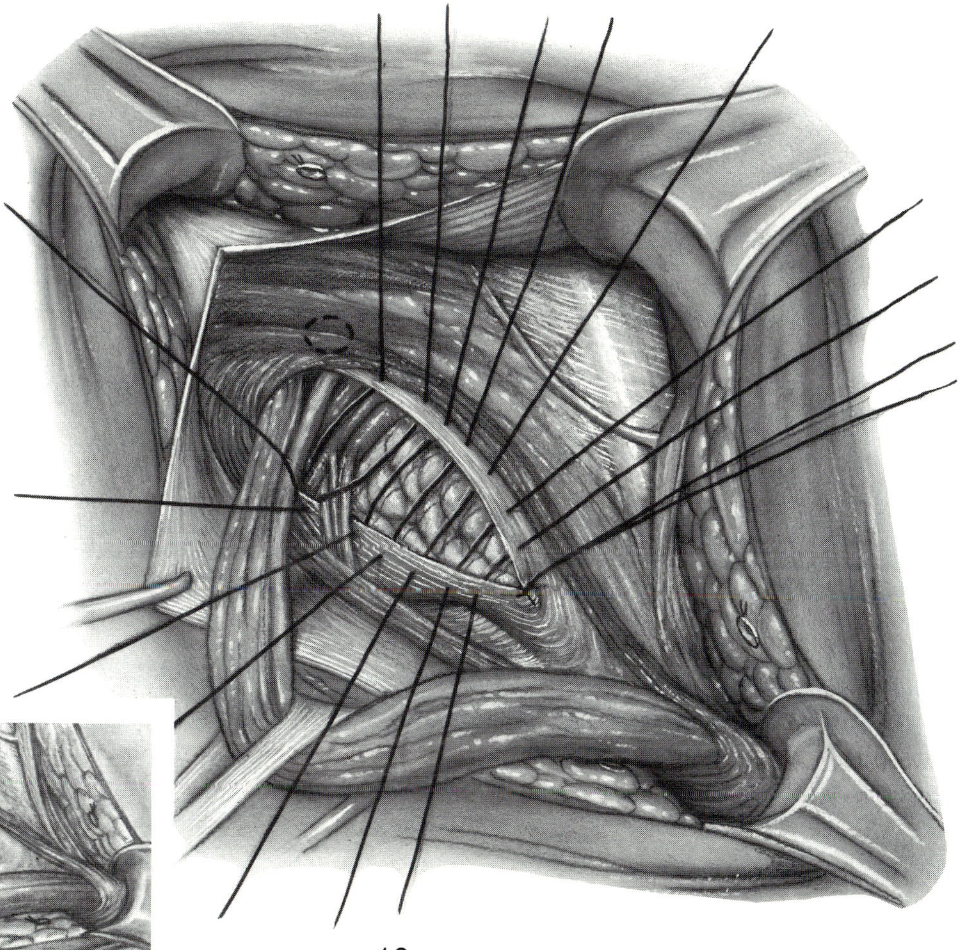

10

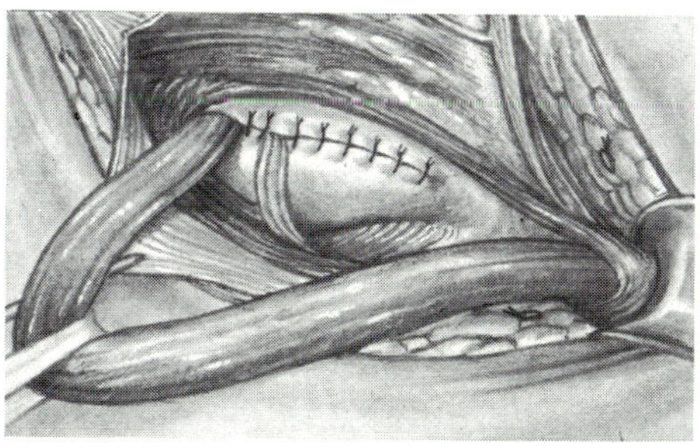

10A

OPERATION 3

REPAIR OF INDIRECT AND DIRECT INGUINAL HERNIAS

Technique of W. J. Lytle

Plate XI
Plate XII
Plate XIII
Plate XIV

The artist, Frank Robinson, visited W. J. Lytle in the Royal Infirmary (Sheffield, England) and witnessed the techniques illustrated here.

1 The neck of an indirect hernial sac has been closed with a pursestring suture, and its transected peritoneal cuff is visible. When the transversalis fascia around the internal ring is adequate and the fascia of the posterior inguinal wall is intact, a snug closure of the internal ring around the cord suffices. To initiate this closure, an interrupted suture of thread or catgut is inserted and tied, to occlude the inner angle of the defect in the transversalis fascia.

2 The inner angle suture is cut and a continuous suture is inserted, loosely at first and later drawn taut, which completes the closure of the defect in the transversalis fascia. The last stitch of this suture includes a portion of the covering of the cord to anchor it to the newly reformed internal ring.

Whenever the transversalis fascia around the internal ring is attenuated, which usually occurs in the outer pillar, the inner pillar is sutured to the deep femoral arch (iliopubic tract) or inguinal ligament, whichever is stronger.

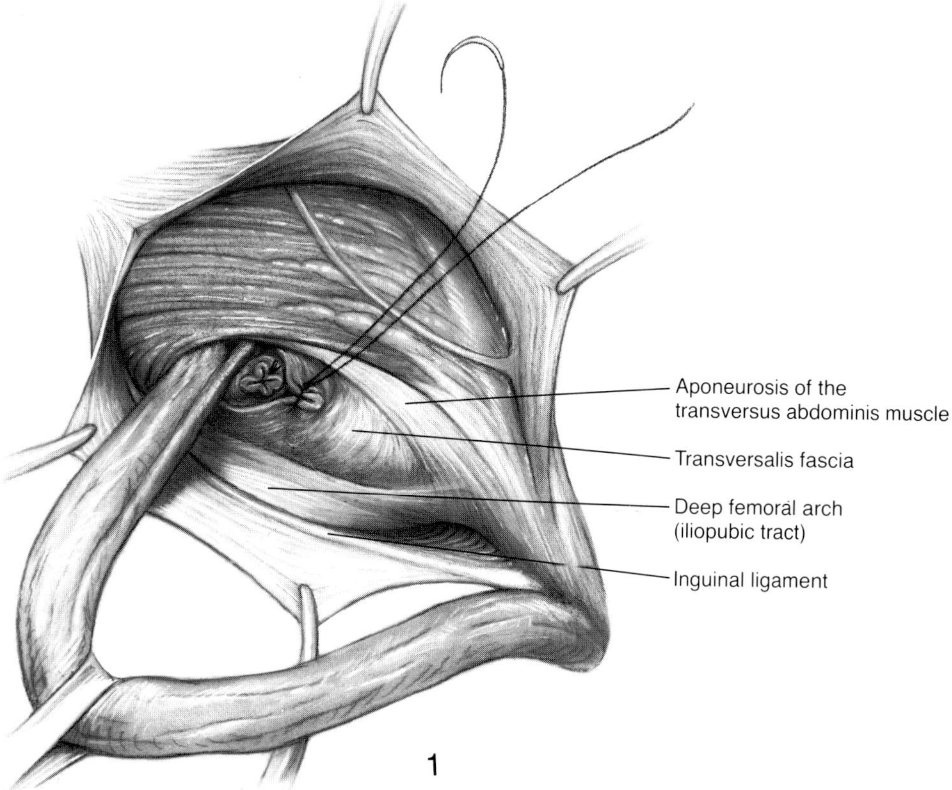
Aponeurosis of the transversus abdominis muscle
Transversalis fascia
Deep femoral arch (iliopubic tract)
Inguinal ligament

1

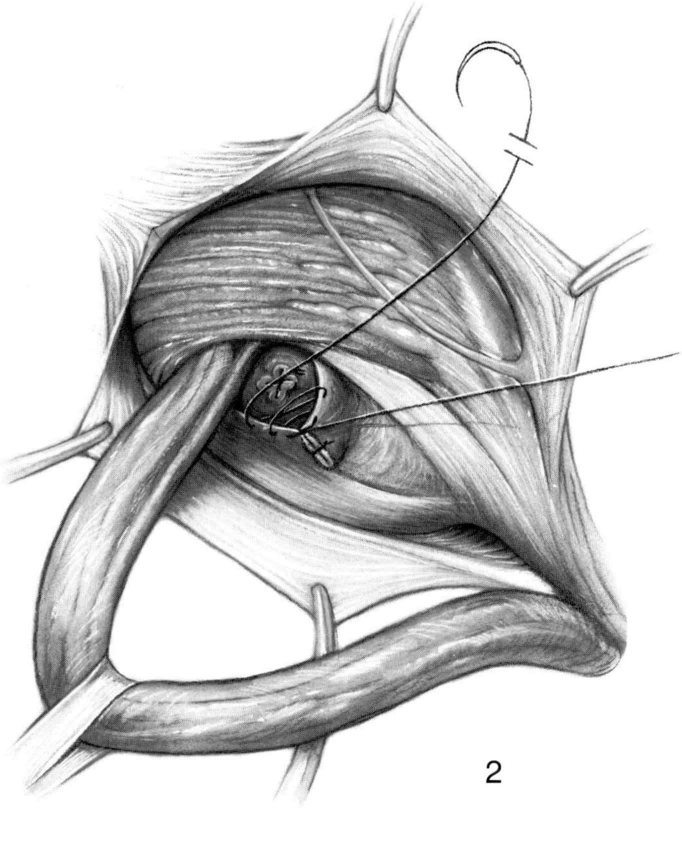

2

REPAIR OF INDIRECT AND DIRECT INGUINAL HERNIAS *Continued*

3, 4, 5 This semidiagrammatic illustration represents Lytle's concept of the composite anatomy in the formation of Gimbernat's ligament. The superficial (medial) or tendinous portion is derived from the inguinal ligament (**3**) and its deep (lateral) or fascial portion from the fascia lata (**4**). The composite formation of Gimbernat's ligament is depicted in **5**.

This illustration clearly shows the concave base or lateral crescentic margin of the deep or fascial portion of Gimbernat's ligament, which forms the medial boundary of the femoral sheath. The site of the femoral hernial orifice in the lower portion of the femoral sheath, through which a femoral hernia protrudes, is in the center (*dark area*) of the concave base. This fixed and narrow medial boundary is the anatomic basis for the invariably small size of a primary femoral hernia.

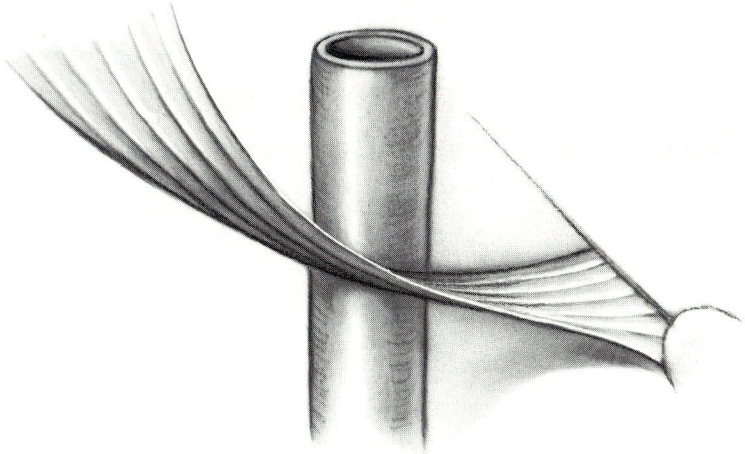

3

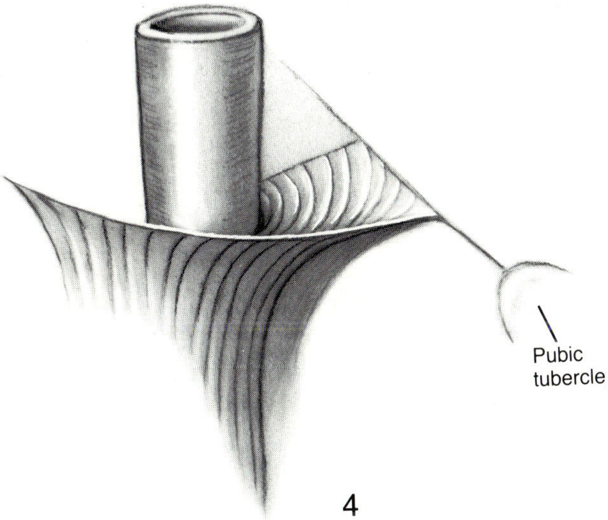

4

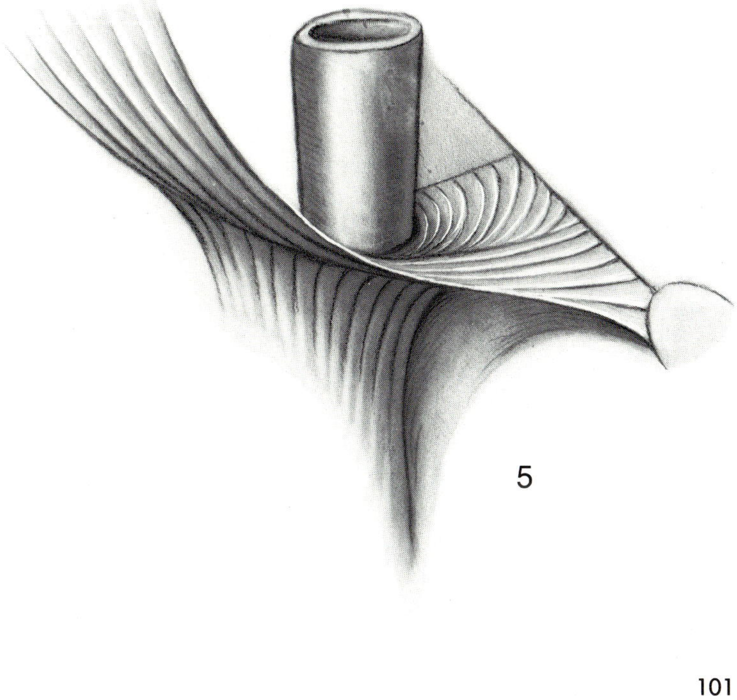

5

6 This illustration depicts in anatomic detail the formation of Gimbernat's ligament and its relationship to the surrounding structures. The *white arrow* indicates the site of the femoral hernial orifice.

7 In this illustration, which complements **6,** the *dotted lines* show the intact femoral canal (A) and the canal breached by a femoral hernia (B). The curved edge of Gimbernat's ligament is at the site of the femoral hernial orifice.

The bold curvilinear striations represent the inguinal ligament and its insertion into the pubic tubercle and adjacent anterior portion of Cooper's ligament to form the superficial or tendinous portion of Gimbernat's ligament. The shaded and interrupted transverse striations, below the inguinal ligament, represent the fascia lata, which twists beneath the inguinal ligament to insert into the posterior portion of Cooper's ligament as the deep or fascial component of Gimbernat's ligament.

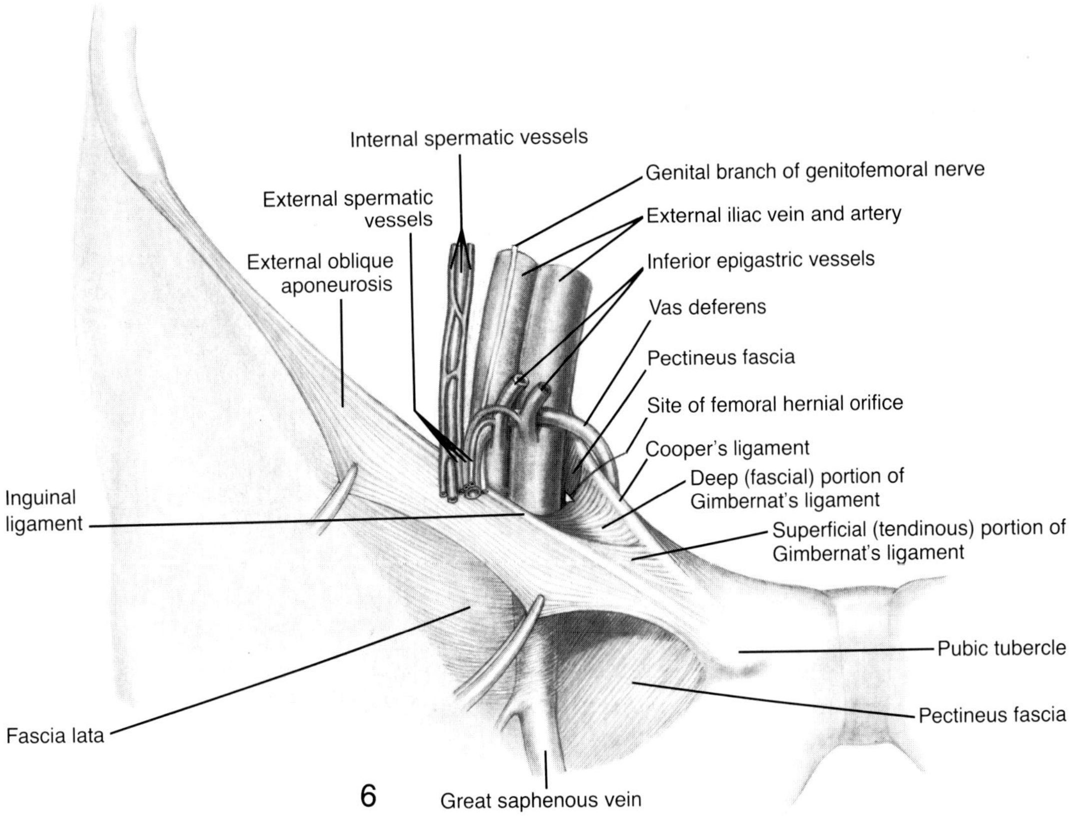
Internal spermatic vessels
Genital branch of genitofemoral nerve
External spermatic vessels
External iliac vein and artery
External oblique aponeurosis
Inferior epigastric vessels
Vas deferens
Pectineus fascia
Site of femoral hernial orifice
Cooper's ligament
Deep (fascial) portion of Gimbernat's ligament
Inguinal ligament
Superficial (tendinous) portion of Gimbernat's ligament
Pubic tubercle
Pectineus fascia
Fascia lata
Great saphenous vein

6

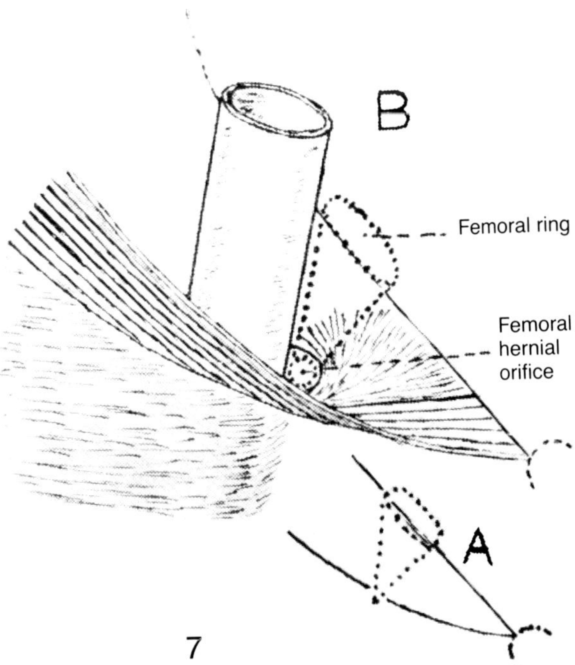
B
Femoral ring
Femoral hernial orifice
A

7

REPAIR OF INDIRECT AND DIRECT INGUINAL HERNIAS *Continued*

8 The overlying frayed fascial layer of the posterior inguinal wall has been excised and the bulge of a direct inguinal hernia, surrounded by preperitoneal fat, is visible. Its relationship to the neighboring structures is also depicted.

For clarity of view, the cremaster muscle, the spermatic cord (internal spermatic vessels and vas deferens), and the more deeply located cremaster vessels and accompanying genital branch of the genitofemoral nerve (not visible) have been resected. For better visibility of their respective transected remnants, ligatures have been omitted.

In the treatment of the bulge, the overlying defect in the fascia of the posterior inguinal wall is repaired by suturing (with 3-0 silk) the cut margin of the transversus aponeurosis to that of the deep femoral arch (iliopubic tract).

9 In this illustration, a large direct hernial sac has been opened and the accompanying hernia of the bladder reduced by scissors dissection. The wide neck of the sac is closed with a nonabsorbable pursestring suture of 3-0 silk and the redundant sac wall excised. Should the fascia of the deep femoral arch prove adequate, the defect in the fascia of the posterior inguinal wall is reconstructed as previously described (see **1**).

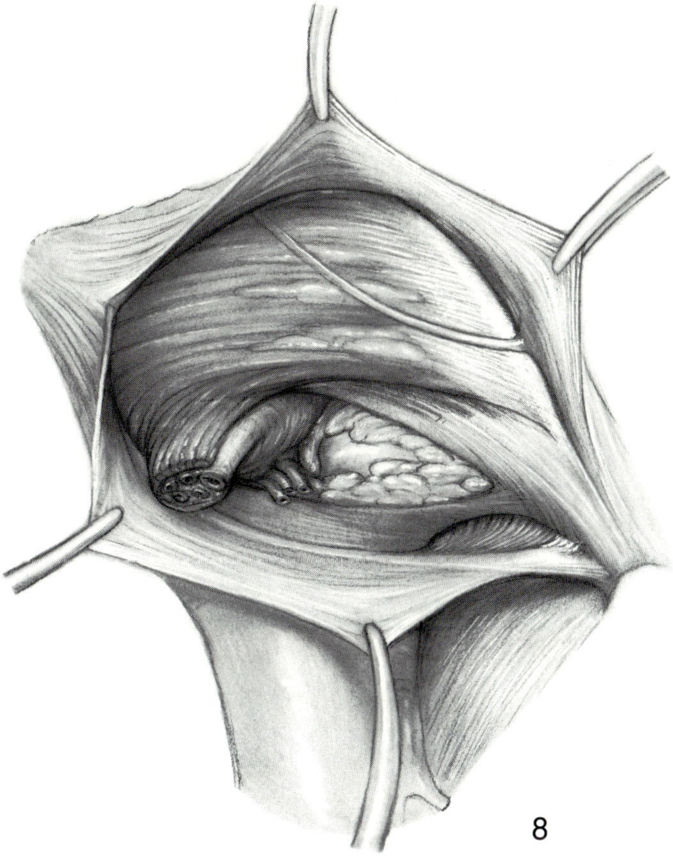

8

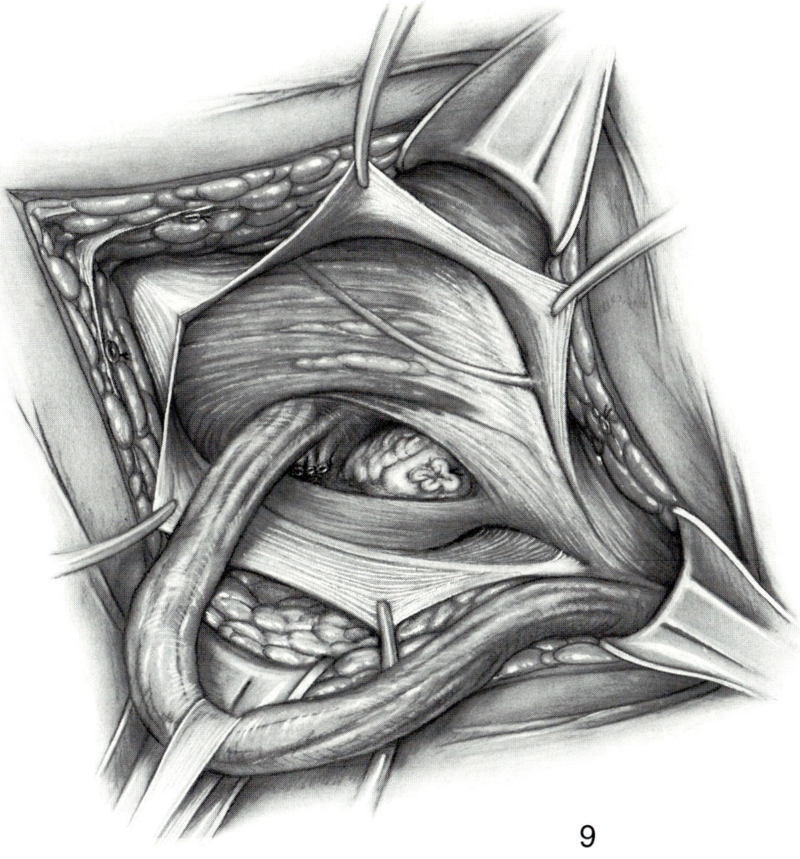

9

REPAIR OF INDIRECT AND DIRECT INGUINAL HERNIAS *Continued*

10 When the fascia of the deep femoral arch is inadequate, a continuous nonabsorbable suture of 2-0 silk is used to close the large fascial defect in the posterior inguinal wall. It is first inserted medially and tied, to obtain a secure closure of the medial angle of the fascial defect. It is then continued laterally, loosely inserted for better visibility, to its midpoint of closure.

Sequentially, the suture is inserted in the fascia of the posterior inguinal wall superiorly and into both portions of Gimbernat's ligament and the inguinal ligament inferiorly. The suture, as it is withdrawn at the site of its midpoint of closure, includes both the deep femoral arch (iliopubic tract) and the inguinal ligament. It continues to do so throughout the remaining lateral closure of the hernial defect.

11 The suture is tightened and terminates laterally in a snug closure of the internal ring around the cord.

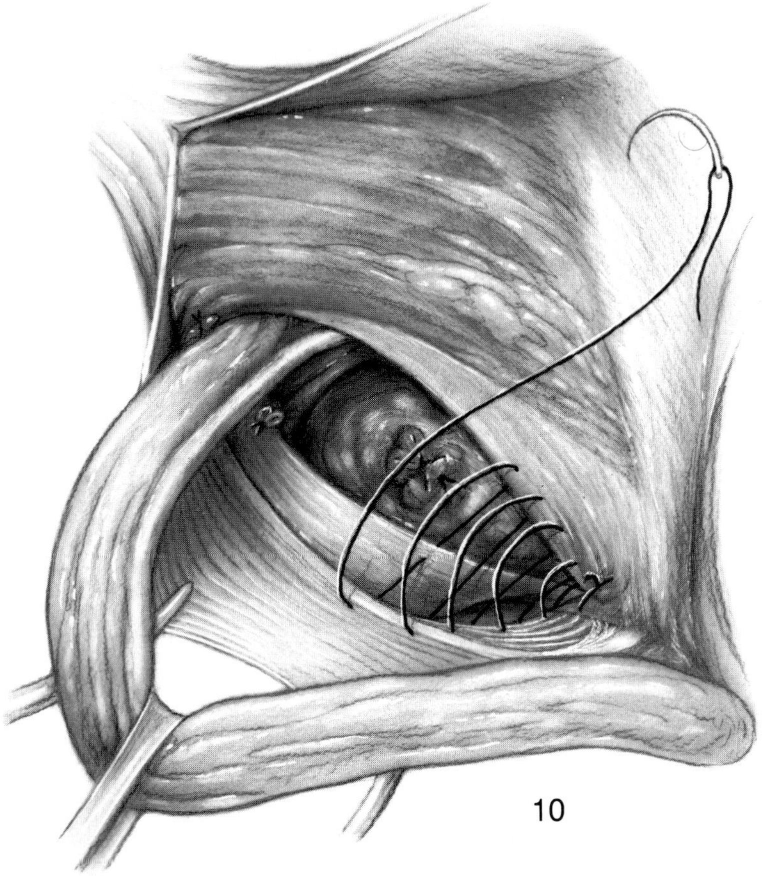

10

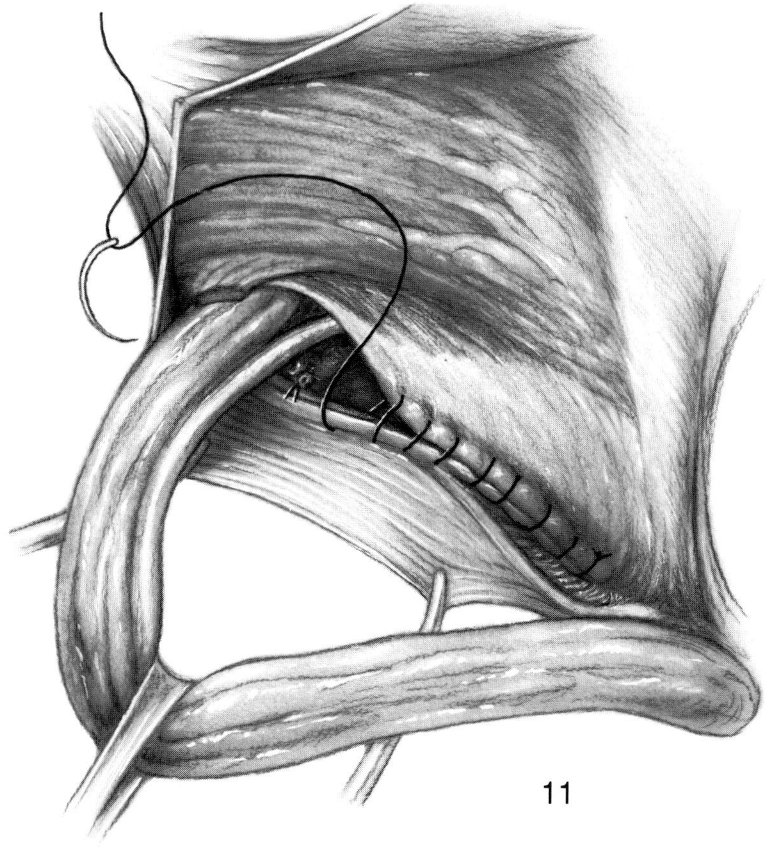

11

REPAIR OF INDIRECT AND DIRECT INGUINAL HERNIAS *Continued*

Technique of Joseph L. Ponka, M.D.

Robinson also visited Joseph Ponka at the Henry Ford Hospital (Detroit) to illustrate his technique for the repair of a large direct inguinal hernia. For ease of comparison, it seemed appropriate that these illustrations should follow those of Lytle's technique for the repair of the same type of hernia. Furthermore, the importance of having one artist as a witness and illustrator of both operations is shown by the standard of excellence of the illustrations.

12 The bulge of the direct inguinal hernia has been reduced by the imbrication of the overlying attenuated fascia of the posterior inguinal wall, using interrupted sutures of 3-0 silk. A relaxing incision in the anterior rectus sheath has been made, preliminary to the insertion of the untied "Master stitch" that is depicted.

This stitch (suture) of 2-0 silk is first inserted through the adjacent margins of the fascia of the posterior inguinal wall at the medial angle of the hernial defect. It is then inserted in sequence through Cooper's ligament (near its site of origin medially), the tendinous portion of Gimbernat's ligament, and the shelving edge of the inguinal ligament. When tied, this suture effects an excellent fascial closure of the medial angle of the hernial defect, which is most important in preventing a recurrence of the hernia.

13 The reconstruction of the fascia of the posterior inguinal wall is continued laterally, using interrupted sutures of 2-0 silk, to approximate the aponeurotic portion of the transversus abdominis muscle superiorly to both the inferior fascial layer of the posterior inguinal wall and the inguinal ligament. This fascial closure of the posterior inguinal wall terminates laterally with the restoration of a "new" internal ring around the exit of the cord.

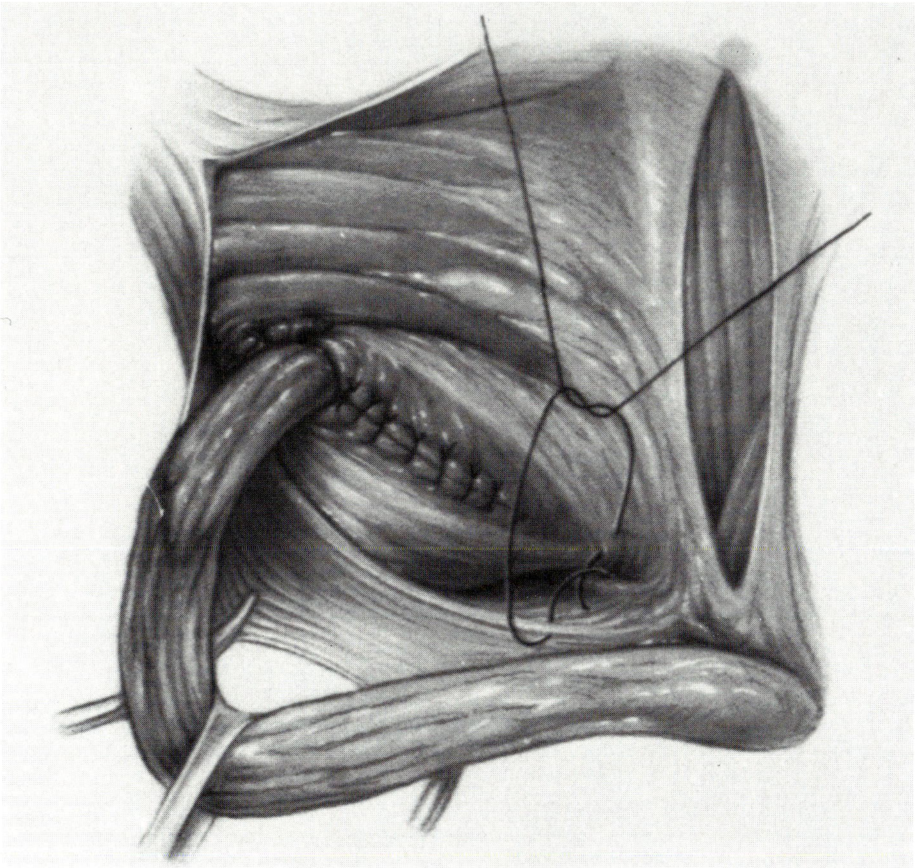

12

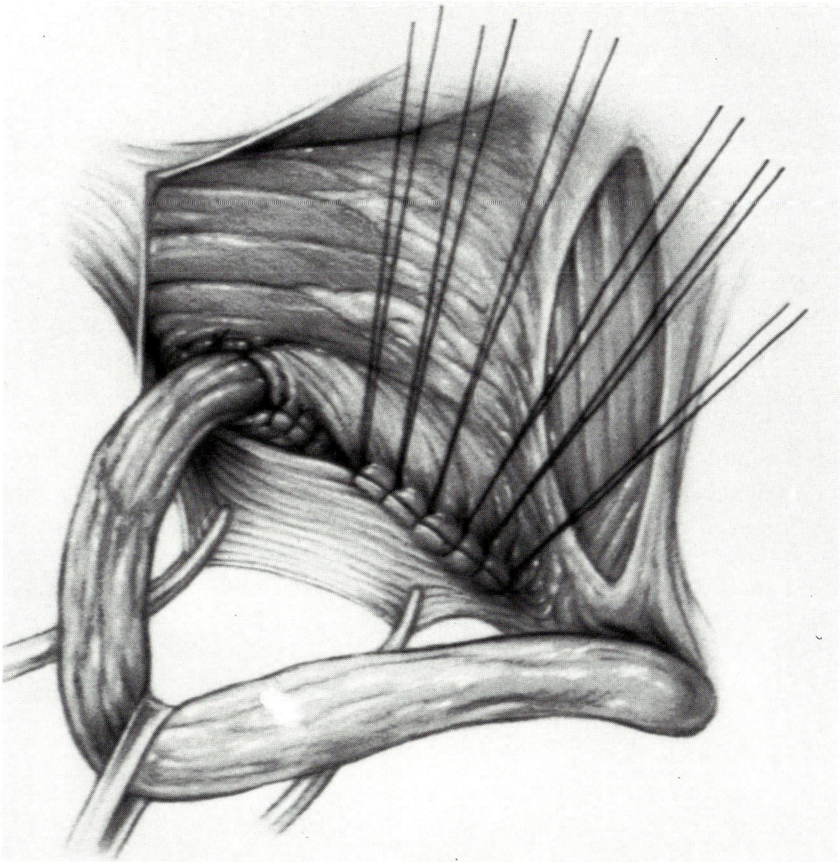

13

OPERATION 4

THE SHOULDICE TECHNIQUE FOR THE ANTERIOR REPAIR OF INGUINAL HERNIAS

GEORGE E. WANTZ, M.D.

Plate XV
Plate XVI
Plate XVII
Plate XVIII

Introduction

The author of this atlas has not used the Shouldice technique in the treatment of inguinal hernias. Accordingly, I am grateful to Dr. George Wantz for kindly accepting the invitation to both discuss and illustrate this technique.

As the result of many visits to the Shouldice Clinic in Toronto, Canada, Wantz changed his own previously well-established technique to conform with that of Shouldice. During the past 17 years he has accumulated an extensive surgical experience in the use of this method, enabling him to present a truly objective and scientifically unbiased evaluation of its merits.

Admittedly, because of my lack of experience with the Shouldice technique, it might seem presumptuous for me to comment on its merits. There are, however, bothersome theoretical objections to its use that I would like to present.

The first is the imbrication of the superior and inferior layers of the fascia of the posterior inguinal wall, or "floor." In doing so, it is frequently necessary to imbricate thinly attenuated fascial layers, which does not enhance the strength of the repair. The experimental studies of Dunphy[1] and Farris, Smith, and Beattie[2] have shown that the end-to-end approximation of freshly cut margins of fascia evokes a much greater fibroblastic response, and therefore a better reparative tissue reaction, than the imbrication of their normal fascial layers. Also, as McVay has stated, "The imbrication of a weak fascia on top of a weak fascia, a strong fascia it doesn't make!"[5]

The second objection is the suturing of the internal oblique muscle and the so-called "conjoined tendon" to the shelving border of the inguinal ligament. These third and fourth layers of repair are both unanatomic and unphysiologic, since they attempt to displace the muscle at a distance from its normal anatomic plane and require it to function under constant tension against an abnormal and unstable site of anchorage—the inguinal ligament. Furthermore, I have never seen a conjoined tendon that was worthy of use as a suture support.

J.L.M

In 1945, Shouldice[6] first reported the inguinal hernioplasty that bears his name. Subsequent to this and later publications, the method has gained widespread acceptance. Its stated advantages are the use of local anesthesia, the short hospital stay, and the infrequency of a hernial recurrence. Accordingly, many Americans have gone to Toronto to have their inguinal hernias repaired by the "Canadian method."

However, many surgeons throughout North America have questioned both the merits of the technique and the excellent results being reported with its use. Yet in recent years it has become increasingly popular in the United States. In 1970 the present author used the Shouldice technique for the first time and became an immediate enthusiast. Since that time to the present, 5250 Shouldice inguinal hernioplasties have been performed.

The technique in the use of this anterior inguinal approach consists of two equally important stages—dissection and repair. The specific techniques employed in dissection are similar to those used in other types of hernial repair. The essential characteristic of the repair is the use of multiple layers of continuous sutures in the closure of the hernial defect. The surgical anatomy of this specific type of repair is depicted in the illustrations. Interestingly, when completed the repair duplicates the original hernioplasty of Bassini.

To both patients and surgeons, the Shouldice hernioplasty is synonymous with the use of local anesthesia. Although local anesthesia is usually acceptable for the elective repair of reducible inguinal hernias in the nonobese patient, the surgeons of Shouldice Hospital deserve most of the credit for the renewal of interest in its more widespread use. A major reason for this interest is that local anesthesia permits the surgeon to evaluate the patient's response to extrinsic painful stimuli. It therefore requires a gentle, precise, and meticulous surgical technique. Accordingly, sharp rather than blunt dissection is mandated.

The disagreeable burning sensation that is felt upon injection of a local anesthetic is due to its low pH and can be eliminated by diluting it with a mixture of 1 ml of bicarbonate of soda solution to 9 ml of lidocaine. However, if the commercially available solution of lidocaine combined with epinephrine is used, the pH is lower and requires additional quantities of bicarbonate of soda; the preferred dilution is 2.5 ml of the bicarbonate of soda solution to 7.5 ml of the combined anesthetic solution.

In the 17-year period from 1970 to 1987, the author has performed 4366 primary Shouldice hernioplasties. There were 55 recurrent hernias in 51 patients for an operative recurrence rate of 1.2% and a patient recurrence rate of 1.14%, respectively. It is strongly believed, however, that recurrence rates are not a valid way to evaluate the success of a hernioplasty. Perfect results are not possible in any type of inguinal hernial operation that is based on the suture repair of the adjoining tissue margins that surround Fruchaud's "myopectineal orifice"[3] (see Plate XVIII). The reason is that the holding power of these tissue margins for sutures varies from patient to patient.

Ideally, the incision in the fascia of the posterior wall of the inguinal canal permits a better evaluation of the fascial margins of the hernial defect and thus provides the best anatomic exposure for the successful suture repair of the hernia. The merits of this dissection are substantiated by the invariably low recurrence rates associated with its use.

There are critics* of the Shouldice hernioplasty who, citing both the mobility of the medial or "suspended" portion of the inguinal ligament and the attenuated frayed fibers of the iliopubic tract, assert that these structures are unsuitable for the anchorage of sutures. These objections are simply not substantiated by the results obtained. Furthermore, the recurrence of a hernia, early or late, is not considered to be the result of the disruption of the sutures from either the inguinal ligament or the iliopubic tract.† Instead, they are new hernias that occur through various sites of progressive deterioration in the fascia that surrounds the myopectineal orifice.

---

*These include Madden and McVay—see their remarks in the Introduction.

†This a priori reasoning of the author seems to imply that any such recurrences, per se, are not related directly to the technique of repair that he describes! (J.L.M.)

THE SHOULDICE TECHNIQUE FOR THE ANTERIOR REPAIR OF INGUINAL HERNIAS

Continued

1 The cremaster muscle is transected with scissors, which is the initial and important step in the exposure of the deep (internal) ring. It is preferable to transect it in the midportion of the inguinal canal, rather than at the level of the pubic tubercle.

2 The medial and lateral segments of the cremaster muscle have been resected and the spermatic cord, previously mobilized by digital dissection, is encircled and retracted up by a Penrose drain. Also, the external spermatic vessels (cremaster vessels) and the site of their parent vessels, the deep epigastrics, are visible. The genital branch of the genitofemoral nerve, which accompanies the cremaster vessels, is hidden from view.

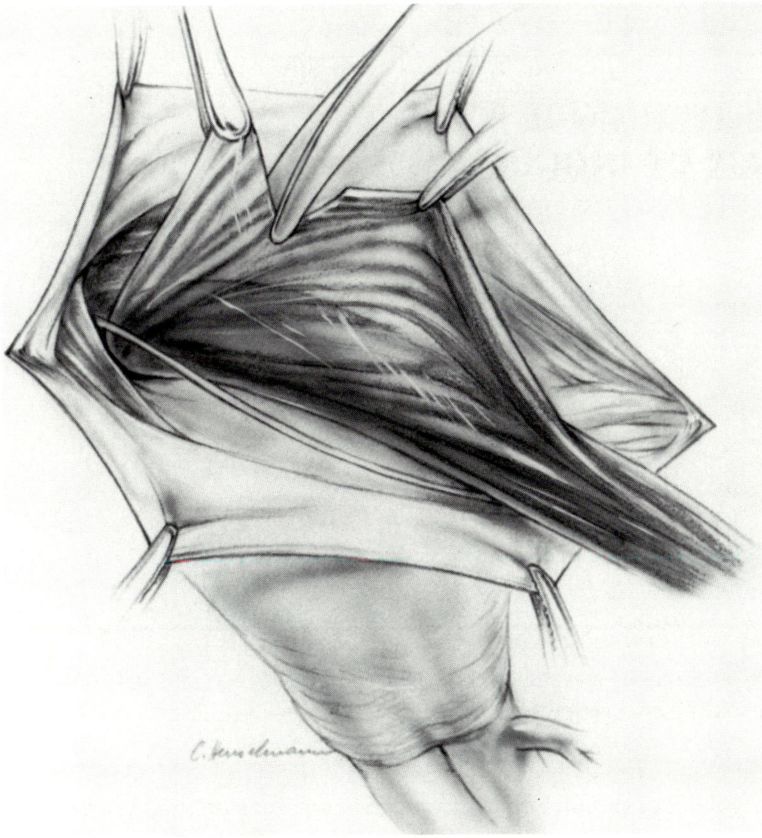

1

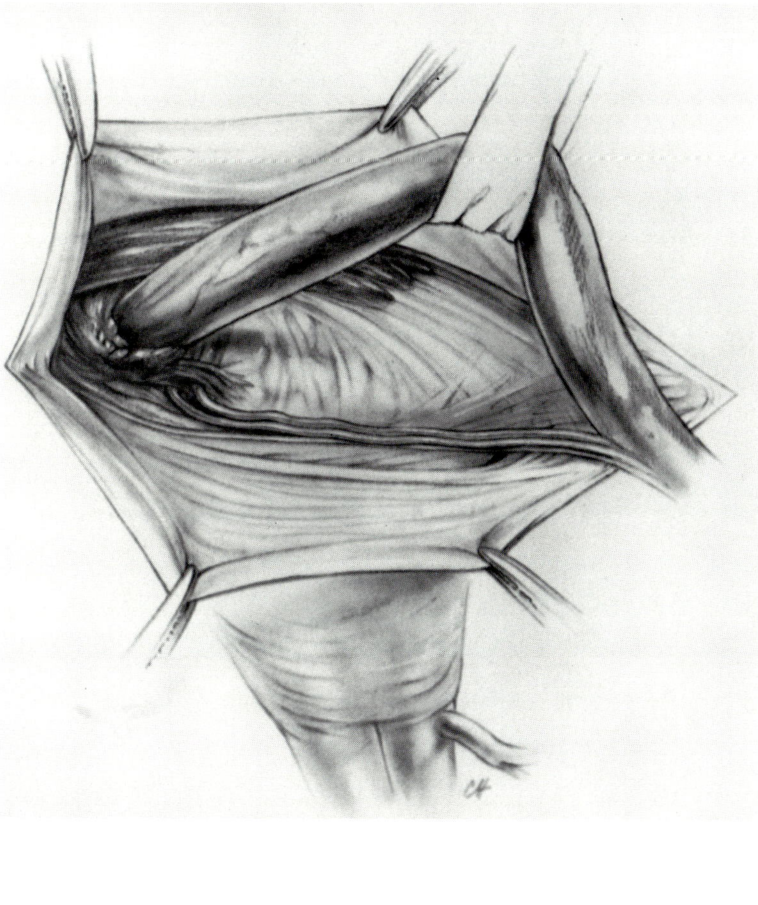

2

THE SHOULDICE TECHNIQUE FOR THE ANTERIOR REPAIR OF INGUINAL HERNIAS
Continued

3 The cremaster vessels and the accompanying genital nerve, because they obscure exposure and hinder repair, have been resected. This may be done with impunity since the blood supply to the testicle is from the internal spermatic artery. Similarly, the genital nerve also may be excised.

By delicate blunt dissection between the reflected portion of the inguinal ligament and the iliopubic tract, the femoral sheath laterally and the lacunar insertion of the inguinal ligament medially are exposed. The resulting space between these two structures is referred to by Madden[4] as the pyriform fossa.

4 The fascia of the posterior inguinal wall, starting at the deep (internal) ring, is severed by scissors dissection. Laterally, the underlying inferior (deep) epigastric vessels and preperitoneal fat are visible.

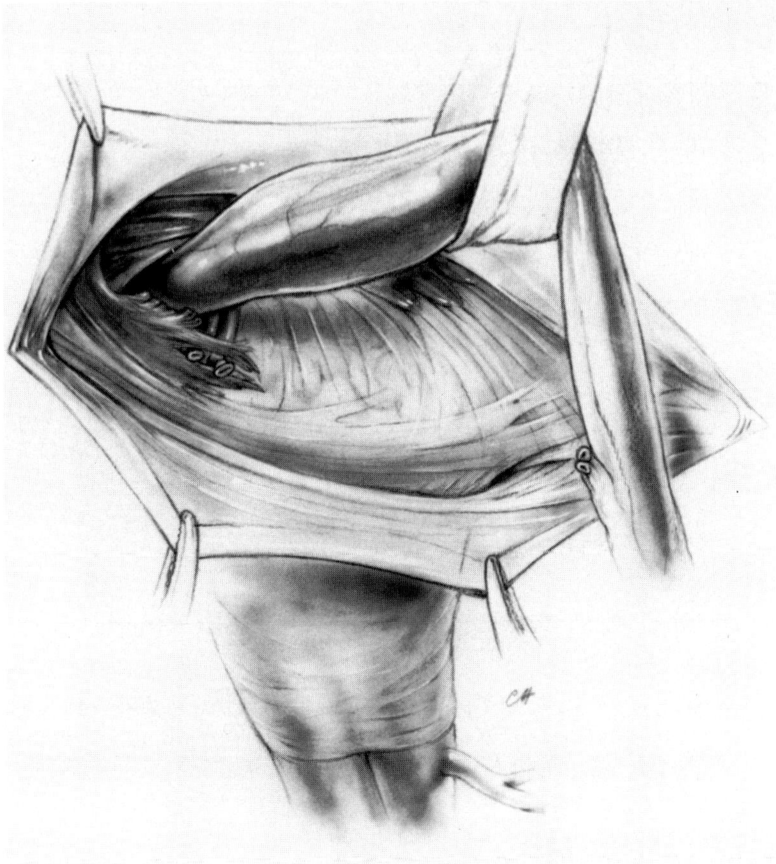

3

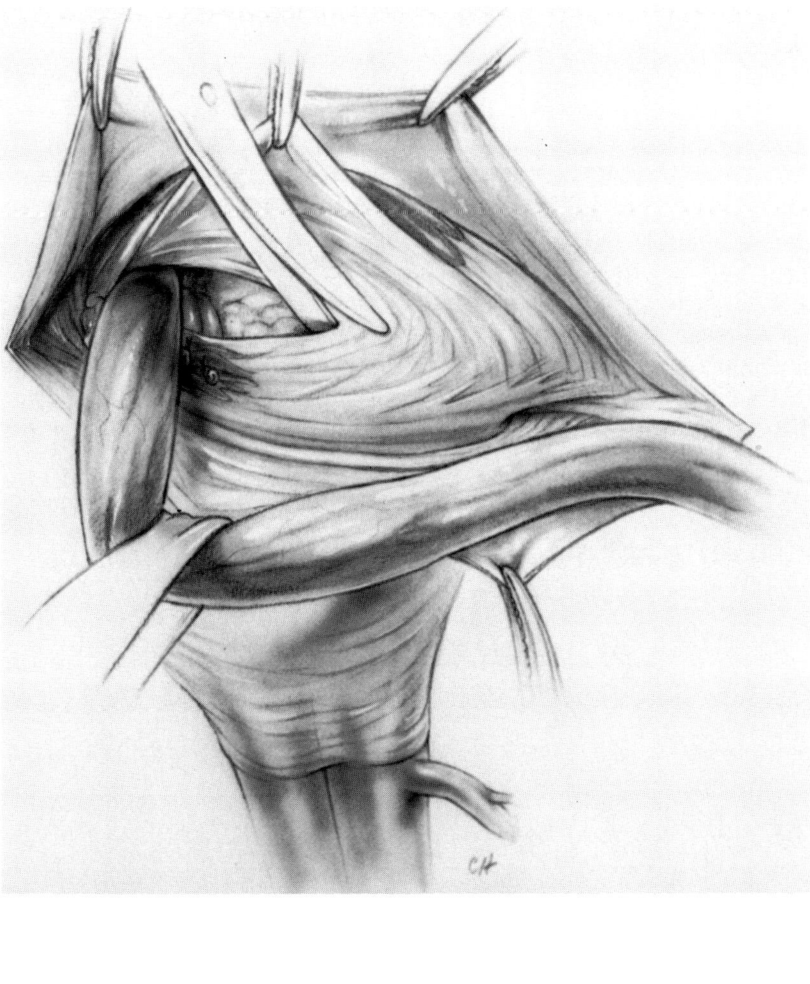

4

THE SHOULDICE TECHNIQUE FOR THE ANTERIOR REPAIR OF INGUINAL HERNIAS

Continued

5 The severance of the fascia of the posterior inguinal wall is completed and its superior segment, the transverse aponeurotic arch, is retracted up with clamps. This segment was previously dissected free of the preperitoneal fat on its undersurface until the rectus muscle was seen.

The large indirect hernial sac has been transected in proximity to its neck and mobilized laterally to the site of convergence of the vas deferens and internal spermatic vessels. The sac may then be ligated, sutured, or simply allowed to retract without closure.

A longitudinal slit is made in the anterior wall of the distal portion of the sac, which remains attached to the cord. This is done to avoid inducing traumatic thrombosis of the pampiniform plexus and its resultant ischemic orchitis and testicular atrophy.

All small indirect, direct, and indirect sliding hernial sacs are simply mobilized by sharp dissection and inverted. The search for a femoral hernia, both above and below the inguinal ligament, completes the dissection.

6 The medial angle of the fascial defect is closed with a nonabsorbable suture of monofilament polypropylene (2-0) that anchors the medial cut margin of the inferior aponeurotic fascial segment to the undersurface of the superior aponeurotic fascial segment. The long strand of this suture is inserted as a continuous suture to unite these two segments with minimal tension. It terminates laterally with the restoration of the deep (internal) ring around the exit of the cord, to complete the first layer of closure of the hernial defect.

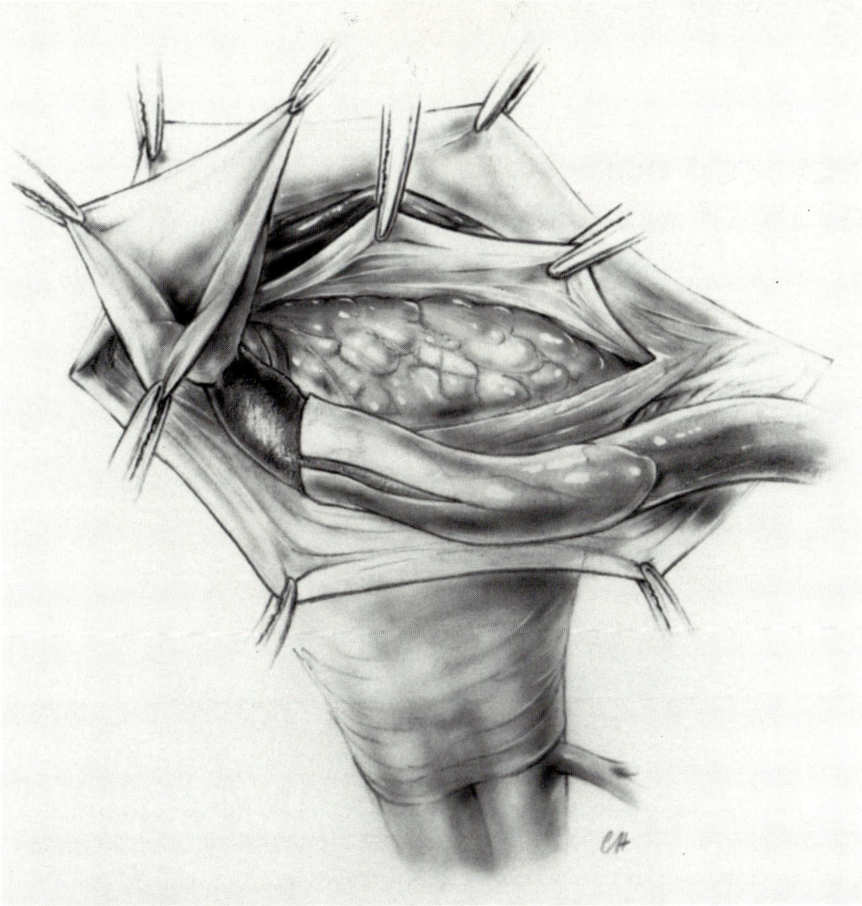

5

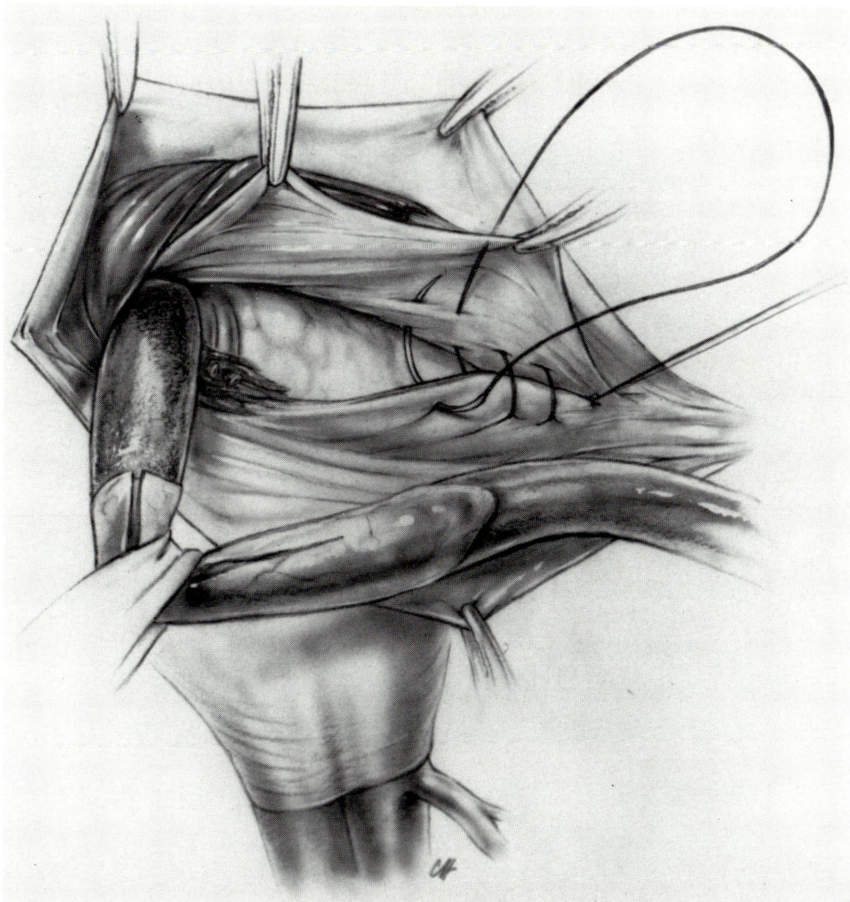

6

7 The suture is returned to its medial angle of origin as it unites the free cut margin of the superior portion to the reflected portion of the inguinal ligament and subsequently to its paddle-shaped insertion into Cooper's ligament at its origin. The imbrication of these two fascial layers with a single continuous suture is the most important part of the operation.

8 The second suture layer of closure is completed, and another continuous suture is inserted as the third layer. This suture, which is started at the deep internal ring, approximates the internal oblique muscle and its conjoined tendon, when present, to the inguinal ligament. The suture line is extended medially as far as the rectus sheath.

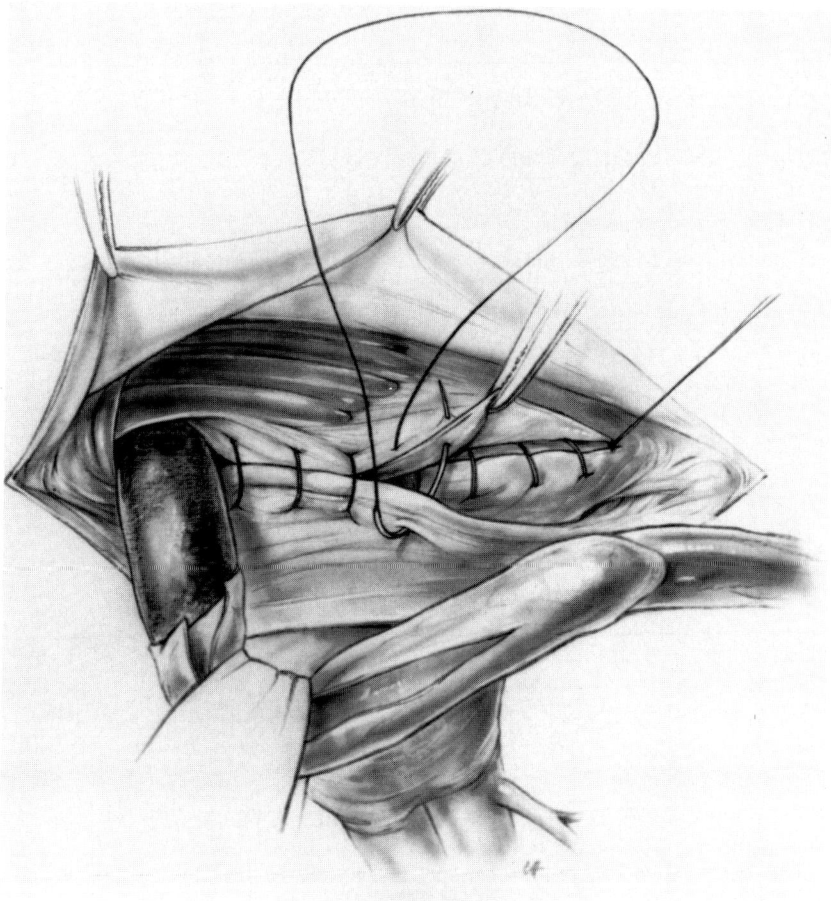

7

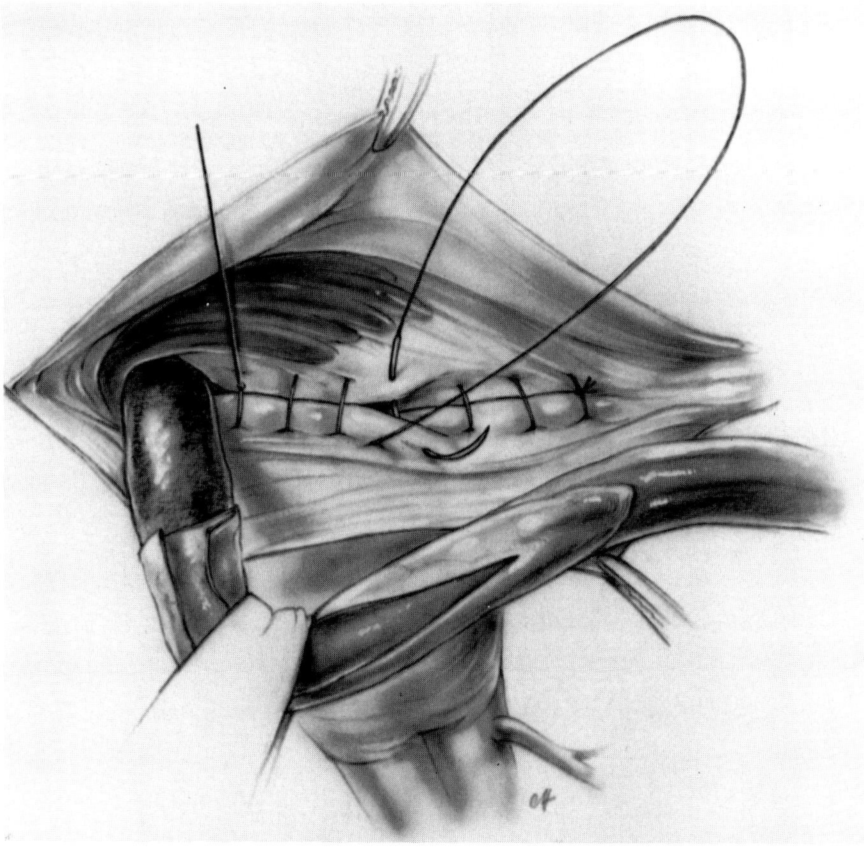

8

THE SHOULDICE TECHNIQUE FOR THE ANTERIOR REPAIR OF INGUINAL HERNIAS

Continued

9 The second suture is returned to its starting point, either on its same line of closure or as a distinct fourth layer as depicted. It is tied to the short strand at its site of origin to complete the four-layer closure of the hernial defect.

10 The aponeurosis of the external oblique muscle is loosely approximated with either absorbable or nonabsorbable continuous sutures. In the restoration of the external ring with the closure of the medial angle, the distal stump of the cremaster muscle is included to "hitch up " the testicle.

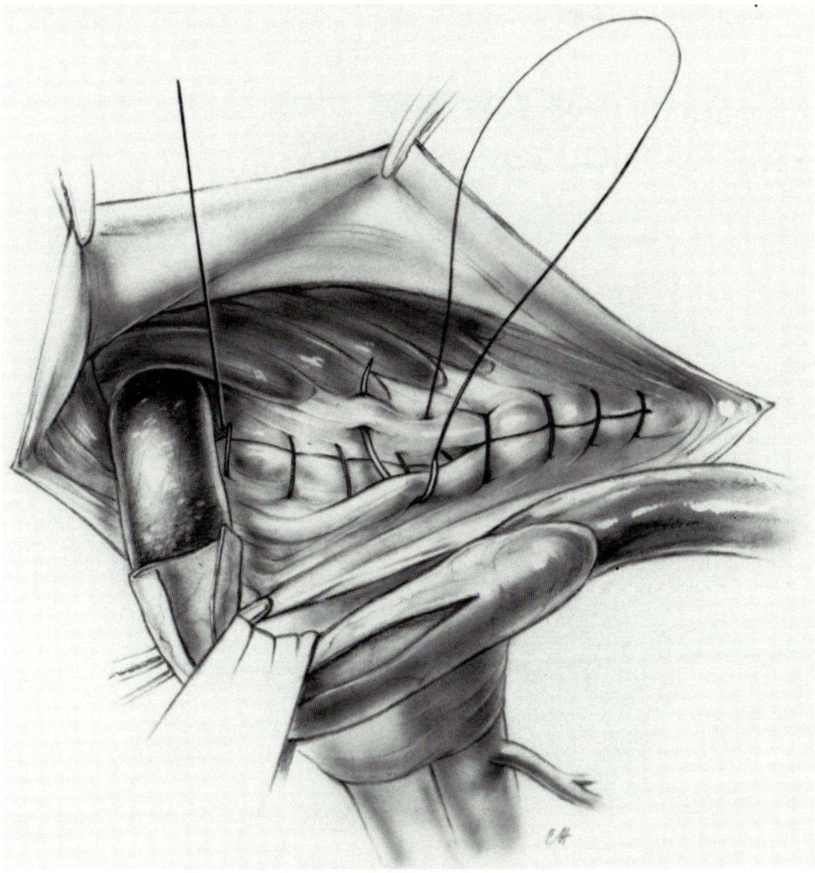

9

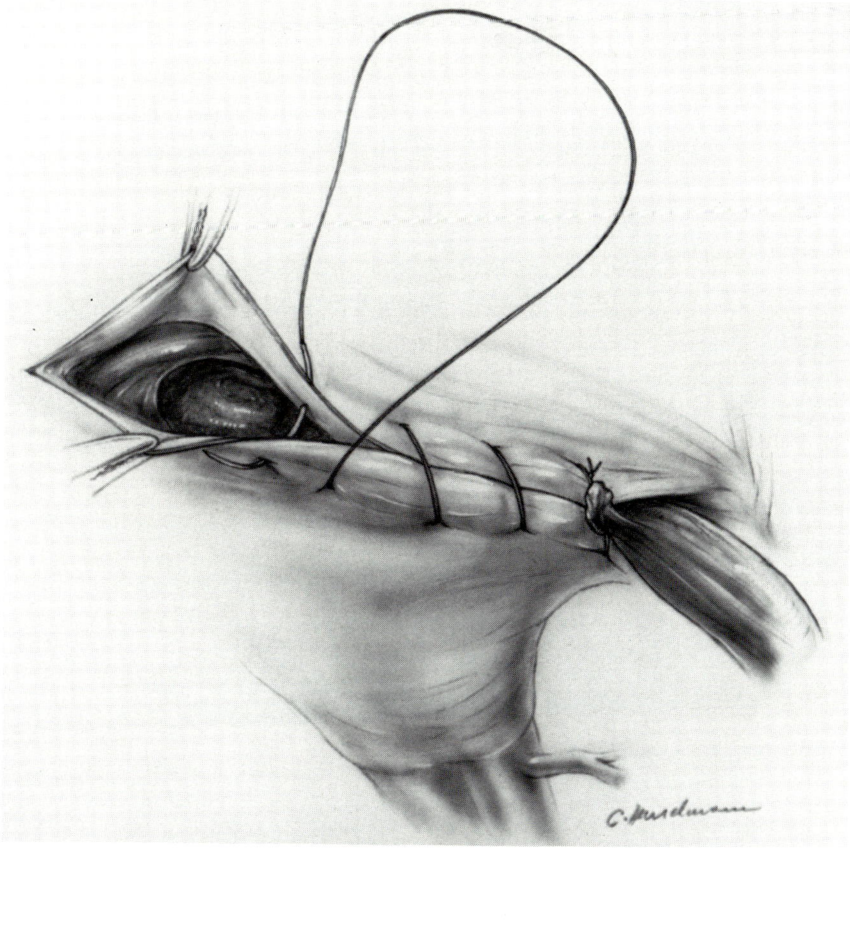

10

THE SHOULDICE TECHNIQUE FOR THE ANTERIOR REPAIR OF INGUINAL HERNIAS
Continued

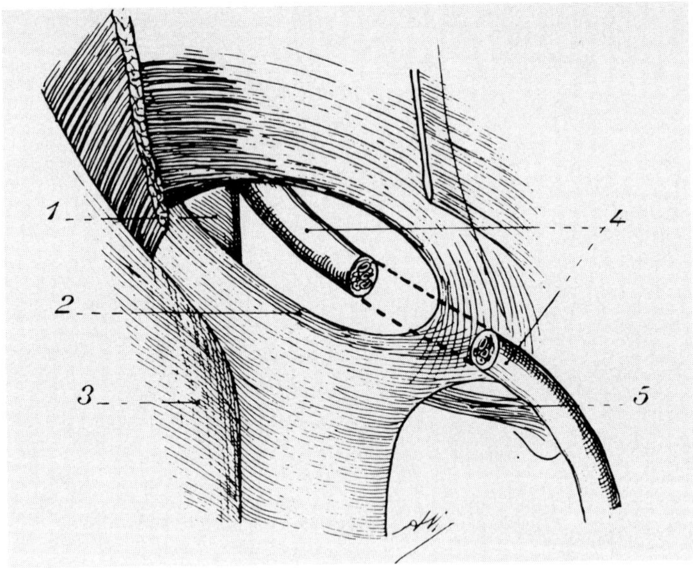

11

11 Fruchaud's diagram of the myopectineal orifice. 1, Free zone of fascia iliaca; 2, iliopubic tract; 3, lower part of fascia iliaca; 4, spermatic cord; 5, Cooper's ligament. The transversalis fascia has been thinned (behind the spermatic cord) and removed. (From Fruchaud H: *Anatomie Chirurgicale des Hernies de l'Aine.* Paris: C. Doin & Cie, 1956, p 301.)

REFERENCES

1. Dunphy JE: On the nature and care of wounds (Moynihan Lecture). Ann R Coll Surg Engl *26*:69–87, 1960.
2. Farris JM, Smith GK, and Beattie AS: Umbilical hernia: An inquiry into the principle of imbrication and a note on the preservation of the umbilical dimple. Am J Surg *98*:236–242, 1959.
3. Fruchaud H. *Anatomie Chirurgicale des Hernies de l'Aine*. Paris: C Doin & Cie, 1956, p 301.
4. Madden JL, Hakim S, and Agorogiannis AB: The anatomy and repair of inguinal hernias. Surg Clin North Am *51*(6):1269–1292, 1971.
5. McVay CB: Personal communication.
6. Shouldice EE: Surgical treatment of hernia. Ont Med Rev *12*:43–69, 1945.

RECOMMENDED READINGS

Berliner SD: Adult inguinal hernia: Pathophysiology and repair. In Nyhus LM (ed): *Surgery Annual, 1983*. Norwalk: Appleton-Century-Crofts, 1983.
Glassow F: The surgical repair of inguinal and femoral hernias. Can Med Assoc J *108*:308–313, 1973.
Glassow F: The Shouldice repair of inguinal hernia. In Nyhus LM and Condon RE (eds): *Hernia,* 2nd ed. Philadelphia: JB Lippincott, 1978.
Glassow F: Inguinal hernia repair using local anesthesia. Ann R Coll Surg Engl *66*:382–387, 1984.
Shearburn EW and Myers RN: Shouldice repair of inguinal hernia. Surgery *66*:450–459, 1969.
Wantz GE: The Canadian repair of inguinal hernias. In Nyhus LM and Condon RE (eds): *Hernia,* 3rd ed. Philadelphia: JB Lippincott, 1989.
Wantz GE: Ambulatory surgical treatment of groin hernia, the prevention and management of complications. In Madden J (ed): *Problems in Surgery*. Philadelphia: JB Lippincott, 1986.

OPERATION 5

COOPER'S LIGAMENT REPAIR OF LARGE INDIRECT AND DIRECT INGUINAL HERNIAS

CHESTER B. McVAY, M.D.

Plate XIX
Plate XX

In the repair of indirect inguinal hernias of small to moderate size, the commonly accepted procedure is high ligation and excision of the sac, associated with simple closure of the defect in the fascia of the posterior inguinal wall.

In large indirect inguinal hernias and in both direct inguinal and femoral hernias, where there is complete disruption of the fascia of the posterior inguinal wall, the Cooper's ligament reconstructive hernioplasty is advocated. It is required, however, only in about 20% of patients with groin hernias of the indirect variety.

1 The large oblong protrusion of the direct inguinal hernia and its complete separation from the cord structures can be seen. The *dashed line* indicates the site of incision for the resection of all of the overlying attenuated fascia of the posterior inguinal wall and related tissue inferiorly.

2 The herniation of the preperitoneal fat and peritoneum through the defect in the fascia of the posterior inguinal wall and its relationship to the surrounding structures are visible. The relaxing incision in the rectus sheath is completed to expose the underlying rectus and pyramidalis muscles.

3 The external iliac vessels and subjacent anterior femoral sheath are retracted laterally, concomitant with the retraction of the hernial protrusion superiorly, to expose Cooper's ligament and the subjacent pectineus fascia that originates from it.

The inguinal ligament can be seen as it courses over the anterior femoral sheath (crural arch) toward its paddle-shaped tendinous insertion into the pubic tubercle.

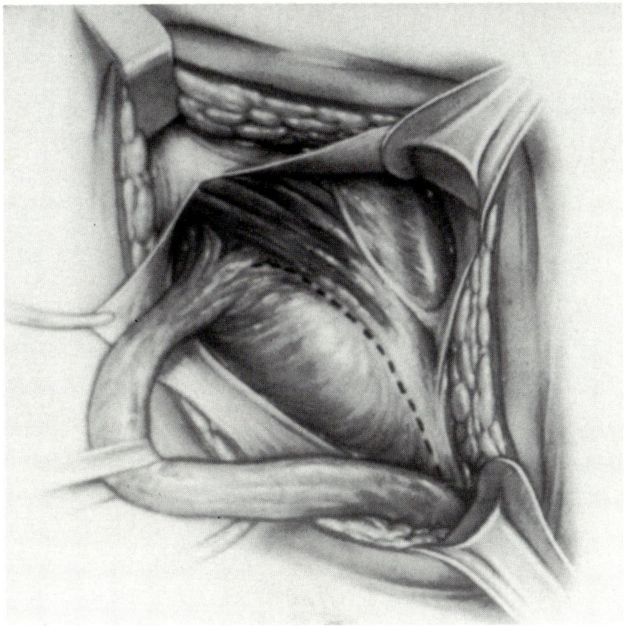

1

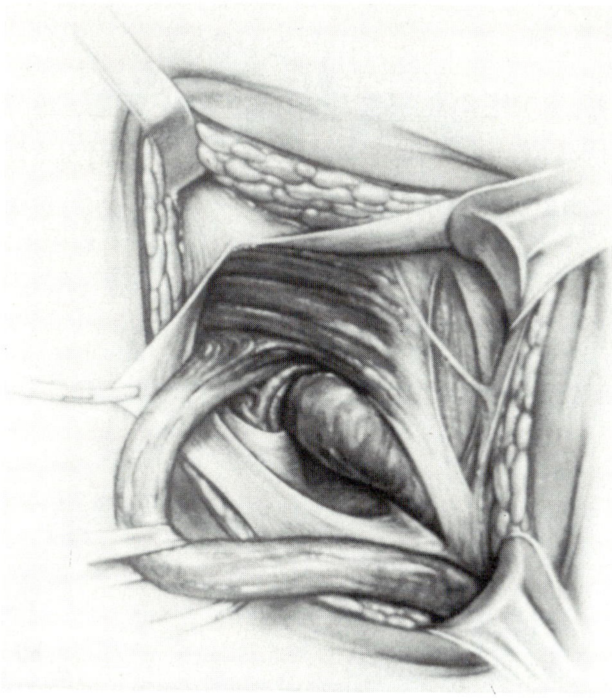

2

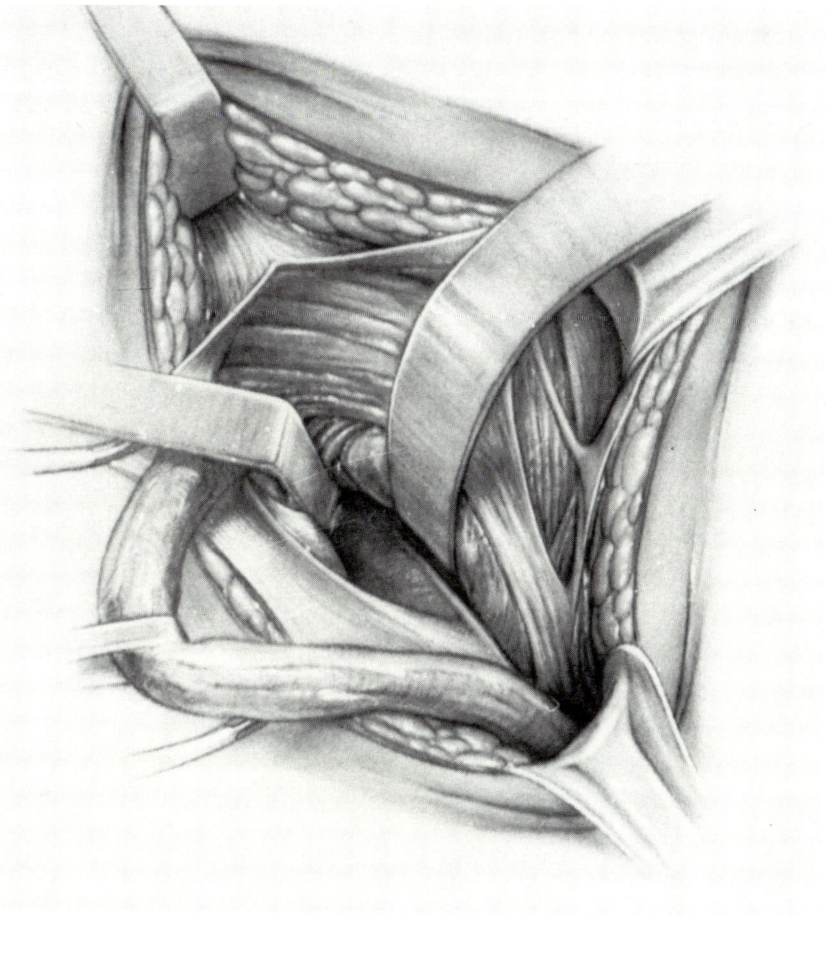

3

COOPER'S LIGAMENT REPAIR OF LARGE INDIRECT AND DIRECT INGUINAL HERNIAS

Continued

4, 4A The hernial protrusion is reduced, and the sutures (2-0 silk) for the reconstruction of the posterior inguinal wall are inserted but not tied. The most lateral of these sutures is the transition suture to restore the medial boundary of the femoral sheath (**4**). It is so named because it marks the transition from the deeply placed Cooper's ligament to the more superficially placed anterior femoral sheath.

This suture, shown in detail (**4A**), is inserted in succession through the musculofascial segment of the transversus abdominis muscle, Cooper's ligament, the pectineus fascia, and the medial wall of the anterior femoral sheath.

5, 5A The previously inserted sutures shown in **4** have been tied and their strands cut, with the exception of the transition suture. The first of the two lateral sutures to be tied is the transition suture, which has restored the medial boundary of the femoral sheath (**5**). For purposes of illustration, this restoration is depicted with the sutures deleted (**5A**). The resulting concomitant closure of the fascial defect at this site limits the potential for a recurrent hernia.

When the three most lateral sutures are tied, a snug fascial closure around the exit of the cord is obtained to complete the fascial reconstruction of the posterior inguinal wall.

The anatomic consequences of the restorative operation are an acutely arched convex border of the newly reconstructed posterior inguinal wall and the accompanying subjacent trough. The mandatory relaxing incision in the rectus sheath permits a fascial closure without undue tension on the suture line.

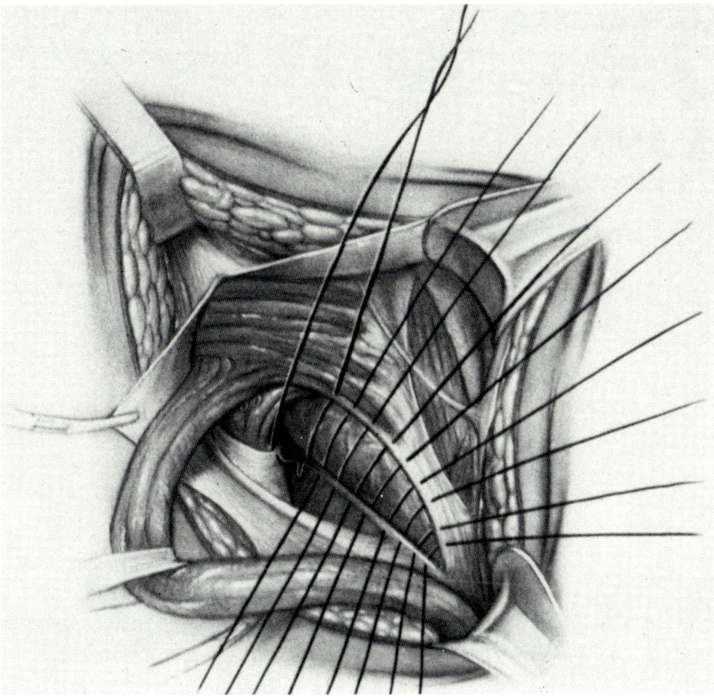

4

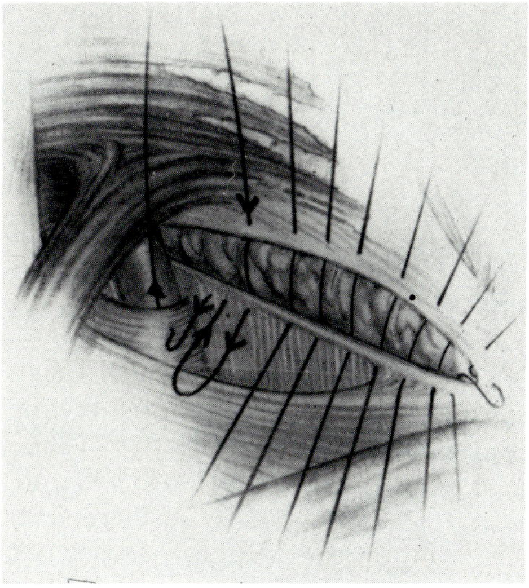

4A

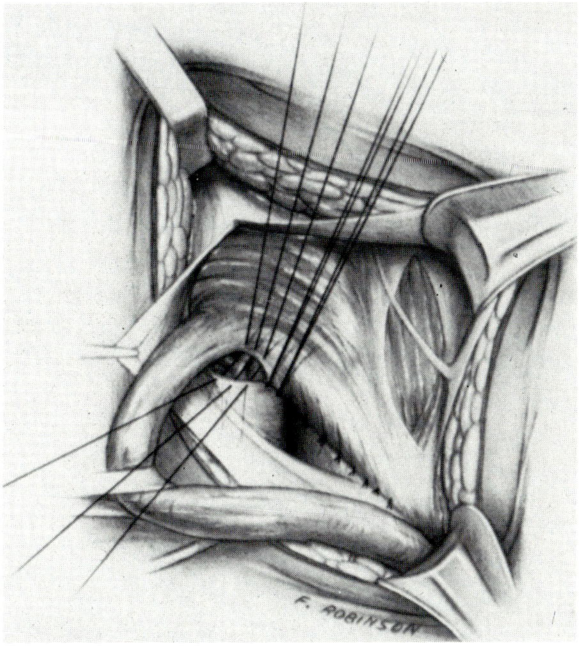

5

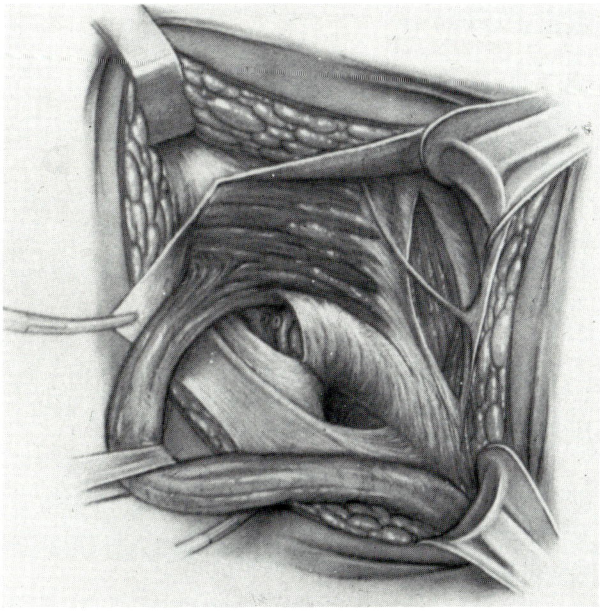

5A

OPERATION 6

COMBINED OPERATION FOR A CONGENITAL INGUINAL HERNIA AND UNDESCENDED TESTICLE

Plate XXI
Plate XXII
Plate XXIII
Plate XXIV
Plate XXV

1 The incision that partly overlies the protuberance caused by the undescended testicle is indicated by the *solid black line*. The empty scrotum on the left side is visible.

2 The skin incision is deepened through Camper's fascia, and the external superficial epigastric vein, doubly clamped, is transected with scissors. The ligated stumps of the external superficial pudendal vein are visible caudad. These vessels are located between Camper's fascia (superficial) and Scarpa's fascia (deep).

3, 4 Scarpa's fascia is incised **(3)**, and the underlying fatty areolar tissue is removed from the surface of the aponeurosis of the external oblique muscle by blunt digital dissection, using a piece of dry gauze **(4)**.

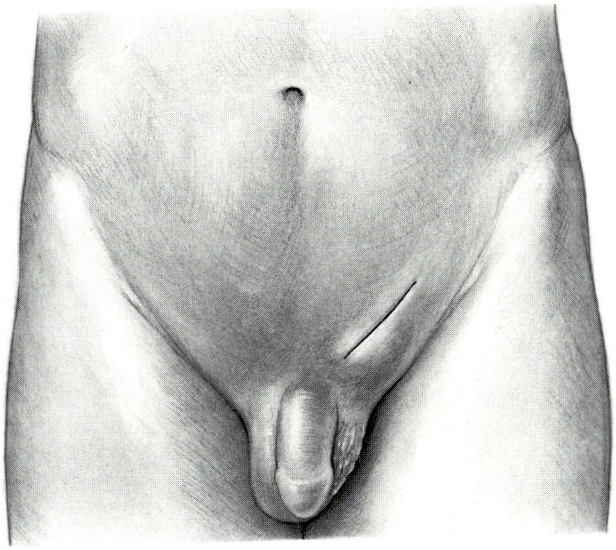

1

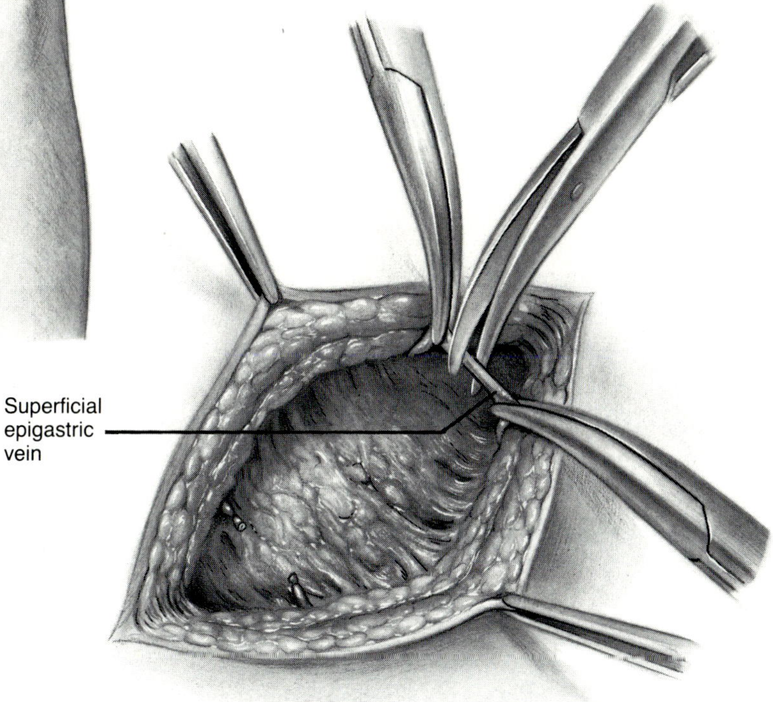
Superficial
epigastric
vein

2

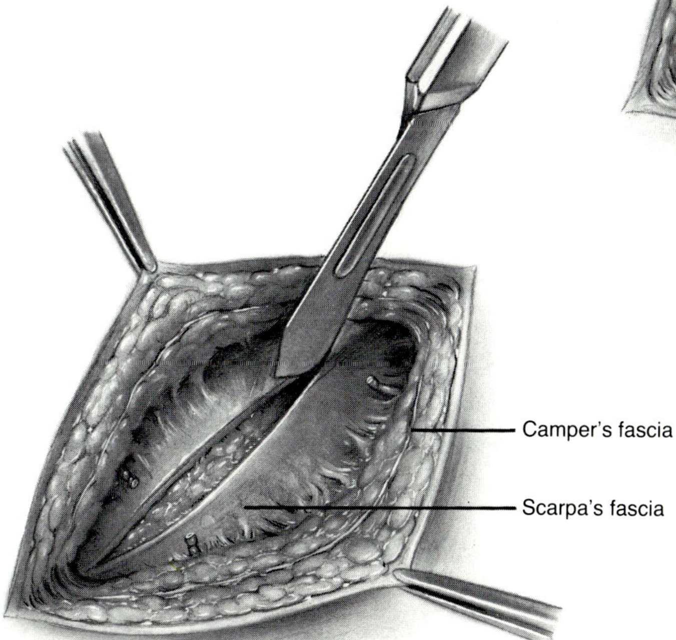
Camper's fascia
Scarpa's fascia

3

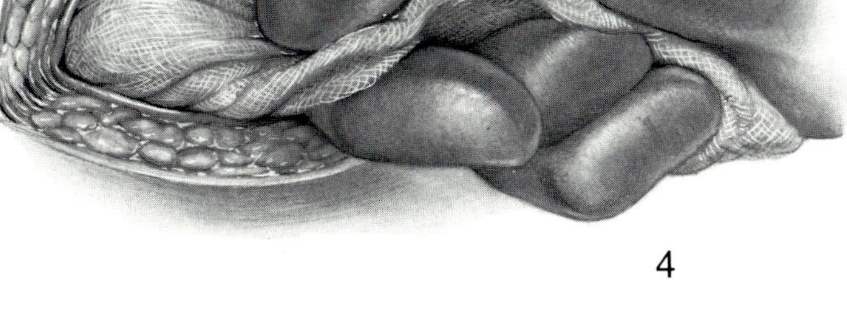

4

COMBINED OPERATION FOR A CONGENITAL INGUINAL HERNIA AND UNDESCENDED TESTICLE *Continued*

5, 6 The wound margins are retracted, and a short incision is made cephalad in the external oblique aponeurosis **(5)** and then extended caudad (*broken line*) through the external ring by a pushing motion with the tips of the partially open scissor blades **(6).** The undescended testicle is protruded through the external ring.

7 The leaflets of the external oblique aponeurosis are retracted, and the underlying structures are exposed. An opening made in the cremaster muscle veil is extended caudad to unroof the dislocated testis, which is held taut by clamp (Babcock) traction through the gubernaculum.

8 The cremaster fibers have been transected distally, which permits the elevation of the cord structures encased by the sac of the accompanying congenital hernia. The sac, held in forceps, is being severed with scissors (*broken line*).

9 The hernial sac is opened anteriorly, and saline is injected between the posterior wall of the sac and the cord structures to facilitate their separation. The *broken line* indicates the incision to be made preparatory to completing the mobilization of the posterior wall of the hernial sac. A portion of omental fat can be seen protruding from the peritoneal cavity.

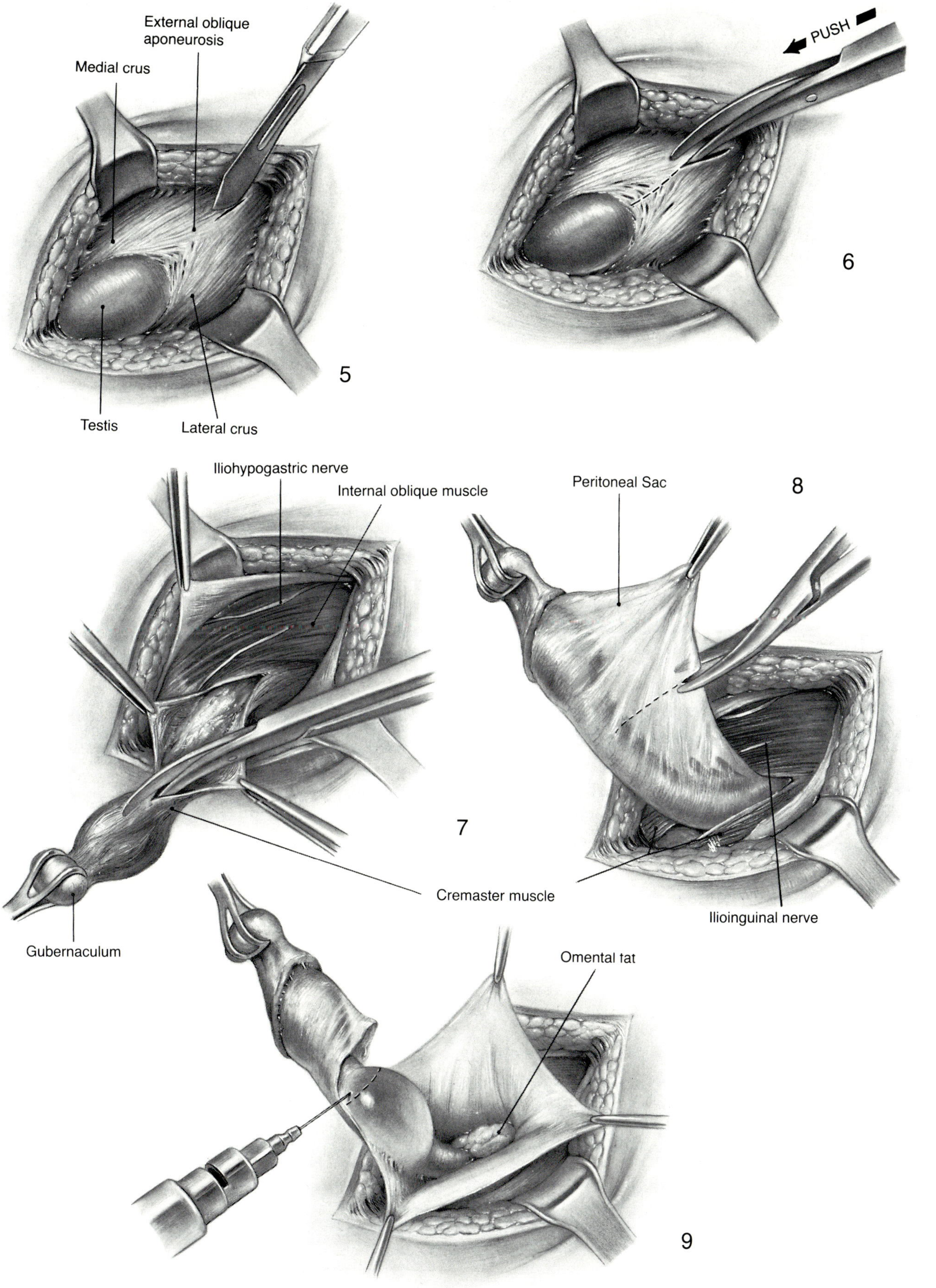
External oblique aponeurosis
Medial crus
Testis
Lateral crus
5
PUSH
6
Iliohypogastric nerve
Internal oblique muscle
Peritoneal Sac
8
7
Cremaster muscle
Gubernaculum
Ilioinguinal nerve
Omental tat
9

COMBINED OPERATION FOR A CONGENITAL INGUINAL HERNIA AND UNDESCENDED TESTICLE *Continued*

10 The partially mobilized posterior wall of the hernial sac is held up in forceps for traction as its separation from the cord structures is completed by scalpel dissection (*broken line*).

11, 12, 13 The neck of the mobilized hernial sac is occluded with a suture ligature of 3-0 silk **(11, 12)**, and the redundant sac tissue is excised **(13)**.

14, 15, 16 The anterior wall of the patent tunica vaginalis is severed with scissors in a longitudinal plane **(14)**, and its everted cut margins are sutured together (3-0 silk) posterior to the testicle **(15, 16)**.

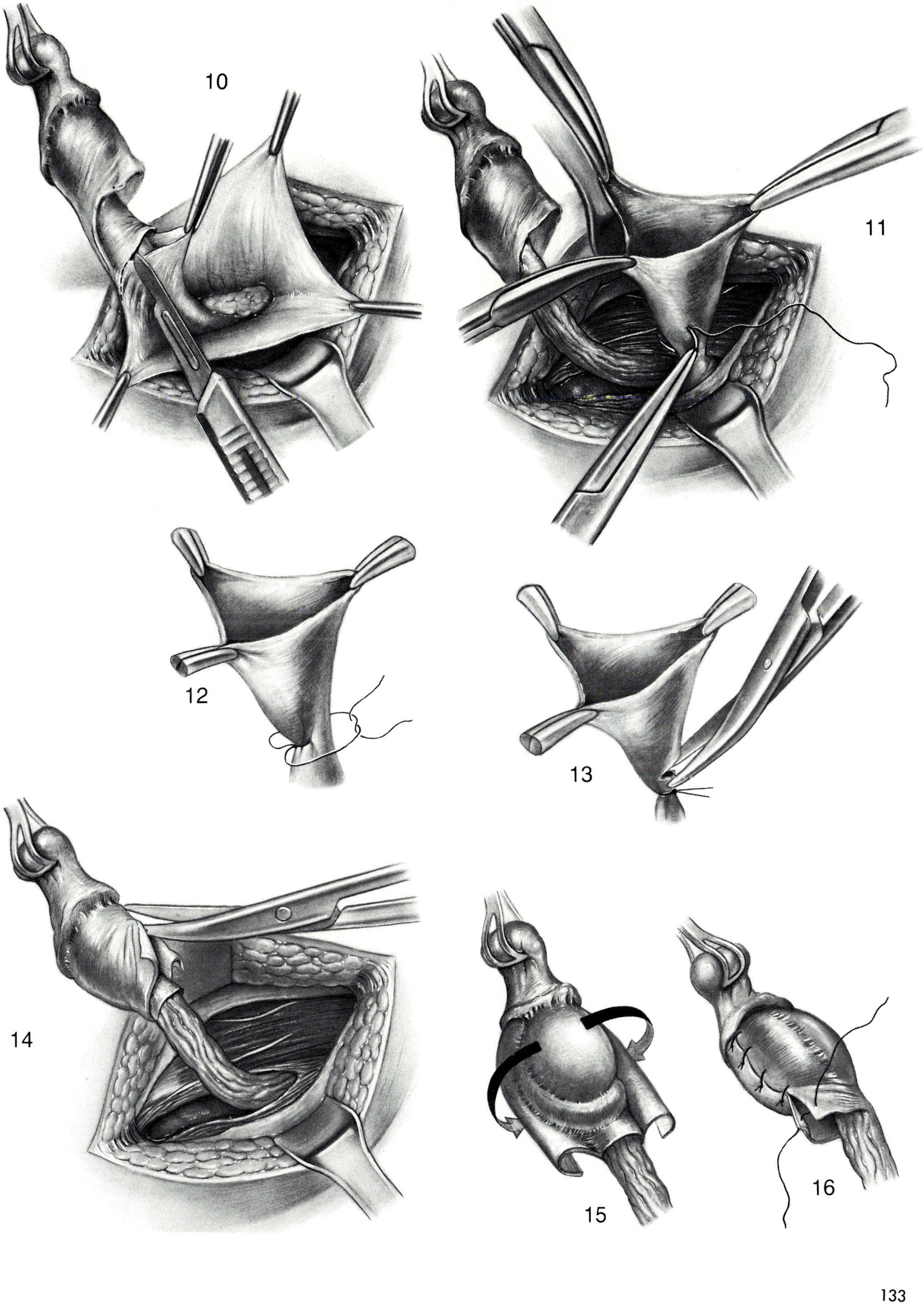
10
11
12
13
14
15
16

COMBINED OPERATION FOR A CONGENITAL INGUINAL HERNIA AND UNDESCENDED TESTICLE *Continued*

17 The vas deferens and the blood vessels that compose the cord structures are "skeletonized" by scissors dissection to obtain the maximum length of the cord.

18 The cord structures are completely mobilized, and the commonly present defect in the transversalis fascia is repaired with interrupted sutures of 3-0 silk. The ligated stump of the hernial sac is visible between the blood vessels laterally and the vas deferens medially. The deep epigastric vessels and their relationship to the cord structures, as well as the defect in the transversalis fascia, are also visible.

19 The closure of the defect in the transversalis fascia is completed, and the strands of a silk (2-0) suture inserted in the gubernaculum have their exit through separate sites in the base of the scrotum. Immediately preceding this step, a scrotal "bed" is made for the testicle by blunt digital dissection from within the incision.

20 The cut margins of the congenitally foreshortened cremaster muscle are approximated anterior to the cord structures. This is usually done after the testicle is placed in the scrotum. The distal segment of the cremaster muscle is visible as a rim of tissue between the lower pole of the testicle and the gubernaculum.

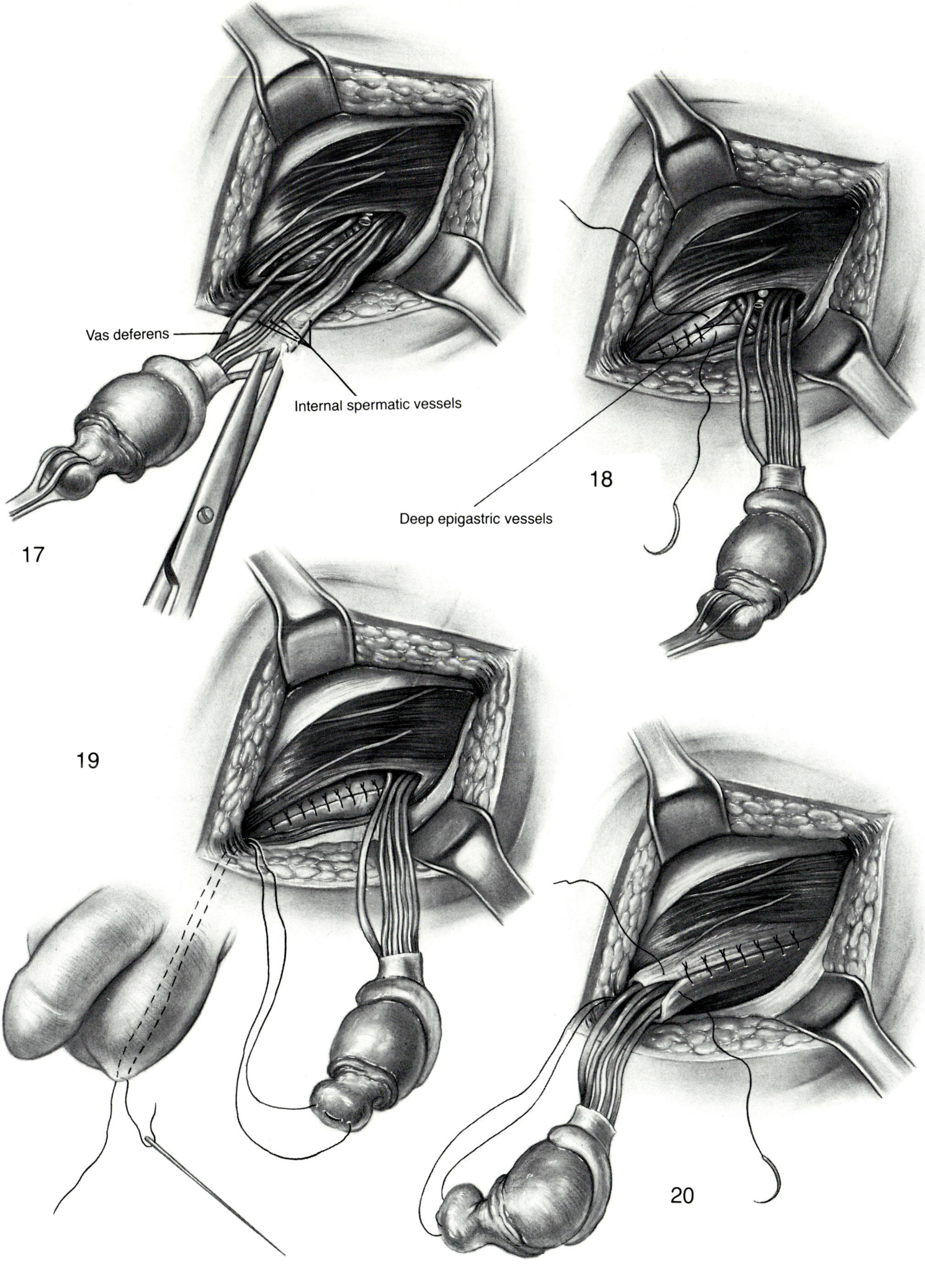
Vas deferens
Internal spermatic vessels
17
18
Deep epigastric vessels
19
20

COMBINED OPERATION FOR A CONGENITAL INGUINAL HERNIA AND UNDESCENDED TESTICLE *Continued*

21 The suture strands are tied to form a loop, which is encircled by a rubber band for traction. When the proper amount of traction is obtained, the rubber band is fixed to the thigh with one or two strips of adhesive. This traction is maintained for five to seven days.

22 The cut margins of the aponeurosis of the external oblique muscle are approximated with interrupted sutures of 3-0 silk. The relationship of the closure of the cremaster muscle to the ilioinguinal nerve may be seen.

23 The subcutaneous fascial layers (Camper's and Scarpa's) are sutured as a single unit with interrupted sutures of 4-0 silk.

24 Skin hooks are inserted into each angle of the incision and the margins approximated with straight (cambric) needles. The needles are withdrawn individually; their suture strands are tied and then cut to complete the operation.

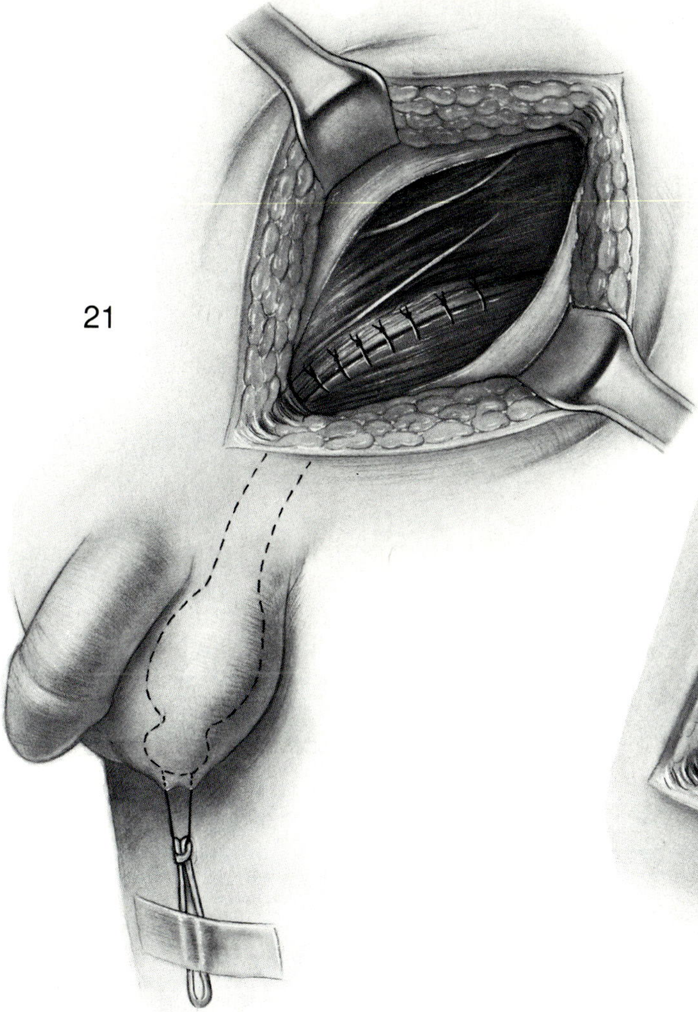

21

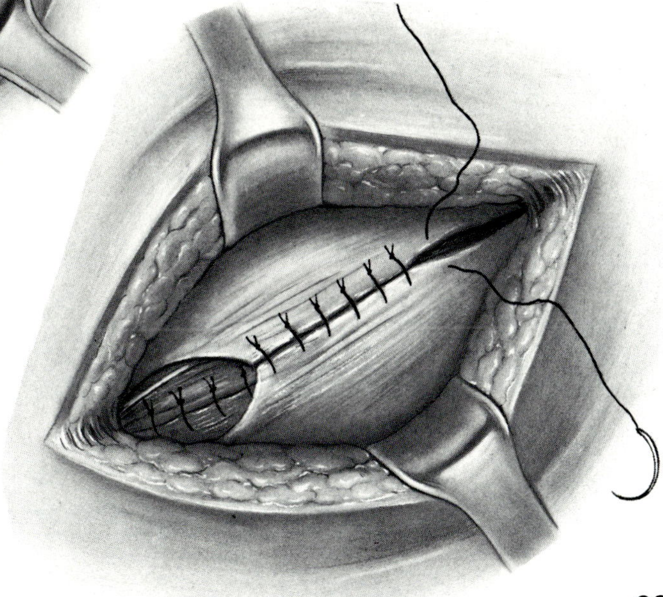

22

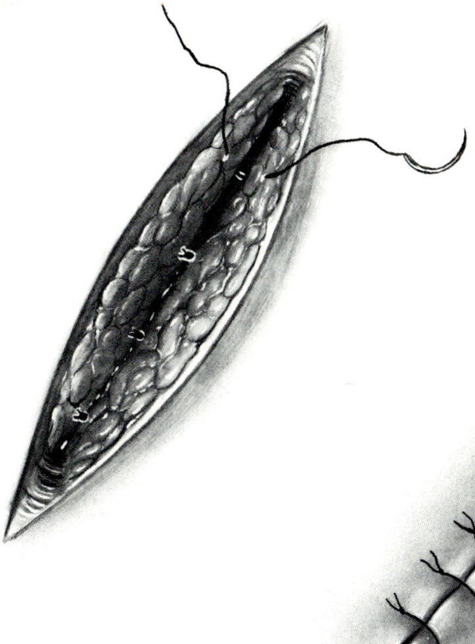

23

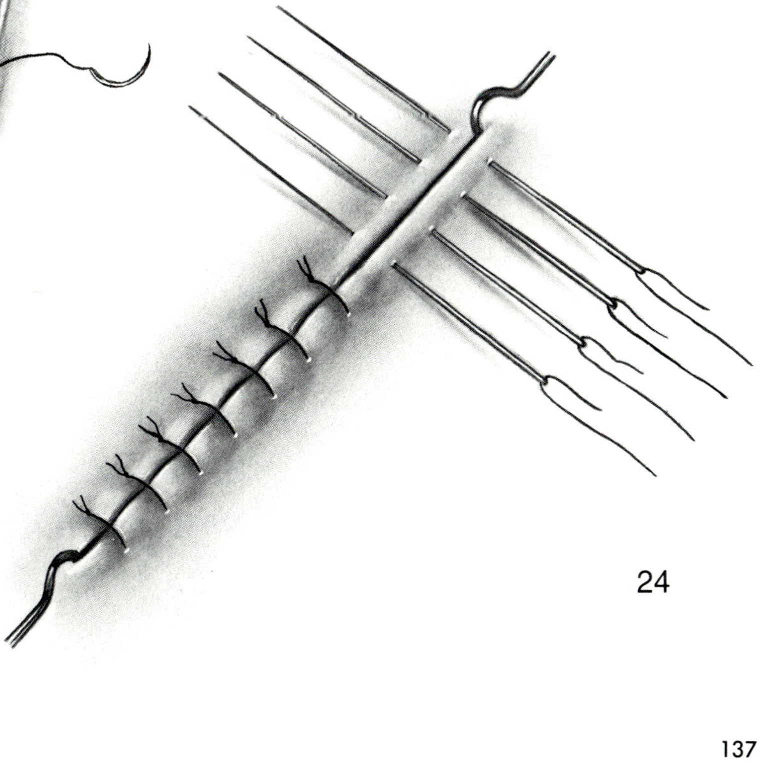

24

OPERATION 7

ANTERIOR REPAIR OF AN INGUINAL HERNIA WITH MARLEX MESH

Technique of Francis C. Usher, M.D.

Plate XXVI

1 The inner border of the rectangular sheath of Marlex mesh is fixed to the undersurface of the internal oblique muscle with interrupted mattress sutures of 2-0 silk.

2 The outer border of the mesh is sutured to the inguinal ligament with simple interrupted sutures of 2-0 silk. The redundant segment of the mesh is subsequently tailored around the cord, which will lie on its new "floor." The overlying leaflets of the external oblique aponeurosis and the subcutaneous fascia and skin are closed serially in layers to complete the operation.

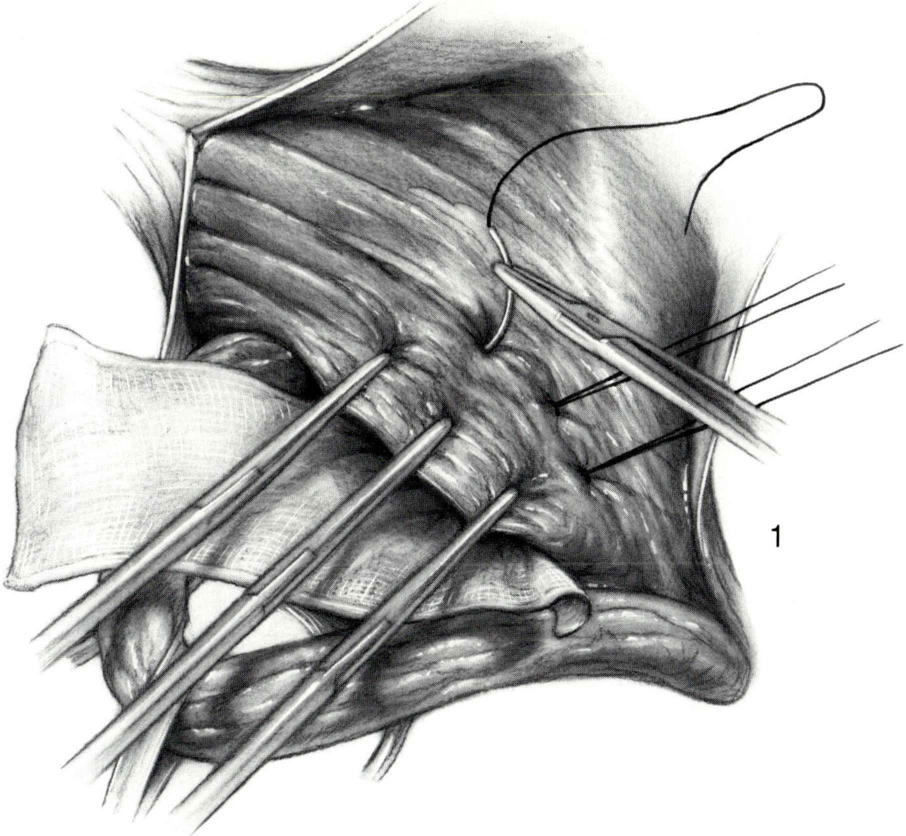

1

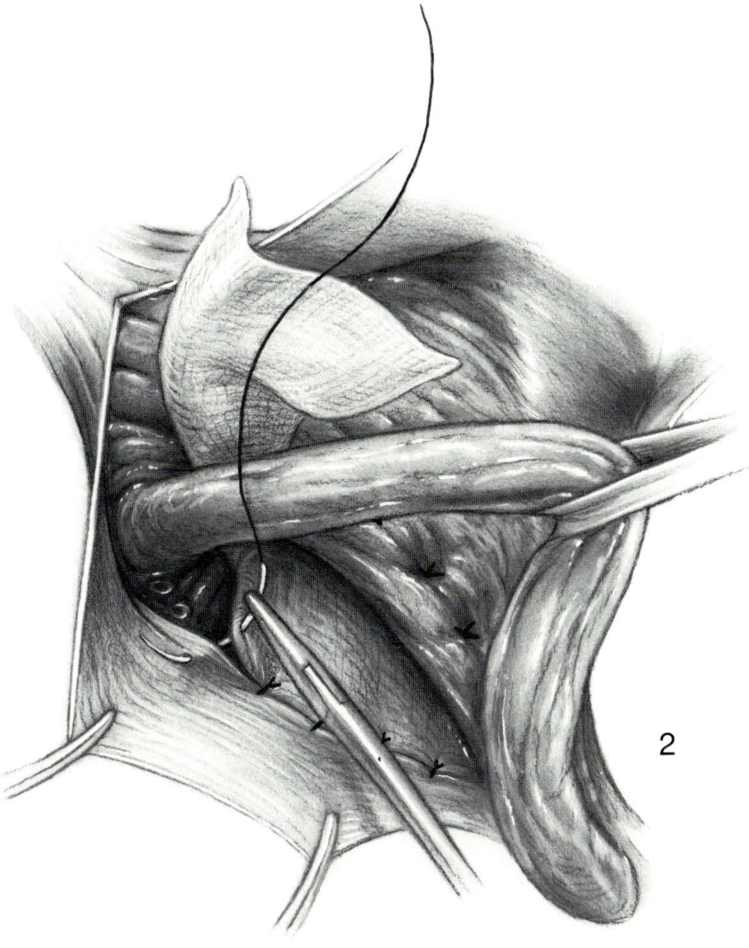

2

OPERATION 8

REPAIR OF A SLIDING HERNIA OF THE SIGMOID COLON

Plate XXVII
Plate XXVIII

A sliding inguinal hernia, by definition, is an incompletely reducible hernia in which a part of the wall of the sac is formed by the protruding viscus—the cecum on the right side, the sigmoid colon on the left side, and, on either side, the urinary bladder.

In every large, incompletely reducible inguinal hernia, particularly in the elderly patient, a sliding hernia should always be suspected. Intraoperatively, its diagnosis is further enhanced when the anatomic findings appear unusual. Such findings should alert the surgeon to the presence of a sliding hernia and help to prevent iatrogenic injuries of varying severity to either the cecum or the sigmoid colon and their respective mesenteries.

1, 2 The anterior wall of the peritoneal sac is excised (**1**), and the opening is extended caudad by scissors dissection (**2**). The elevated, convex, peripheral margin of the sac is formed by the underlying sigmoid colon.

3 The opening in the anterior wall of the hernial sac is completed, exposing the loop of sigmoid colon and its mesentery, which form the posterior wall of the sac. The *dashed lines* on each side of the sigmoid colon indicate the planes of scissors dissection in the formation of the free peritoneal flaps for the construction of the new posterior wall of the sac.

4 The inner peritoneal flap is mobilized, and scissors dissection of the outer flap is begun (*dashed line*).

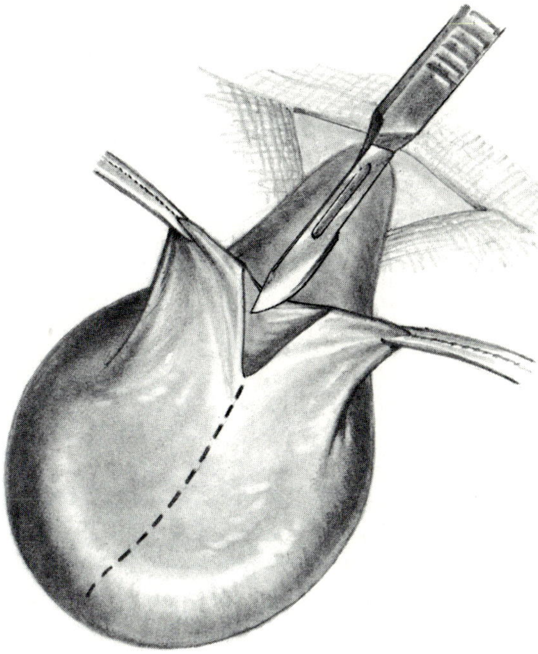

1

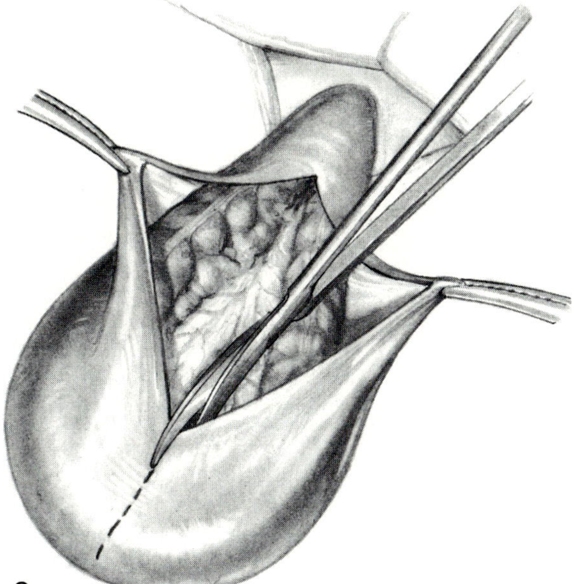

2

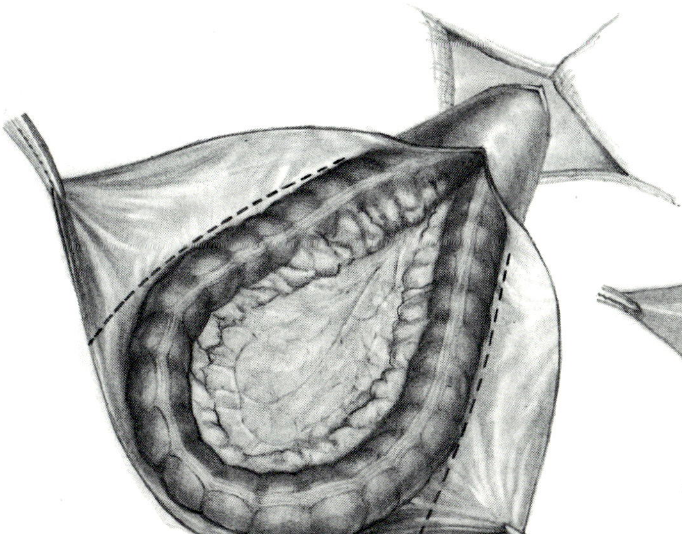

3

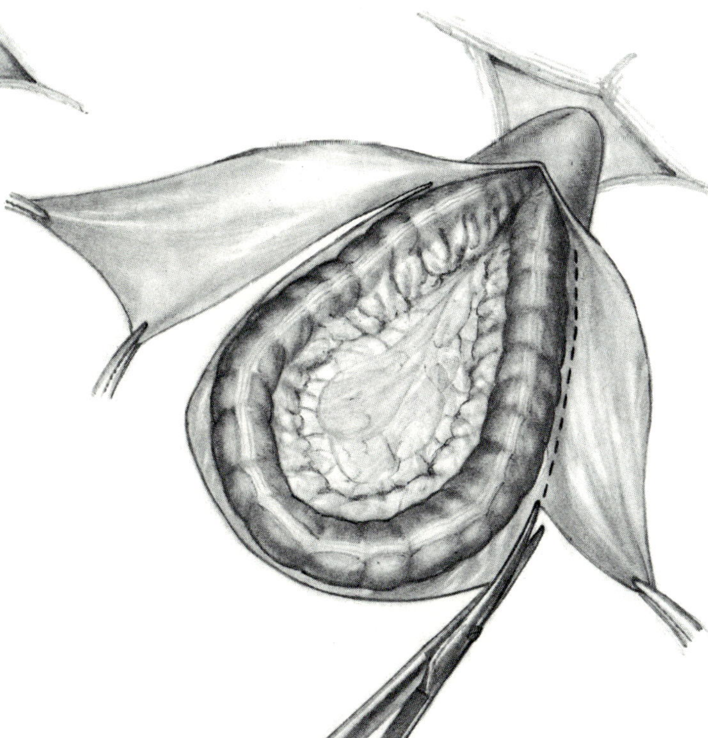

4

5 Formation of the free peritoneal flaps is completed, and combined instrumental and manual reduction of the sigmoid colon into the peritoneal cavity is initiated.

6, 7 Digital manipulation is used to complete the reduction of the loop of sigmoid colon **(6).** Before the reduction is completed, the free cut margins of the peritoneal flaps are approximated with interrupted sutures of 3-0 silk **(7).**

8, 9 A pursestring suture of 3-0 silk, for closure of the neck of the peritoneal sac, is inserted **(8)** and tied concomitantly with the instrumental reduction of the remnant of the sigmoid colon into the peritoneal cavity **(9).**

10 The neck of the sac is obliterated. The redundant portion is excised and its "cuff" oversewn with several interrupted figure-of-eight mattress sutures of 3-0 silk.

Reconstruction of the fascia of the left posterior inguinal wall is performed as described in Operation 10 (Repair of a Sliding Hernia of the Cecum) (Plate XLII, Fig. 7). The overlying tissue layers are then closed sequentially to complete the operation.

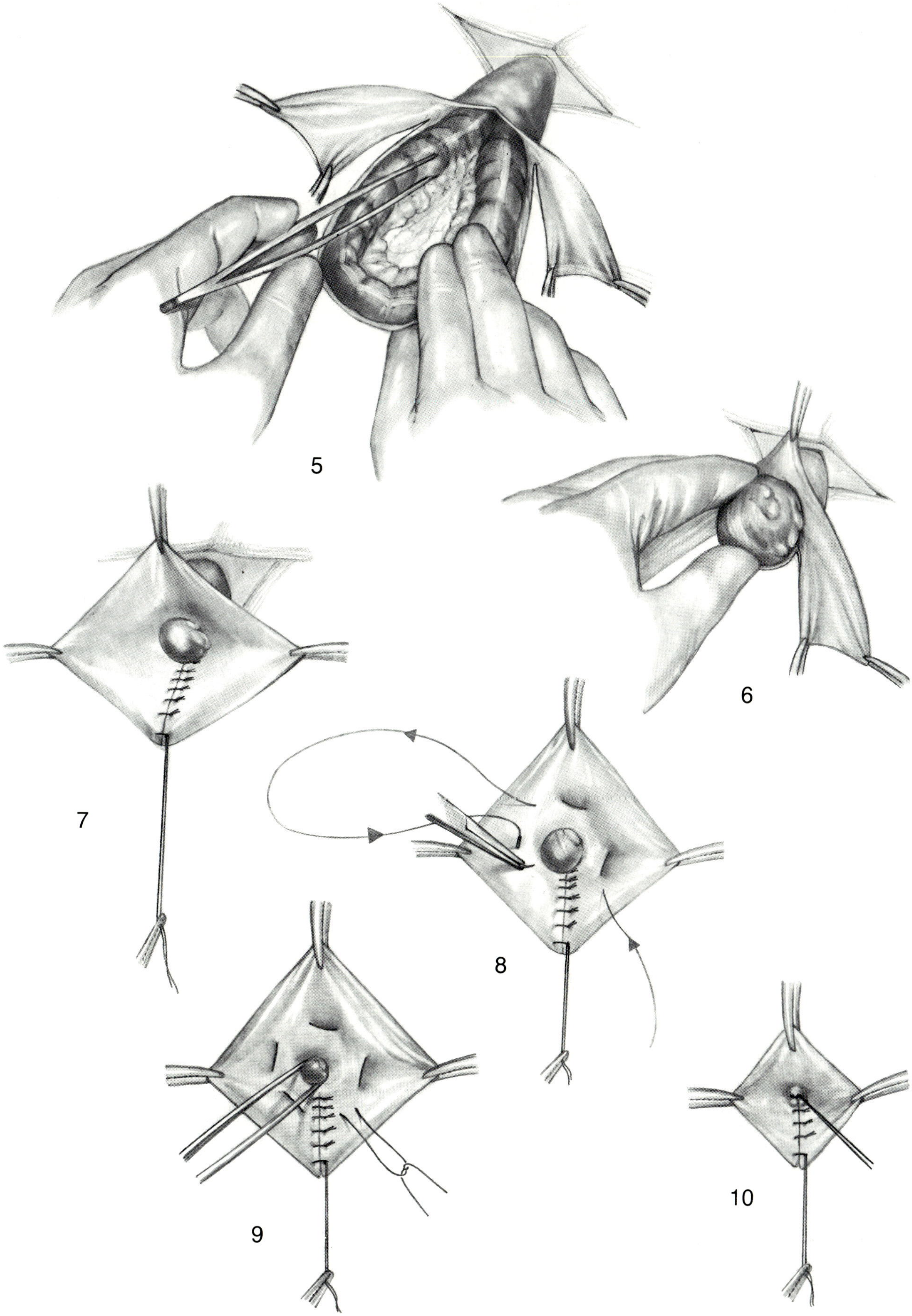
5
6
7
8
9
10

SLIDING HERNIAS OF THE SIGMOID COLON AND CECUM: INTRAOPERATIVE PHOTOGRAPHS

Plate XXIX
Plate XXX
Plate XXXI
Plate XXXII
Plate XXXIII
Plate XXXIV
Plate XXXV
Plate XXXVI
Plate XXXVII
Plate XXXVIII

1, 2 In this sliding hernia of the sigmoid colon in an 81-year-old man, preoperative frontal (**1**) and oblique (**2**) views show a long oval left inguinoscrotal hernia.

3 The aponeurosis of the external oblique muscle and the protuberance of the hernia through the external (subcutaneous) ring are visible.

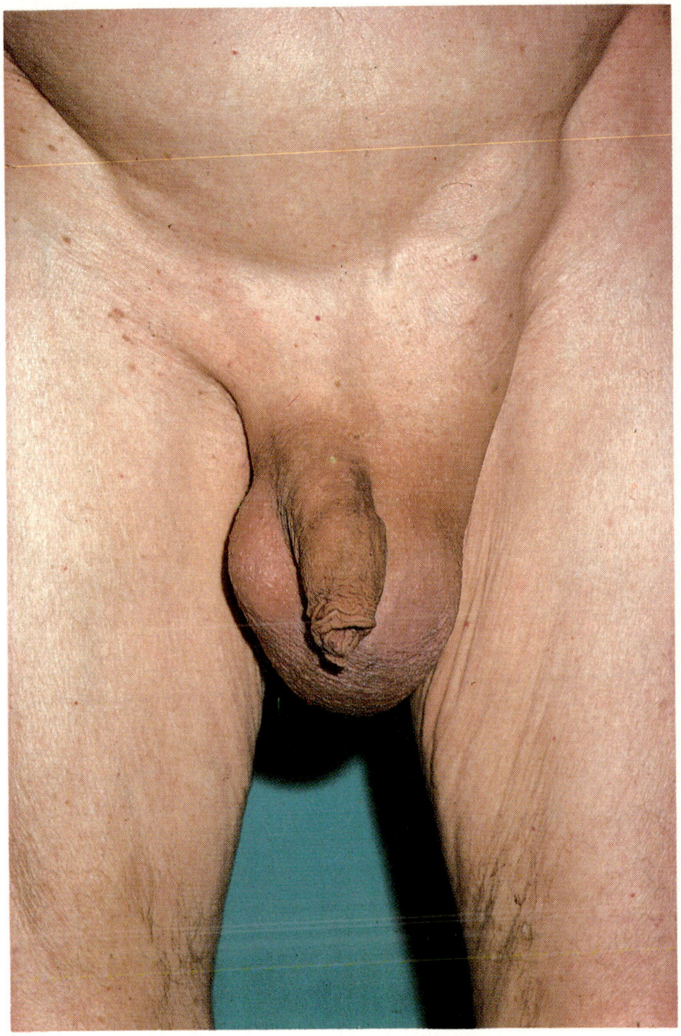

1

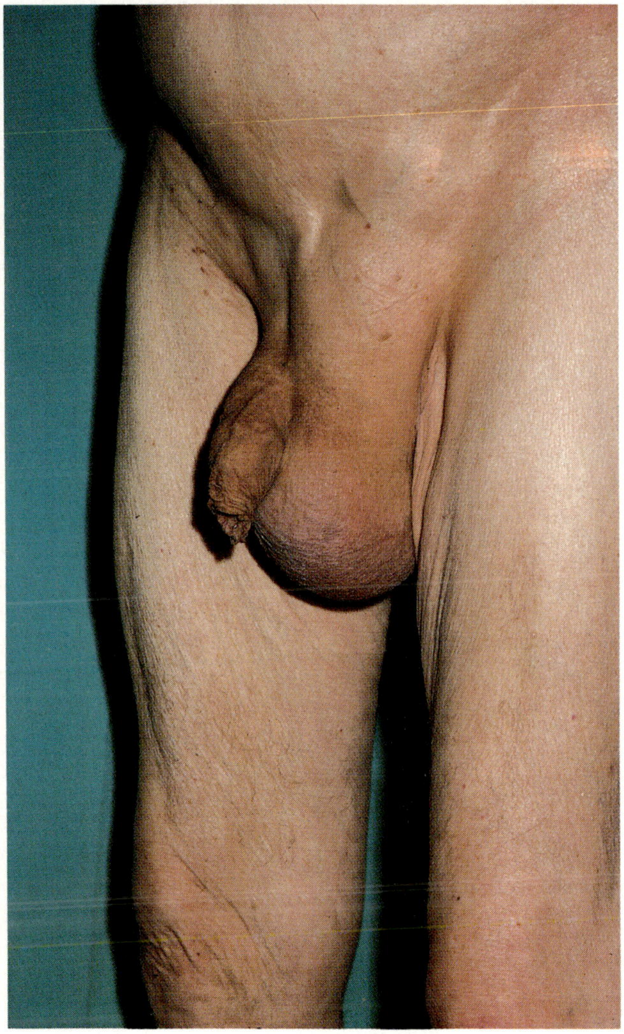

2

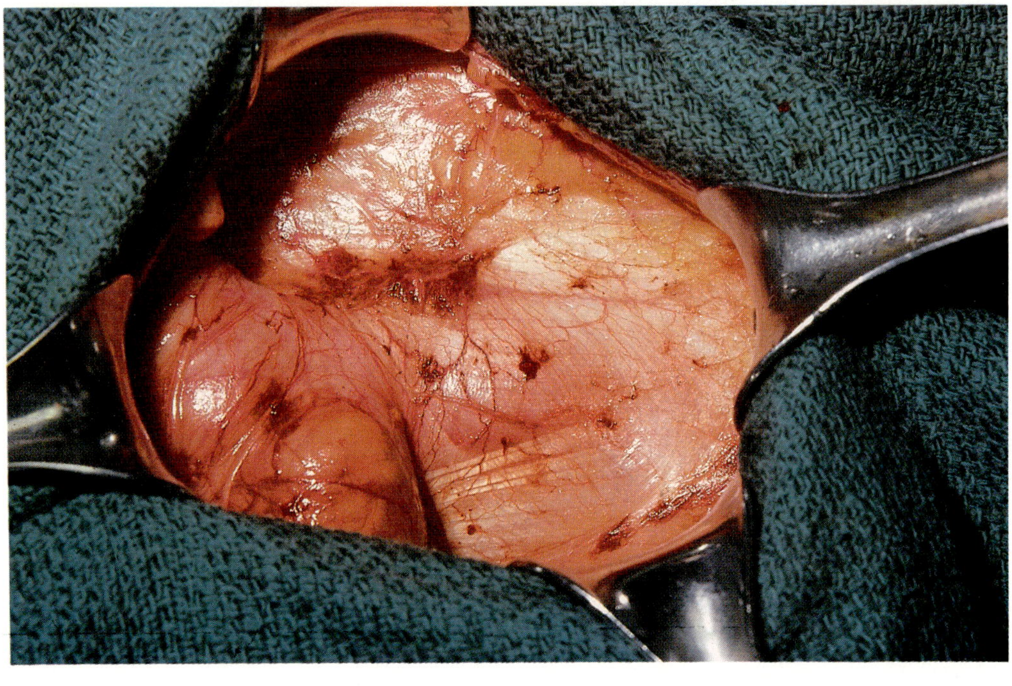

3

4 The external ring is opened to expose the sliding hernia of the sigmoid colon. The right index and middle fingers are placed behind the hernia; as it is elevated against the overlying anterior wall of the hernial sac, the bulge of the sigmoid colon, which forms its posterior wall, is shown in bas-relief.

5 The anterior wall of the sac, held in forceps, is incised with a scalpel.

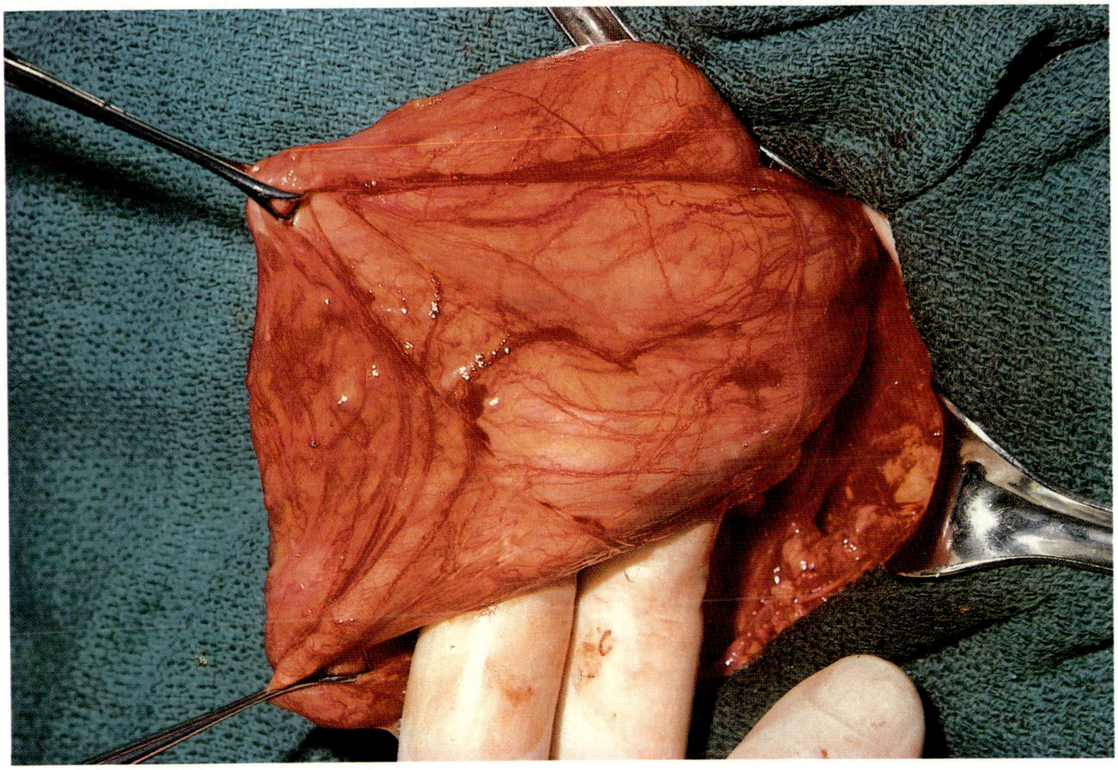

4

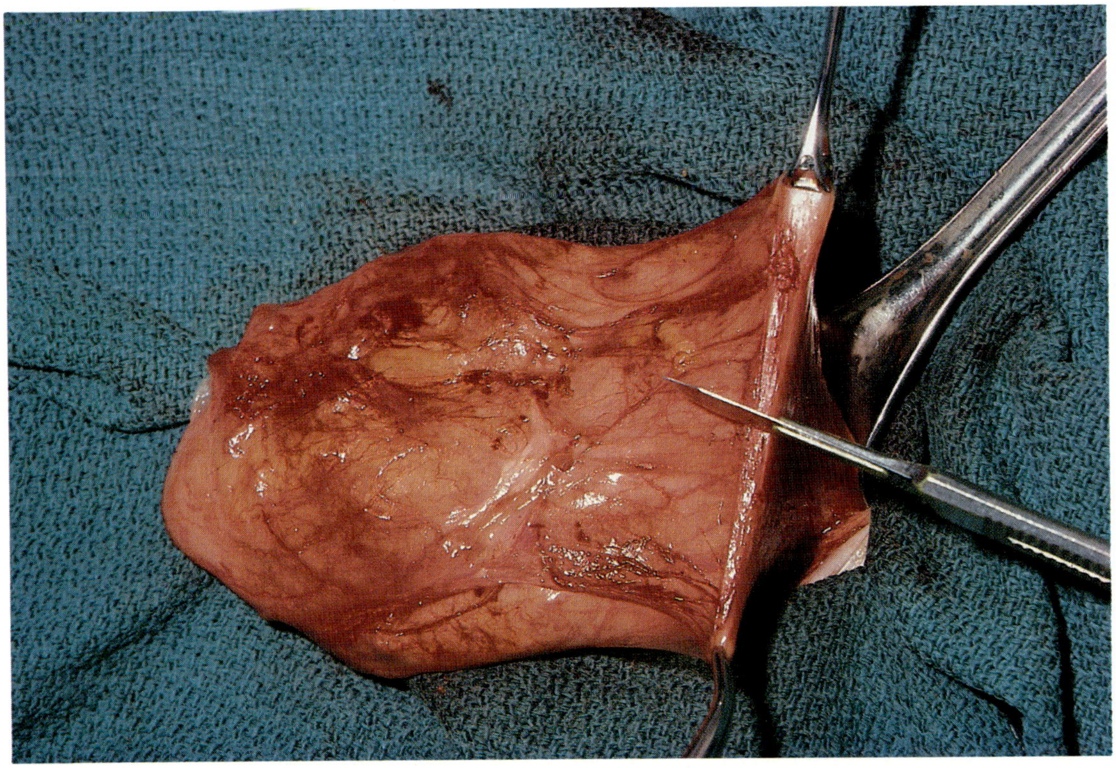

5

6, 7 The peritoneal sac is entered **(6)**, and the opening is extended caudad by scissors dissection **(7)** to expose the sliding hernia of the sigmoid colon.

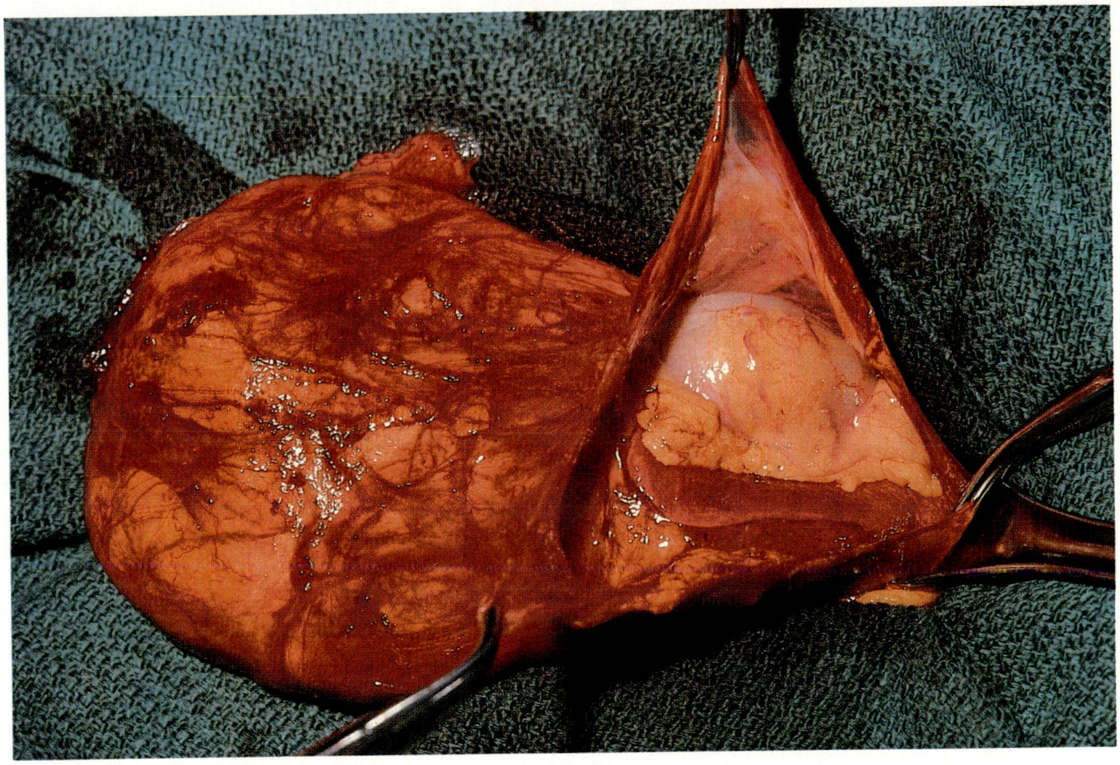

6

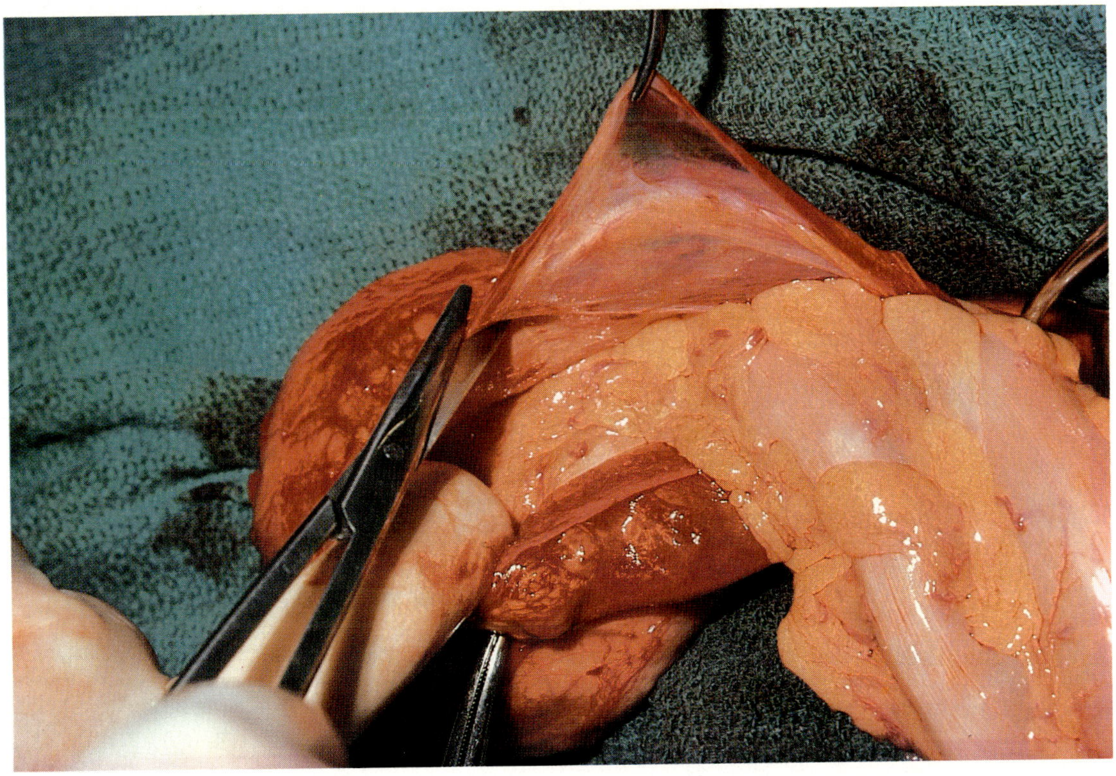

7

SLIDING HERNIAS OF THE SIGMOID COLON AND CECUM: INTRAOPERATIVE PHOTOGRAPHS *Continued*

8, 9, 10 The lateral juxtacolonic peritoneal flap is mobilized by scissors dissection **(8, 9)**, as is the medial flap **(10)**.

11 Mobilization of the juxtacolonic peritoneal flaps is completed, and their relationship to the detached cephalad portion of the sliding hernia of the sigmoid colon is seen.

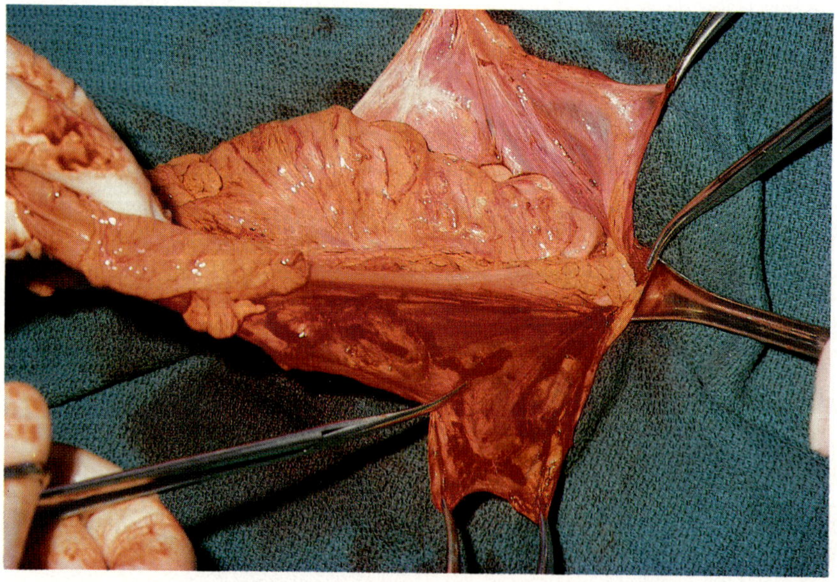

8

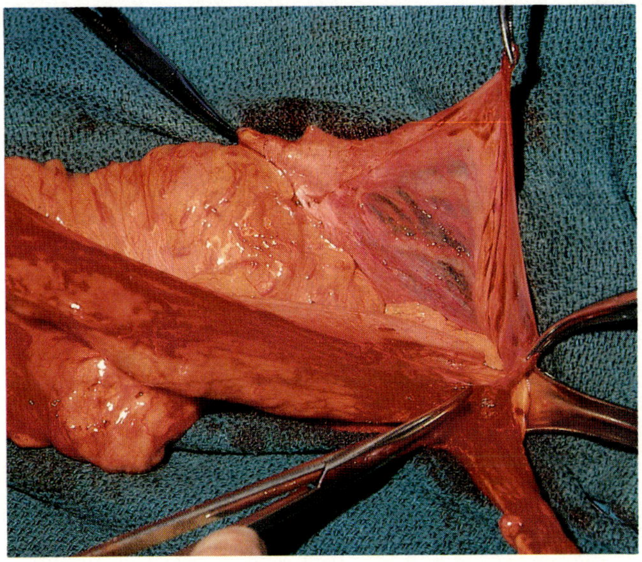

9

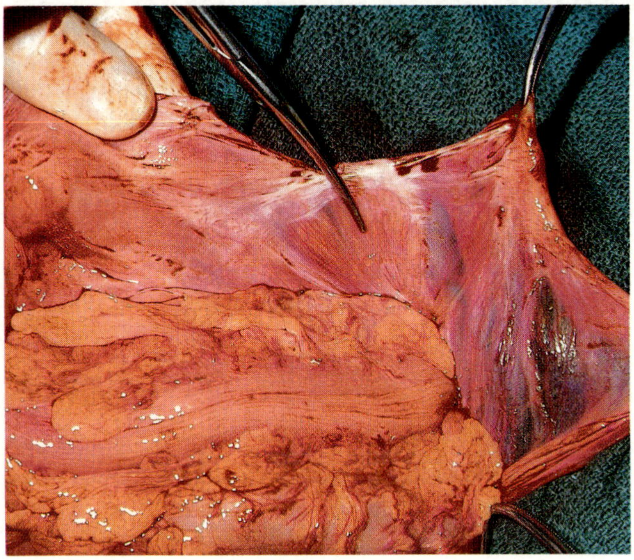

10

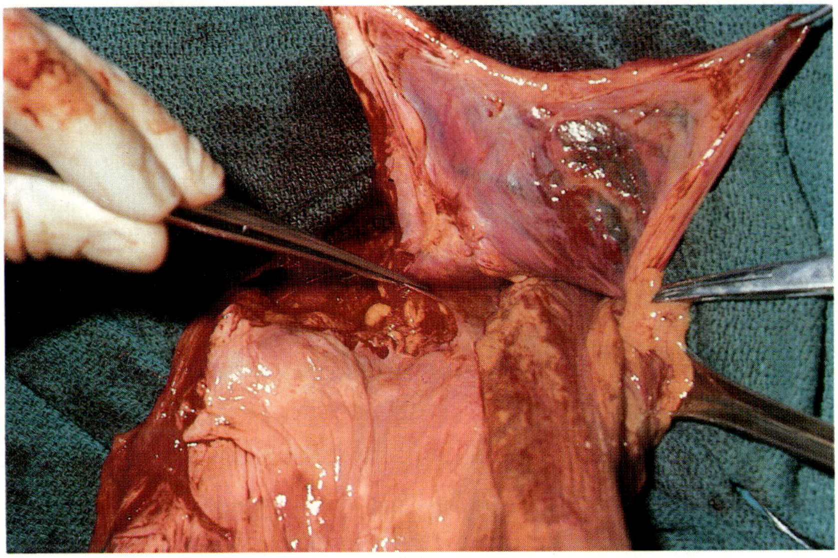

11

12, 13, 14, 15 The whole of the detached sliding hernia of the sigmoid colon and its mesentery is shown (**12**), preparatory to its reduction into the peritoneal cavity by progressive instrumental and digital manipulation (**13, 14, 15**).

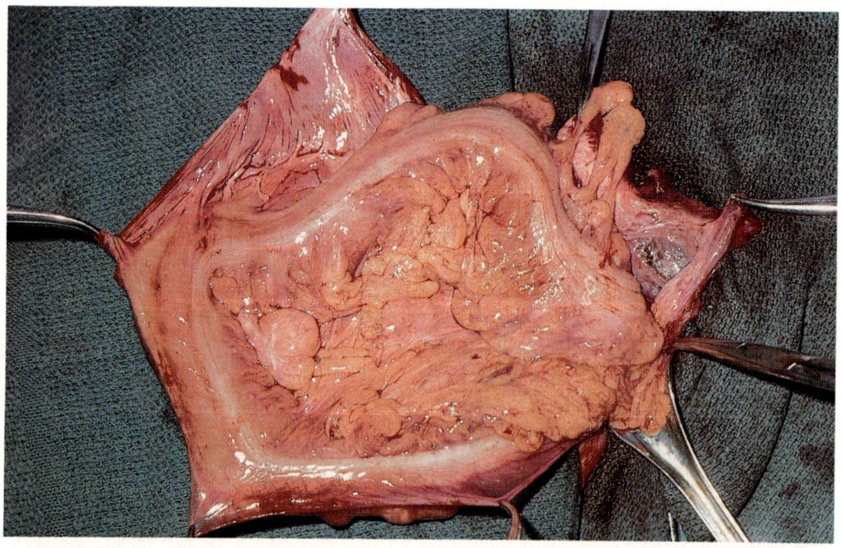

12

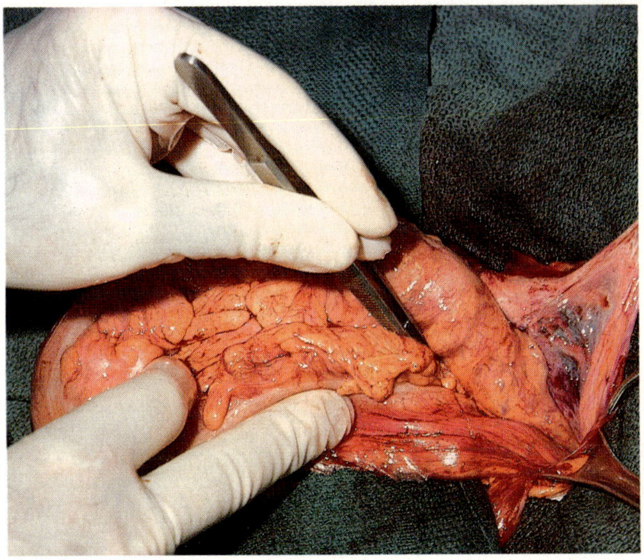

13

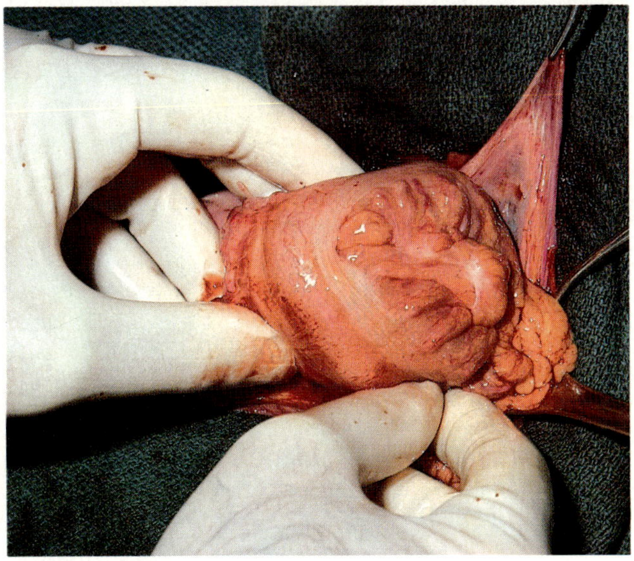

14

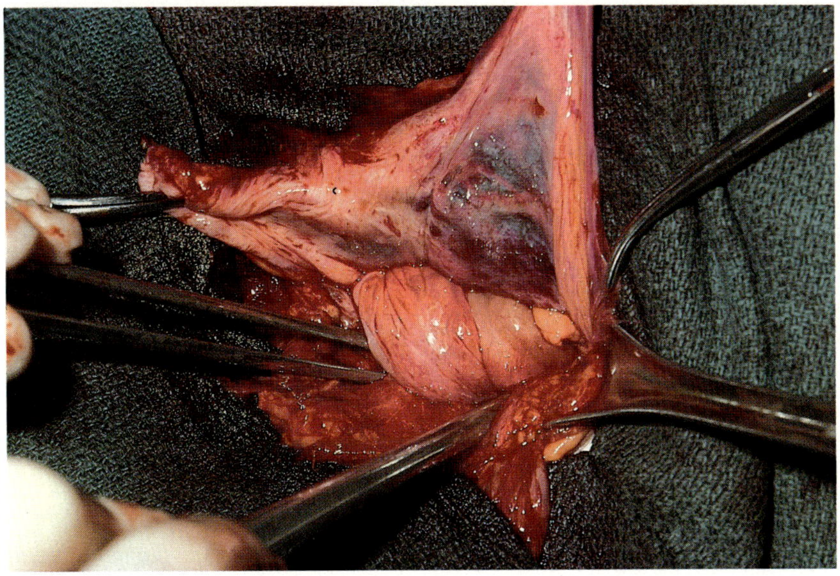

15

16 The sliding component of the sigmoid colon is reduced, and the new posterior wall of the hernial sac is formed by suturing together the cut margins of the previously mobilized medial and lateral peritoneal flaps. The line of suture is indicated by the inner and outer intact strands of silk (4-0) sutures.

17, 18, 19 A pursestring suture (3-0 silk) is inserted from the inside of the sac **(17, 18)**; when completed, it is tied as the forceps, which maintained the reduction of the sigmoid colon, is simultaneously withdrawn **(19).**

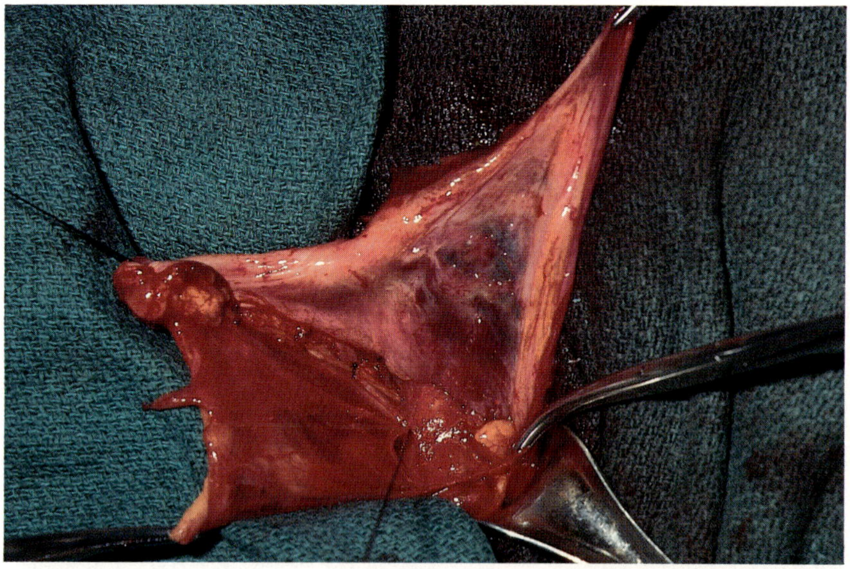

16

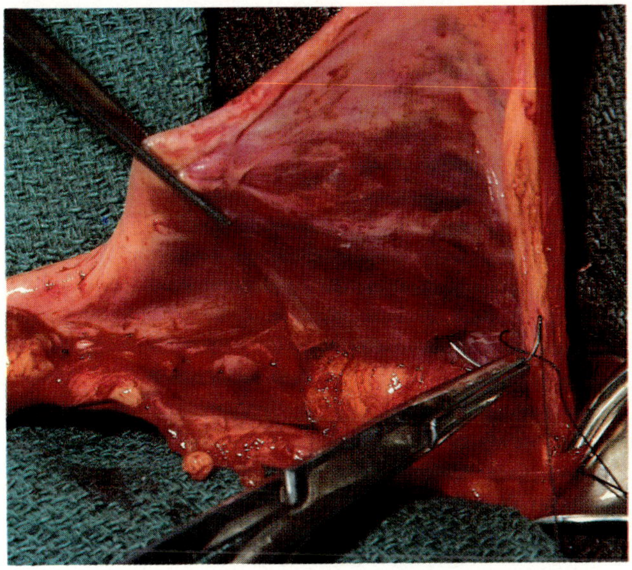

17

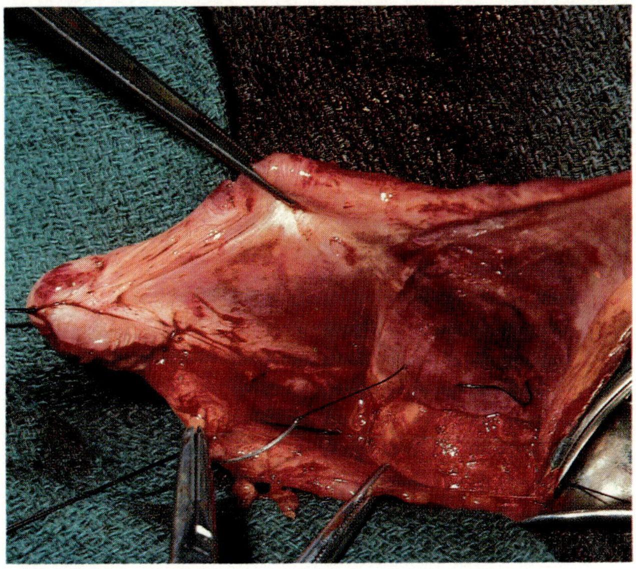

18

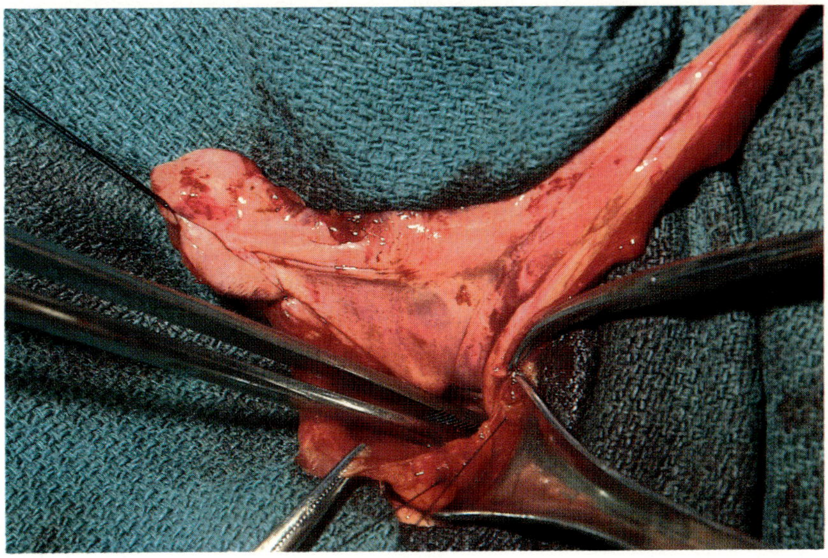

19

SLIDING HERNIAS OF THE SIGMOID COLON AND CECUM: INTRAOPERATIVE PHOTOGRAPHS *Continued*

20 The closure of the neck of the sac is completed, and the strands of the suture are drawn taut for better exposure. After the strands are cut, the redundant portions of the wall of the new sac are resected and their cut margins approximated to reinforce the peritoneal closure.

21, 22, 23 The attenuated fascia of the posterior inguinal wall **(21)** is excised **(22),** and the crown suture is inserted to close the medial angle of the defect in the fascia of the posterior inguinal wall **(23).**

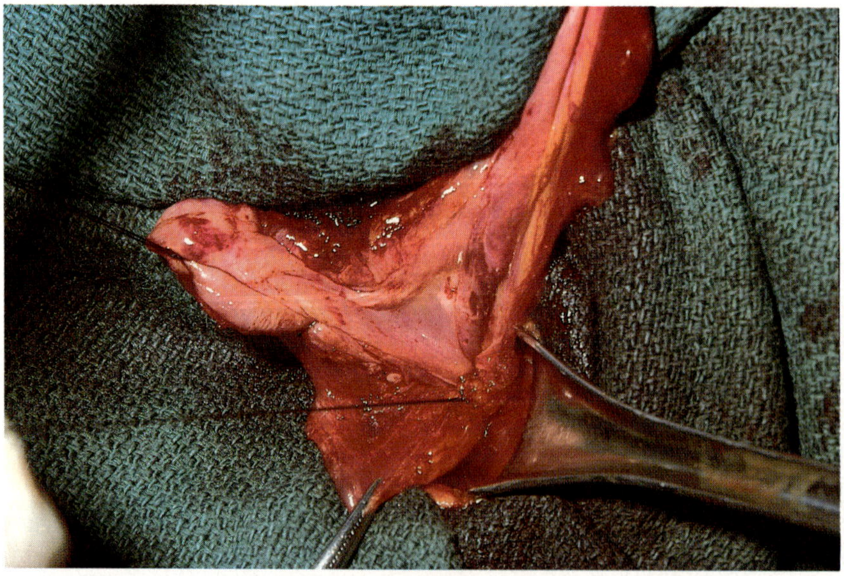

20

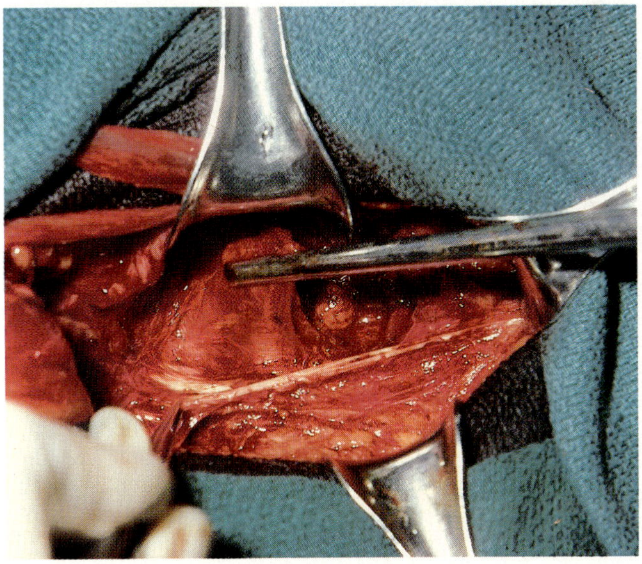

21

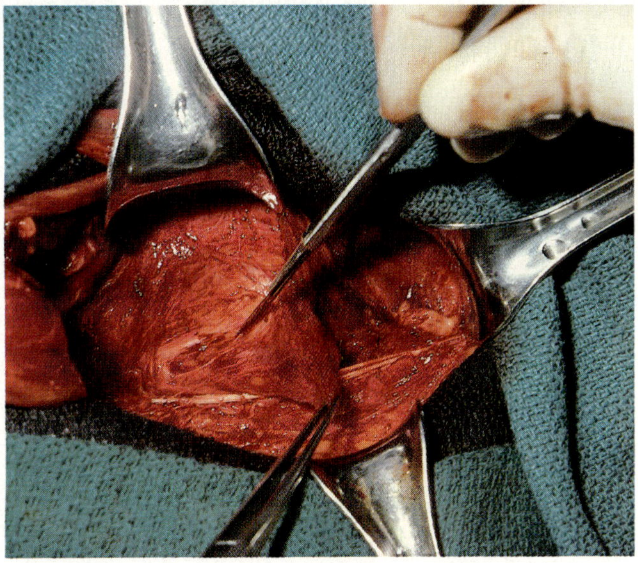

22

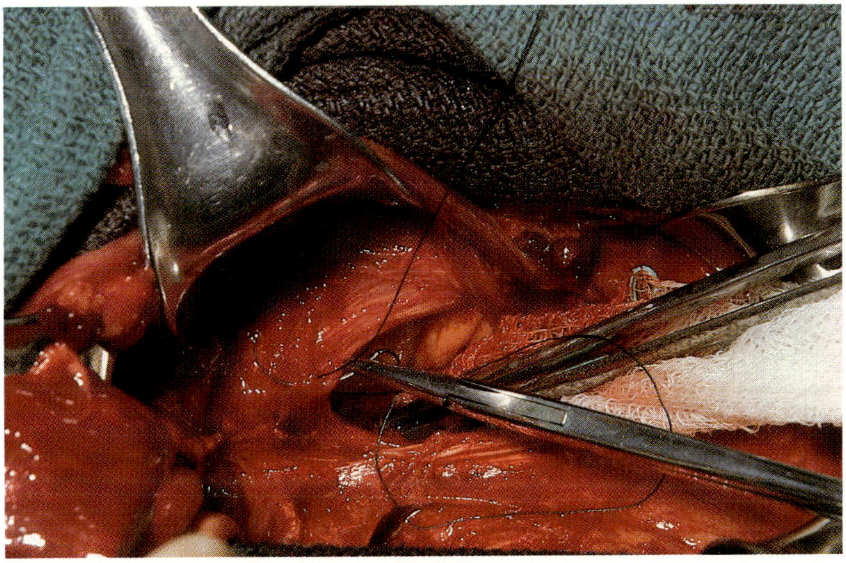

23

24 The superior segment of the fascia of the posterior inguinal wall is sutured to its inferior segment (iliopubic tract), the holding power of which is excellent, using interrupted sutures of 3-0 silk. The location of the forceps holding the inferior segment marks the site of its outward angulation as it continues laterally over the underlying true femoral sheath and encased vessels to form the anterior femoral sheath. The convex outline and white markings of this sheath are visible immediately lateral to the forceps.

Medial to and below the forceps is the pyriform fossa, the lateral boundary of which is formed by the medial wall of the femoral sheath. The horizontal white line, coursing medially, is the shelving edge of the inguinal ligament, which forms the inferior boundary of the pyriform fossa. The fossa's superior boundary is the inferior segment of the fascia of the posterior inguinal wall, which is held taut by both the untied sutures medially and the forceps laterally. The floor of the fossa, which is not visible, is formed by the fascial part of Gimbernat's ligament.

25 The single-layer reconstruction of the fascia of the posterior inguinal wall is completed. The suture strands medially are those of the crown suture; the middle strands represent the normal anatomic transition suture, which is not associated with a trough deformity of the posterior inguinal wall; and the most lateral strands are those of the suture that secures the snug closure of the internal ring around the exit of the spermatic cord. The internal oblique muscle superiorly and the inguinal ligament inferiorly have only a contiguous anatomic relationship to the fascial reconstruction of the posterior inguinal wall.

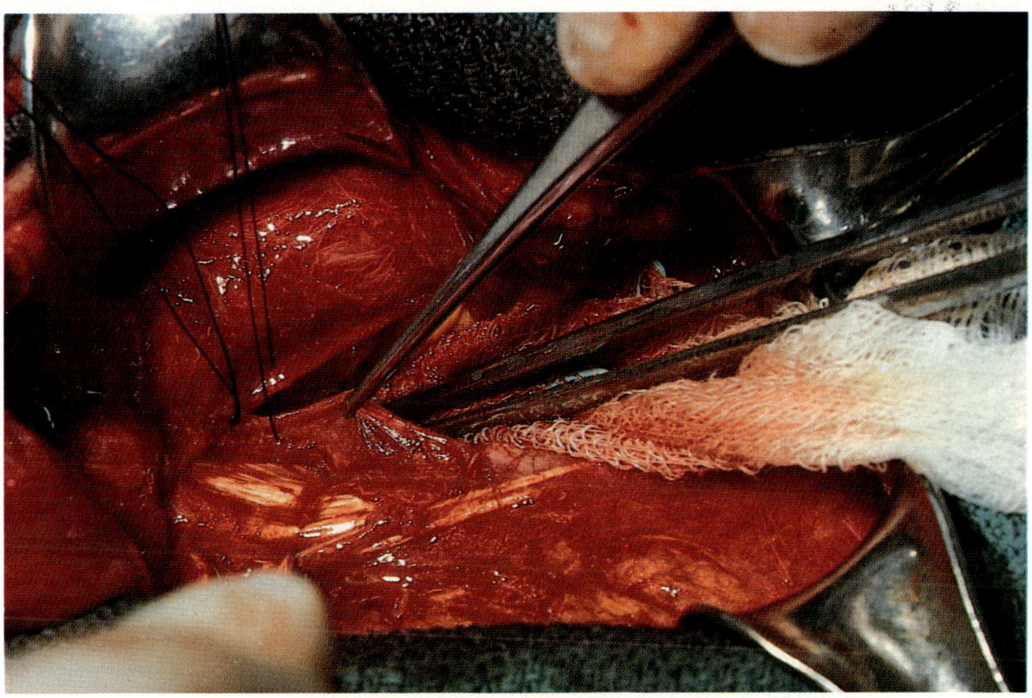

24

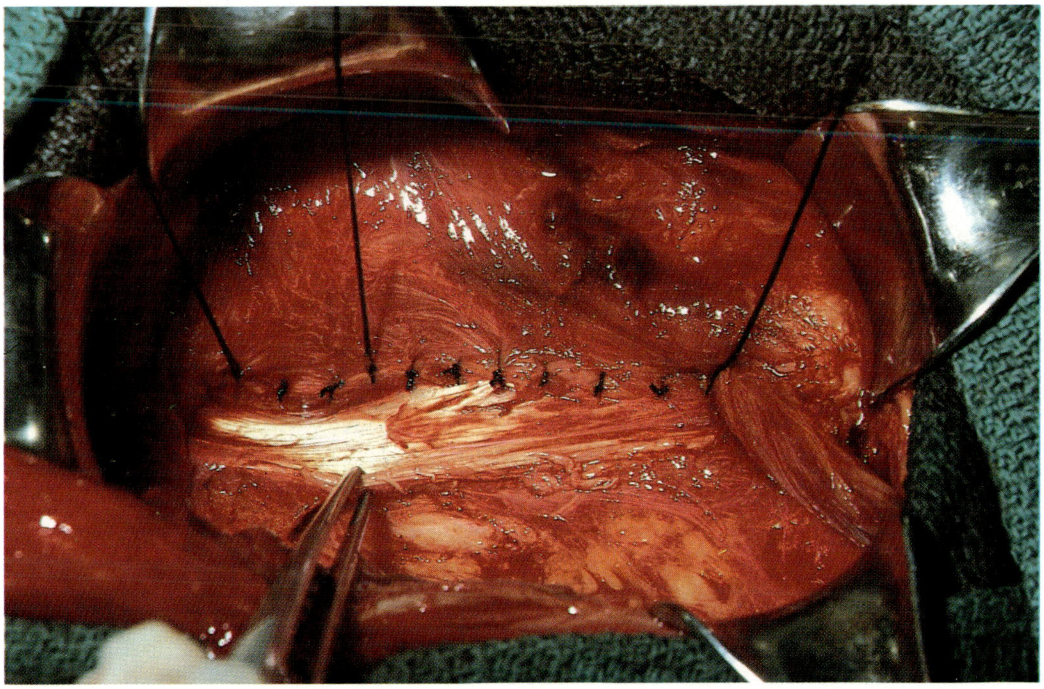

25

SLIDING HERNIAS OF THE SIGMOID COLON AND CECUM: INTRAOPERATIVE PHOTOGRAPHS *Continued*

26 This view of a sliding hernia in a 56-year-old man shows the sigmoid colon, which forms the posterior wall of the hernial sac.

27 This enlargement of the preceding photograph shows more clearly the internal closure of the neck of the newly formed peritoneal sac.

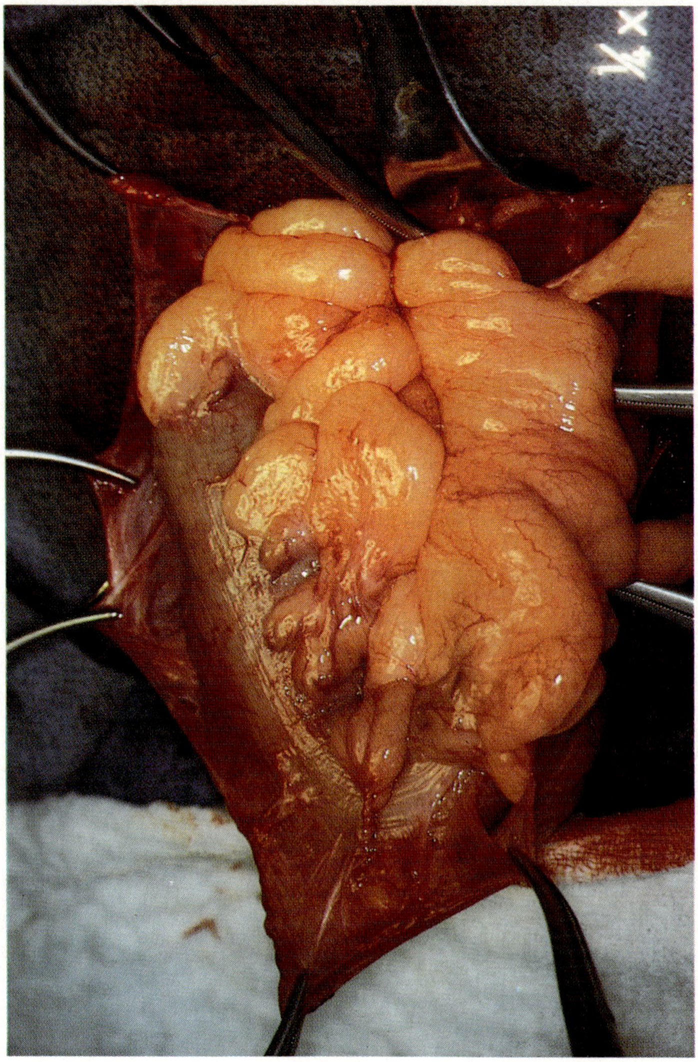

26

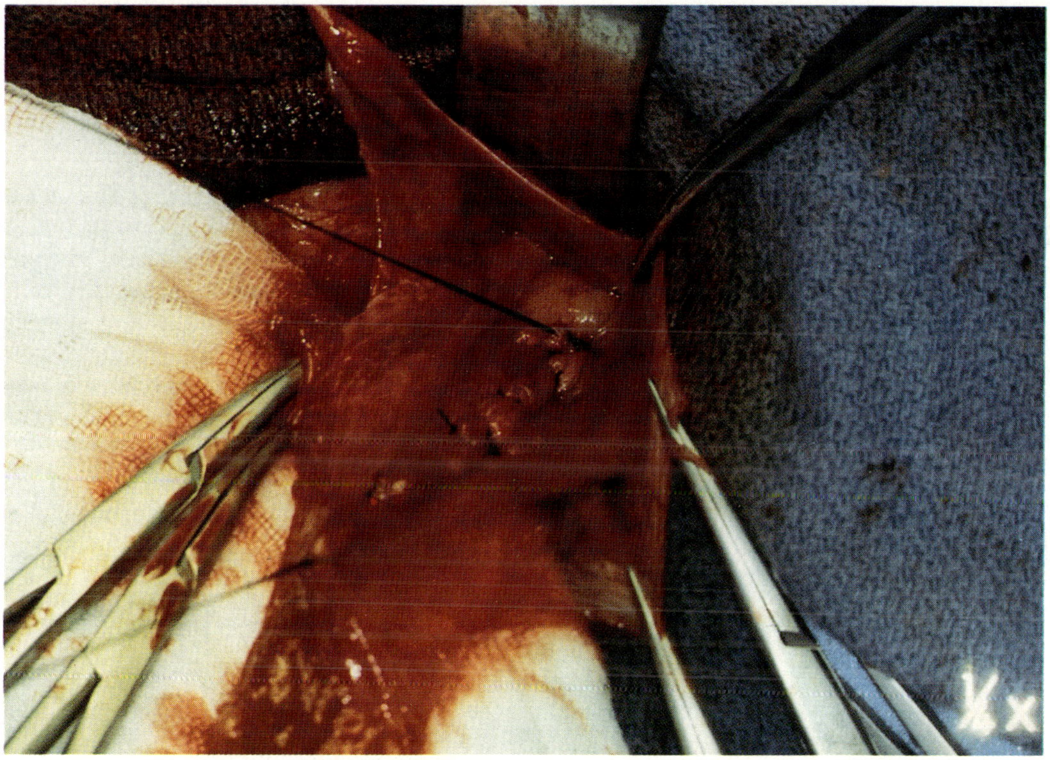

27

SLIDING HERNIAS OF THE SIGMOID COLON AND CECUM: INTRAOPERATIVE PHOTOGRAPHS *Continued*

28 The same technique described for the repair of a sliding hernia of the sigmoid colon (Operation 8) is used in the treatment of a sliding hernia of the cecum.

This intraoperative photograph shows a sliding hernia of the cecum in a 62-year-old man. The hernial sac, held taut in clamps, is elevated to show the bulge of the cecum, which forms its posterior wall. A preperitoneal lipoma of the spermatic cord, held in forceps, is also shown.

29 The herniated ileocecal segment and appendix are shown after the anterior wall of the peritoneal sac is opened and the paracecal peritoneal flaps are formed. Following the reduction of the hernial contents into the peritoneal cavity, the opposing cut margins of the peritoneal flaps are sutured to establish a new posterior wall of the hernial sac.

The neck of the sac is closed by the insertion of a pursestring suture (3-0 silk) from within the sac, and its redundant portion is excised. A single-layer reconstruction of the fascia of the posterior inguinal wall, depicted in **25,** is then done.

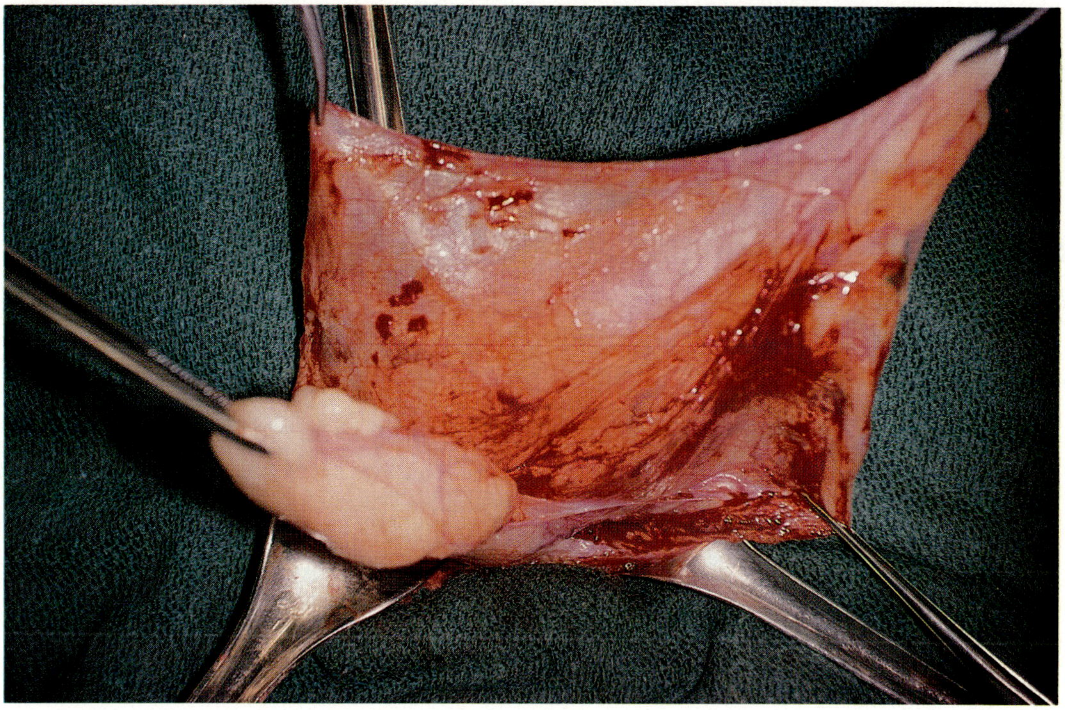

28

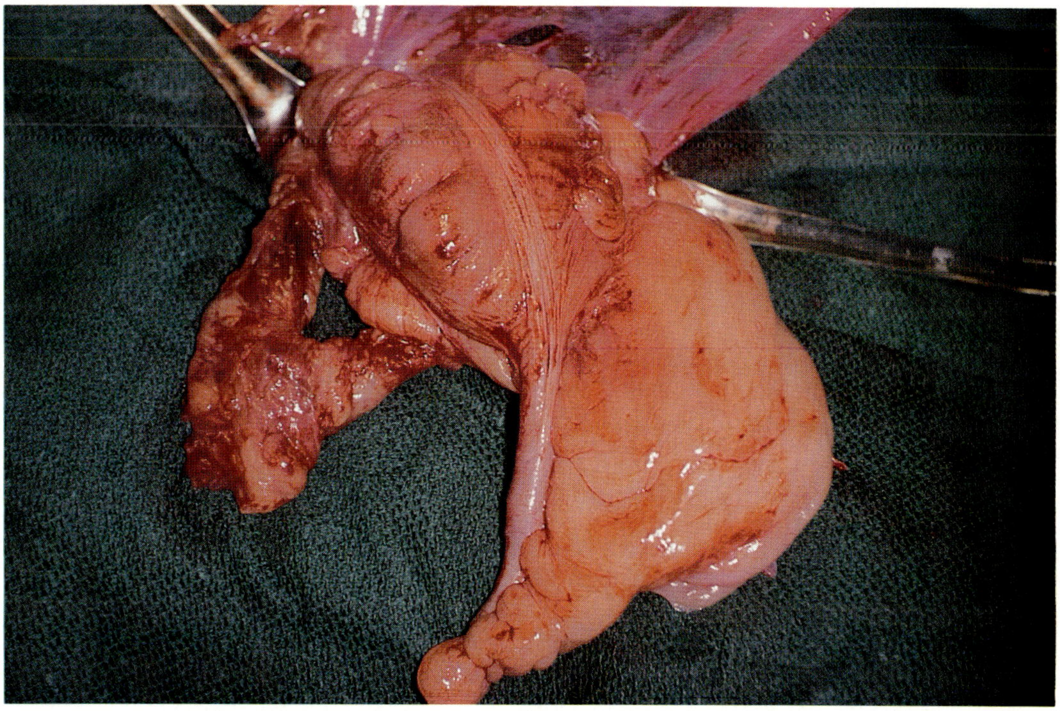

29

OPERATION 9

REPAIR OF A SLIDING HERNIA OF THE SIGMOID COLON

Technique of Carrington Williams

Plate XXXIX
Plate XL

The surgical technique illustrated here is a modification of the La Roque transperitoneal repair. The relative simplicity of this method, the fact that it is based upon a clear understanding of the anatomic pathologic changes that occur in a sliding hernia, and the technical ease of reduction of the hernia make it an ideal operation.

1 Downward traction is maintained on the intact anterior wall of the sac to show more clearly the outline of the underlying sigmoid colon, which forms the posterior wall of the sac. The line of incision (*dashed line*) in the anterior wall of the sac is shown.

2 The sac is opened, and the sliding hernia of the sigmoid colon, which forms its posterior wall, is exposed.

3 The cephalad *(a)* and caudad *(b)* limits of the incision in the anterior wall of the sac are indicated. The superior leaflet of the external oblique aponeurosis is retracted for better exposure of the internal oblique muscle. The incision in this muscle, immediately superior to the iliohypogastric nerve, is shown by the *dashed line*.

4 The incision is deepened through the underlying internal oblique and transversus abdominis muscles to expose the line of incision in the anterior parietal peritoneum.

5 The peritoneal cavity is entered, and, by a combination of manual traction from above and digital manipulation from below, the sliding hernia component of the sigmoid colon is withdrawn from the cavity.

6 Withdrawal of the sliding hernia of the sigmoid colon from the peritoneal cavity is completed. The opening in the anterior wall of the sac is now seen as an opening in the visceral peritoneum of the sliding hernia of the sigmoid colon, with the letters *a* and *b* reversed from their positions in **3**.

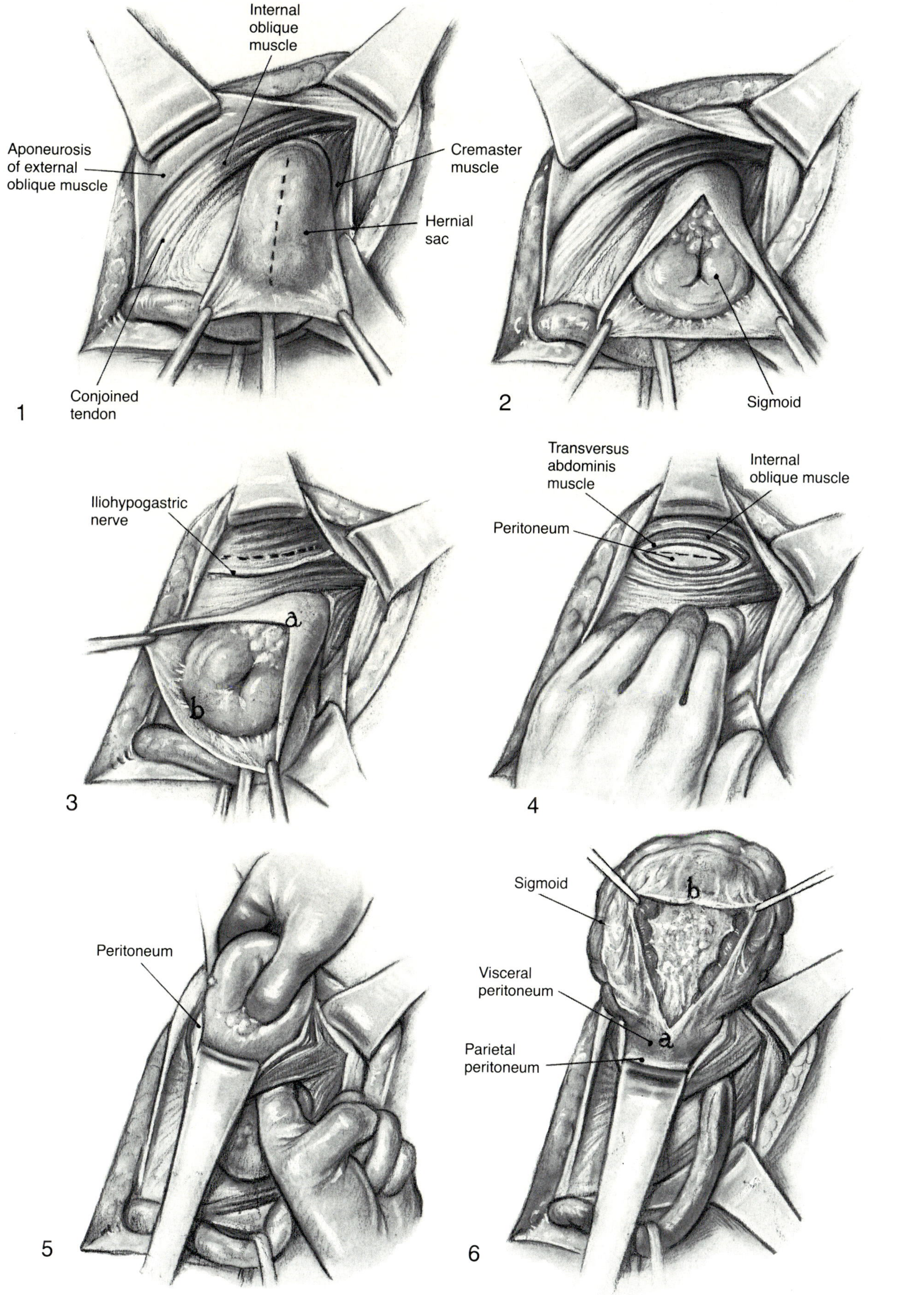
Internal oblique muscle
Aponeurosis of external oblique muscle
Cremaster muscle
Hernial sac
Conjoined tendon
1
2
Sigmoid
Iliohypogastric nerve
a
b
3
Transversus abdominis muscle
Internal oblique muscle
Peritoneum
4
Peritoneum
5
Sigmoid
b
Visceral peritoneum
a
Parietal peritoneum
6

7 The redundant "sac" of the mesosigmoid is resected and the free margins are approximated, using a continuous suture of 4-0 chromic catgut. Fixation of the sigmoid colon to the adjacent parietal peritoneum is not performed.

8 The closure of the peritoneal incision is completed, and the overlying muscle layers are approximated with interrupted sutures of 3-0 chromic catgut. The elliptical defect in the fascia of the posterior inguinal wall is closed with interrupted sutures of 3-0 silk. Its relationship to the deep epigastric and cremaster vessels is visible.

The spermatic cord will be placed onto the reconstructed posterior inguinal wall, and the overlying cremaster veil, external oblique aponeurosis, subcutaneous fascia, and skin closed in layers to complete the operation.

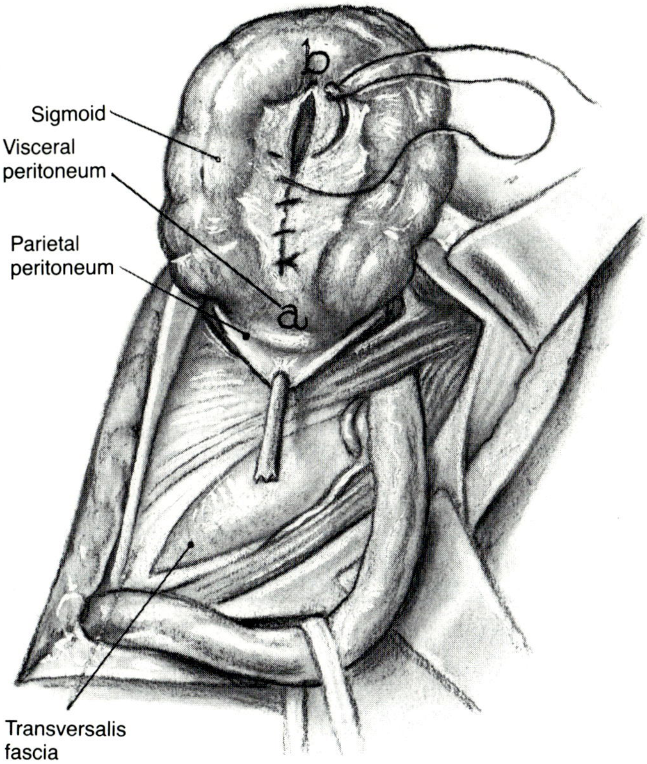
b
Sigmoid
Visceral peritoneum
Parietal peritoneum
a
Transversalis fascia

7

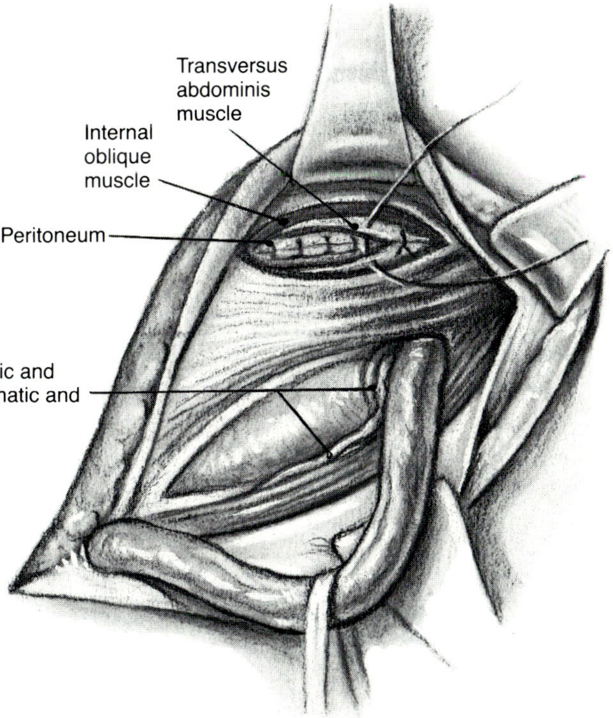
Transversus abdominis muscle
Internal oblique muscle
Peritoneum
Deep epigastric and external spermatic and pubic vessels

8

OPERATION 10

REPAIR OF A SLIDING HERNIA OF THE CECUM

Plate XLI
Plate XLII
Plate XLIII

1 The intact hernial sac is grasped in clamps and retracted up to show the posterior aspect of the sliding hernia of the cecum.

2 In this magnified view of the opened sac and the sliding hernia of the cecum that forms its posterior wall, the incisional lines (*dashed lines*) for the simultaneous mobilization of the cecum and formation of the paracecal peritoneal flaps are shown.

3 The peritoneal flaps have been mobilized, and the reduction of the cecum into the peritoneal cavity is gently performed with the thumb and index finger.

4, 5 The base of the cecum, held in tissue forceps, is displaced up; as traction and counter-traction on the peritoneal sac and its flaps, respectively, are maintained, the initial suture (3-0 silk) in the construction of the new posterior wall of the hernial sac is inserted **(4)**. The suture is tied and traction is applied to its strands as the succeeding interrupted sutures (3-0 silk) are inserted in sequence **(5)**.

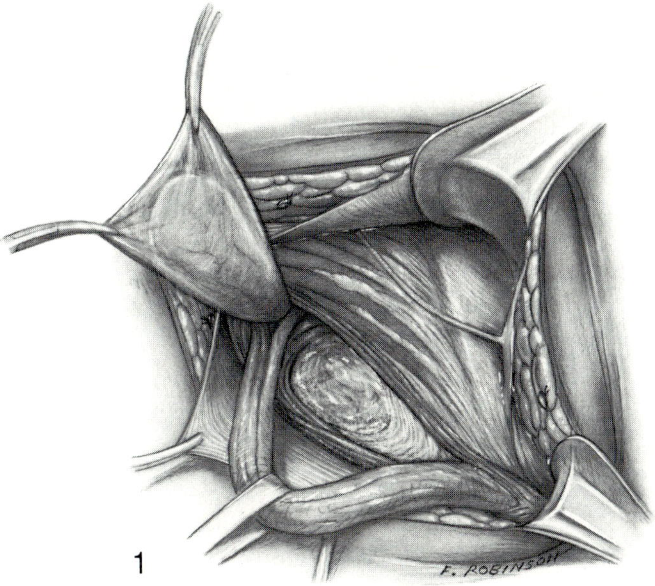

1

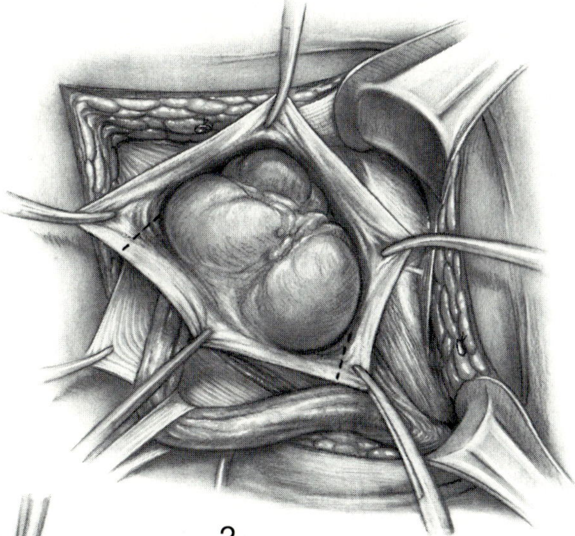

2

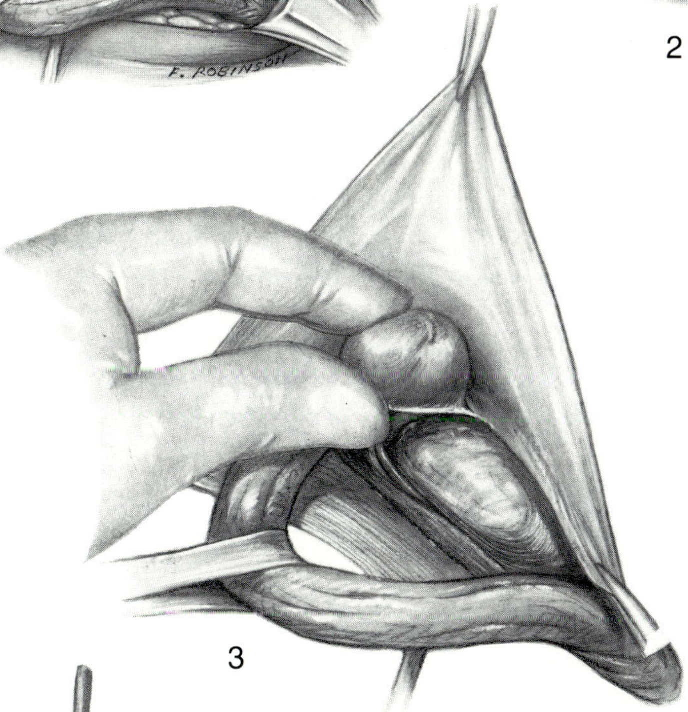

3

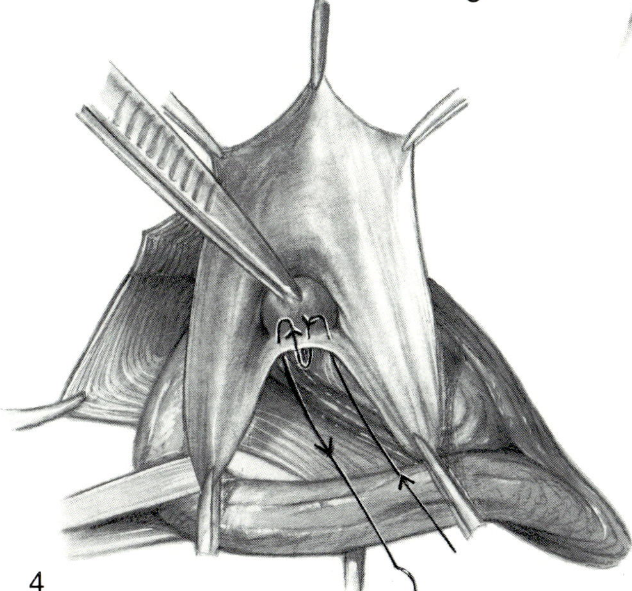

4

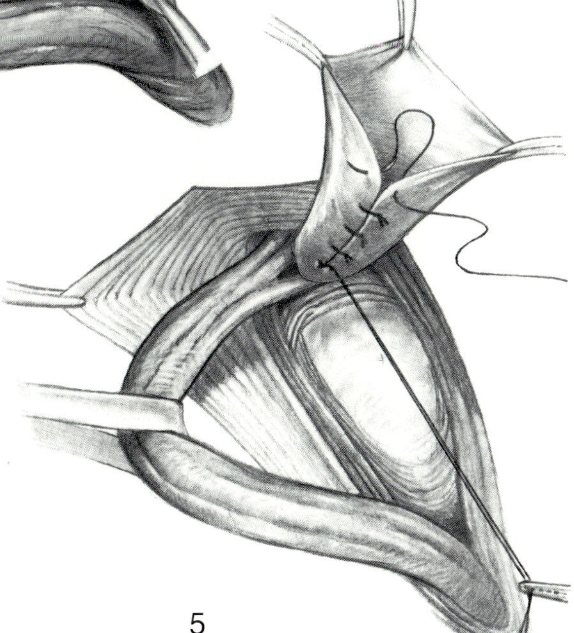

5

REPAIR OF A SLIDING HERNIA OF THE CECUM *Continued*

6, 6A The last suture in the construction of the posterior wall of the hernial sac is inserted **(6)**; when it is tied, the lower angle suture is cut **(6A)**.

6B, 6C, 6D After it has been ensured that the sac is empty, the needle of a swaged-on transfixion suture of 3-0 silk is inserted through its neck **(6B)**. The suture is tied behind and then in front **(6C)**. The insertion of the transfixion suture is completed, and the redundant portion of the peritoneal sac is resected with scissors at the level indicated by the *dashed line* **(6D)**.

7 The cuff of the ligated neck of the sac, retracted beneath the internal oblique muscle, is indicated by the *circular dashed line*. The fascia of the posterior inguinal wall is reconstructed by suturing its superior (medial) segment to its inferior (lateral) segment (iliopubic tract).

The first or crown suture (3-0 silk) is inserted and tied to close the medial angle of the fascial defect. For technical expediency, the rest of the sutures (3-0 silk) are inserted separately and untied; later they are tied in sequence from medial to lateral.

The relationship of the fascial reconstruction, both to the underlying preperitoneal fat and to the normal site of exit of the cremaster vessels (which is not through the internal ring), is visible. Its relationship to the pyriform fossa medially and the anterior femoral sheath laterally is also seen.

When the closure of the fascial defect in the posterior inguinal wall is completed, the spermatic cord is replaced on its newly constructed floor, and the overlying anatomic layers are closed sequentially to complete the operation.

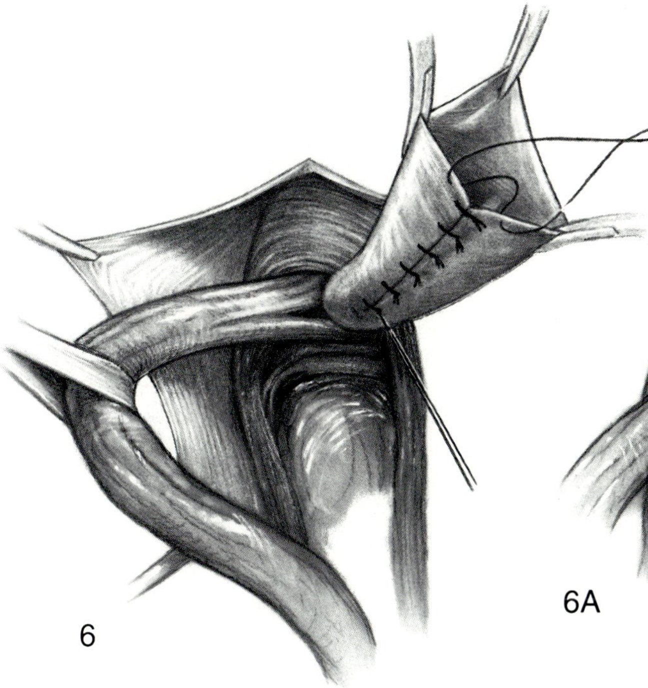

6

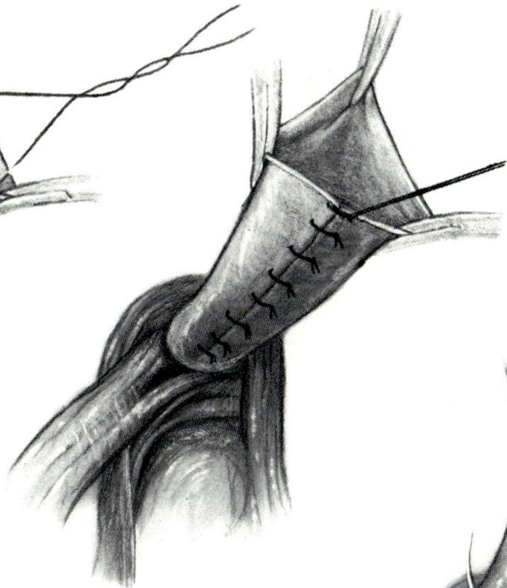

6A

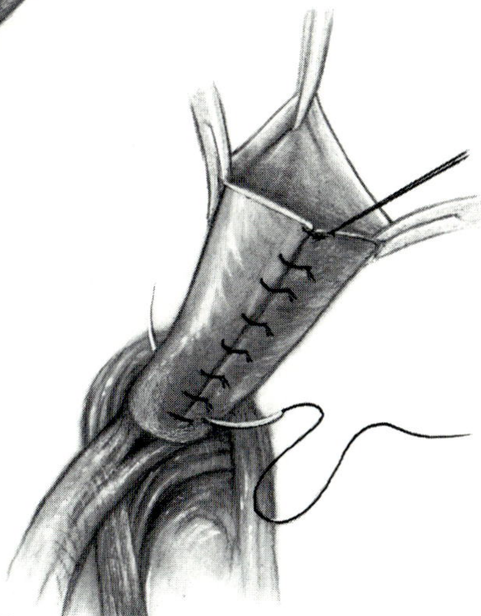

6B

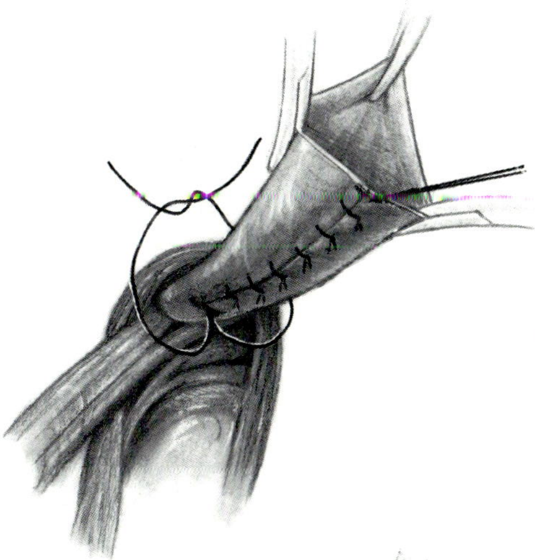

6C

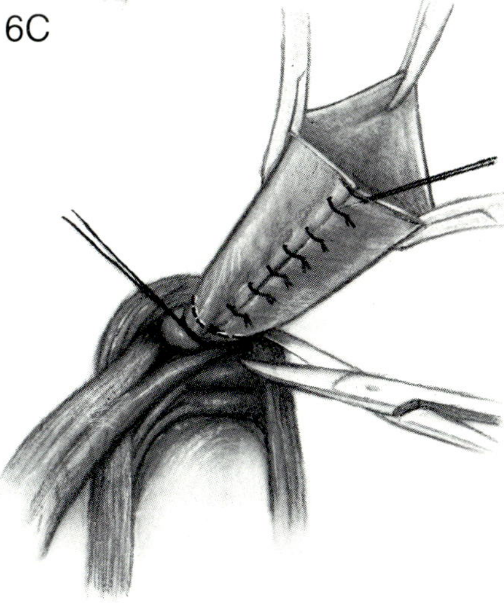

6D

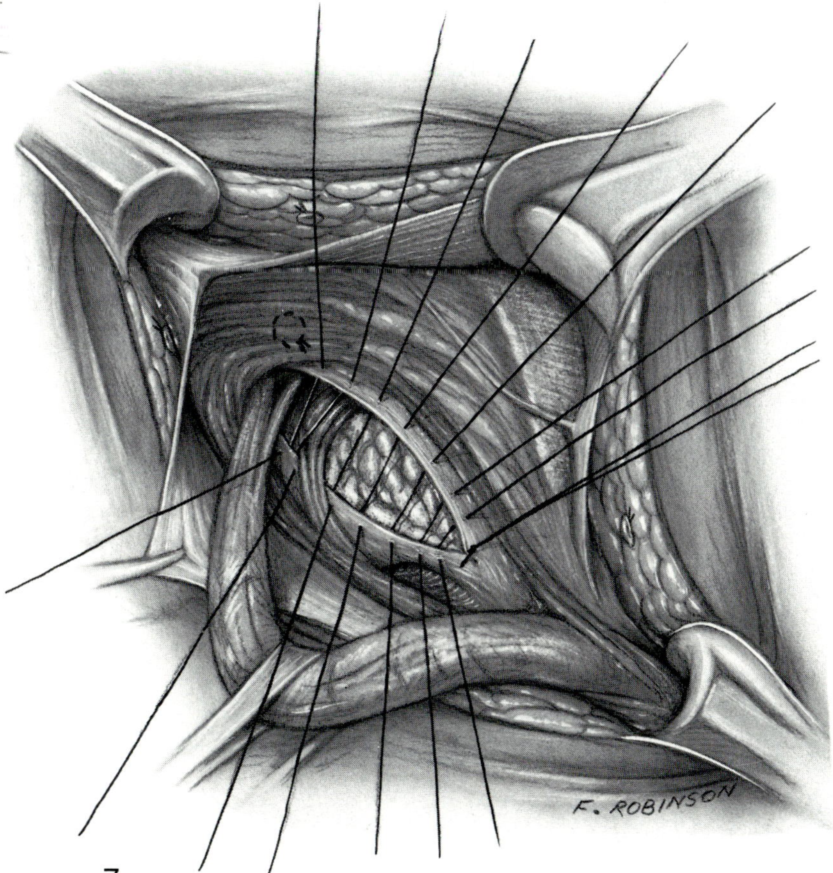

7

REPAIR OF A SLIDING HERNIA OF THE CECUM *Continued*

8, 8A The construction of the new posterior wall of the sac is completed, and a pursestring suture (3-0 silk), starting from and finishing on the outside of the neck of the sac, is inserted **(8)**. If preferred, however, this suture may be inserted from the inside of the sac **(8A)**.

9 The pursestring suture is gradually tightened *(arrows)* as the cecum, held in tissue forceps, is replaced within the peritoneal cavity.

10, 11, 12 The repositioning of the cecum is completed, and the pursestring suture is tied **(10)**. The redundant portion of the newly formed sac is excised with scissors **(11)**, and the retraction of its sutured cuff beneath the internal oblique muscle is indicated by the *circular dashed line* **(12)**.

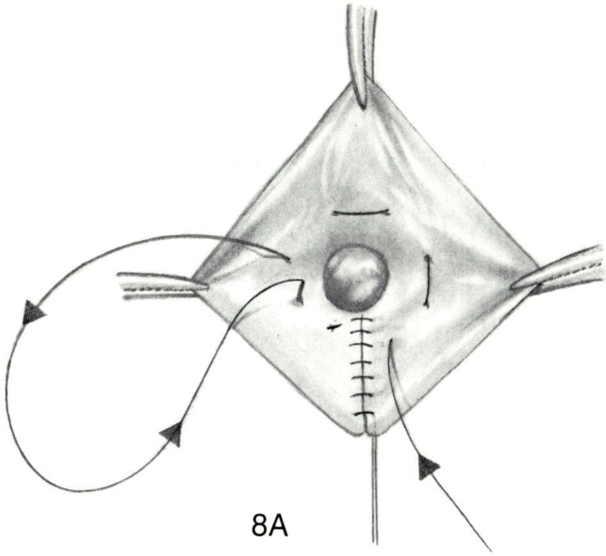

8A

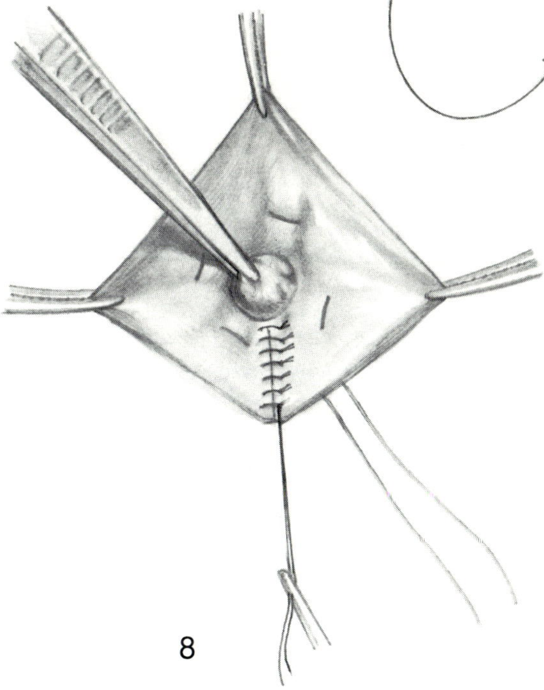

8

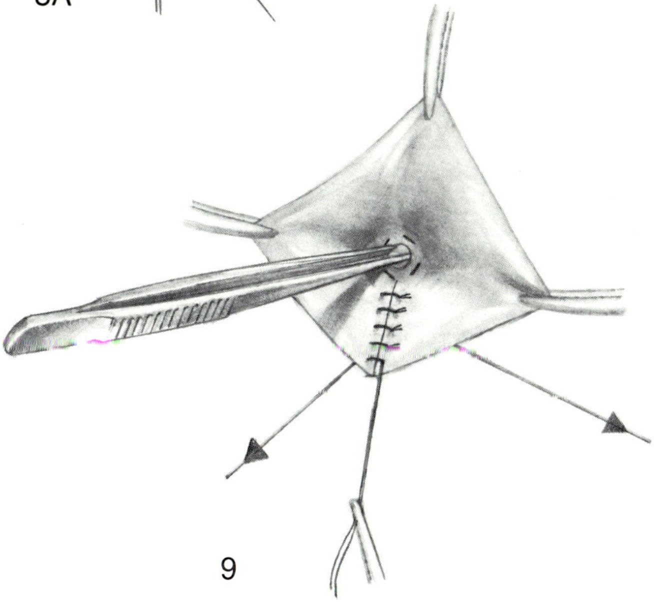

9

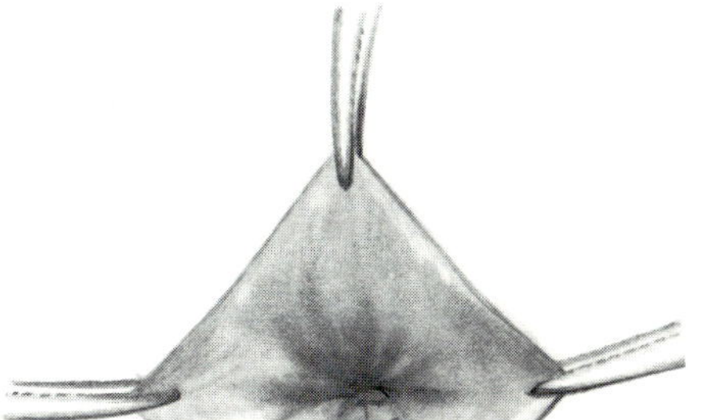

10

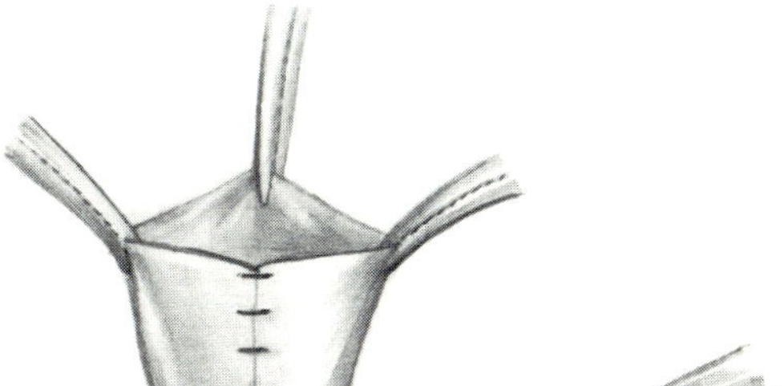

11

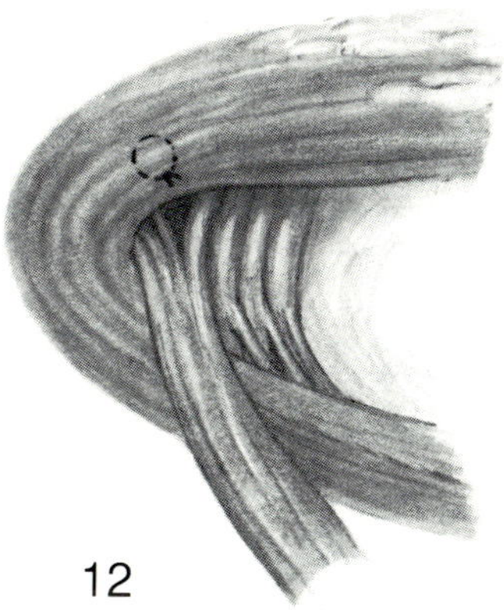

12

OPERATION 11

FEMORAL ("LOW") APPROACH TO REPAIR OF A FEMORAL HERNIA

Plate XLIV
Plate XLV
Plate XLVI
Plate XLVII

1 The site of the transverse incision overlying the summit of the femoral hernia is indicated by the *dashed line*. The hernia depicted is larger than is commonly seen. In fact, the small size of strangulated femoral hernias not infrequently precludes their correct diagnosis.

2 A portion of the hernial sac is held in tissue forceps; as downward traction is maintained, it is mobilized from the surrounding fatty tissue layer by scalpel dissection (*dashed line*).

3 After the sac is opened, repeated attempts by digital manipulation to reduce the contained segment of omentum into the peritoneal cavity may prove unsuccessful.

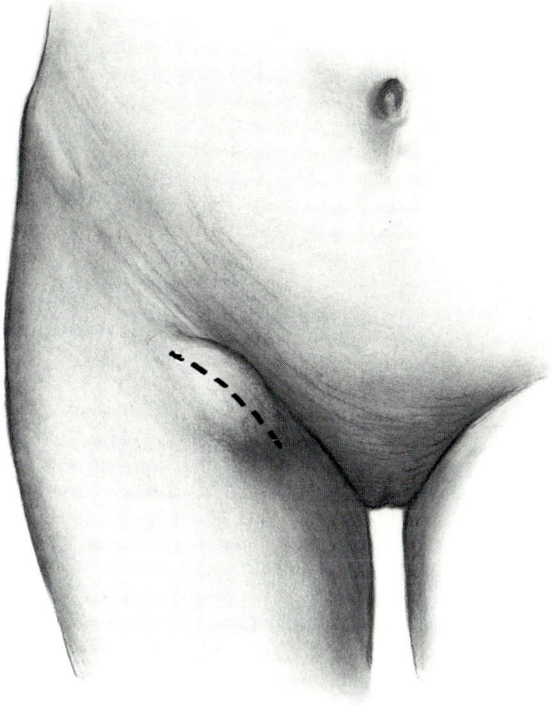

1

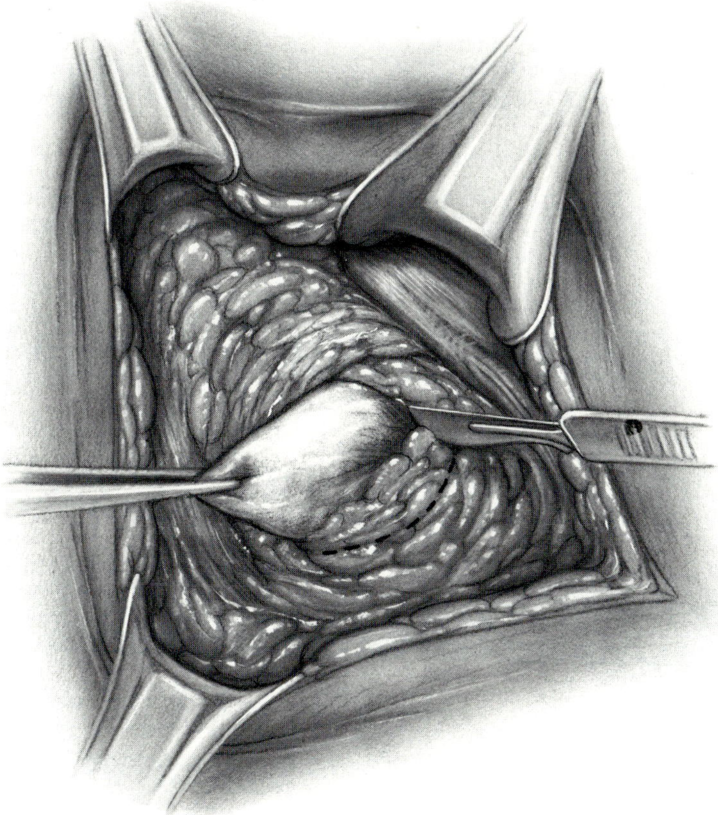

2

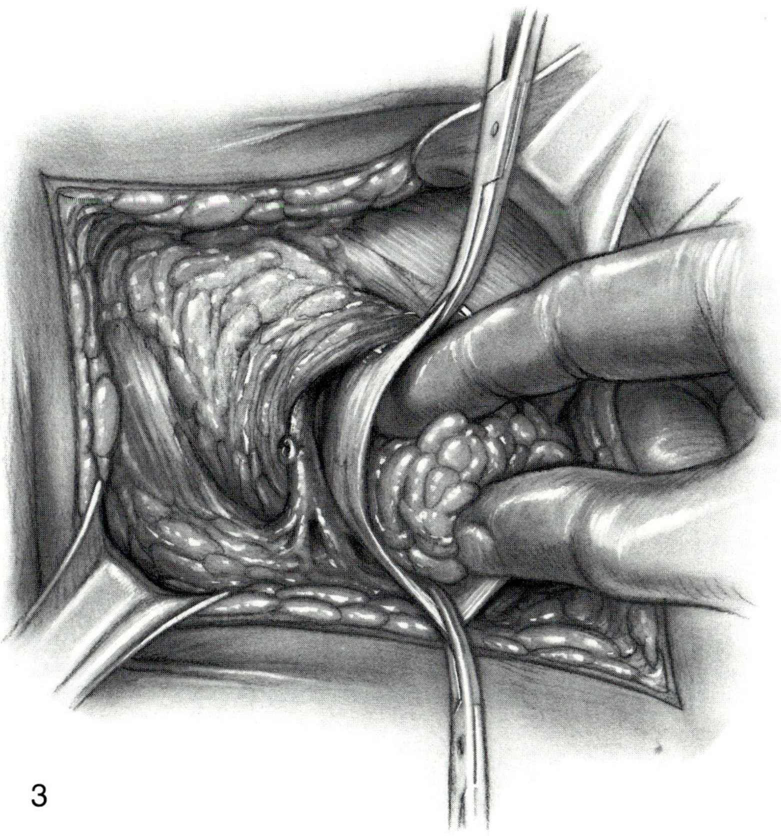

3

FEMORAL ("LOW") APPROACH TO REPAIR OF A FEMORAL HERNIA *Continued*

4, 4A When the hernia is irreducible, a small incision is made in the lateral crescentic margin of Gimbernat's ligament to facilitate the reduction of the herniated omentum **(4)**. For purposes of illustration, this technique is represented semidiagrammatically **(4A)**.

4B, 4C The relationship of Gimbernat's ligament to the neck of the femoral hernia is shown from below. The planned incision in this ligament (*dashed line*) to release the constriction of the neck of the sac is shown **(4B)**, as well as the completion of the incision and reduction of the contents of the sac **(4C)**.

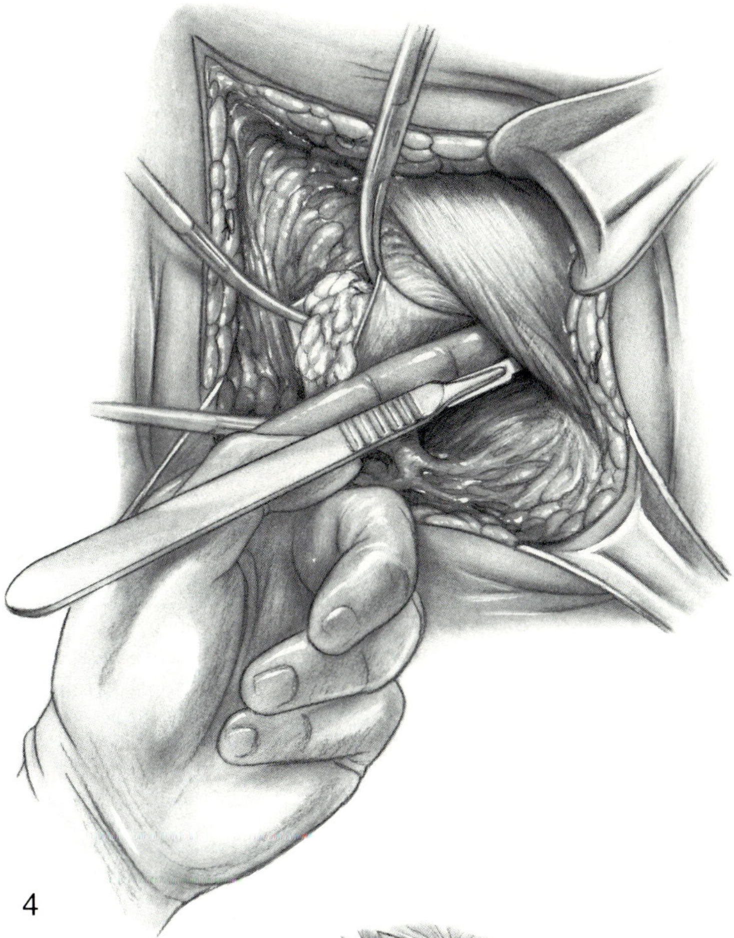

4

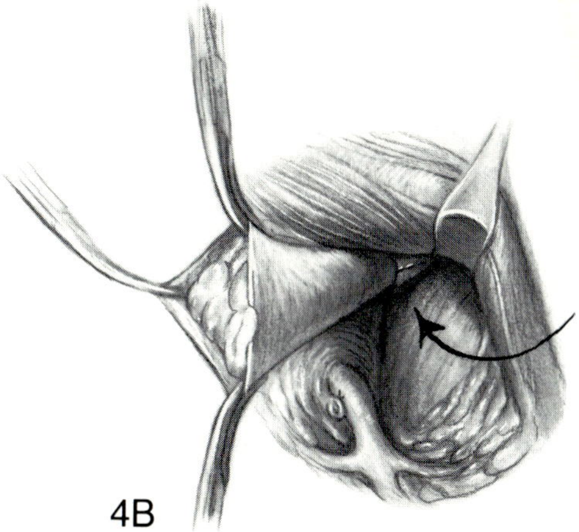

4B

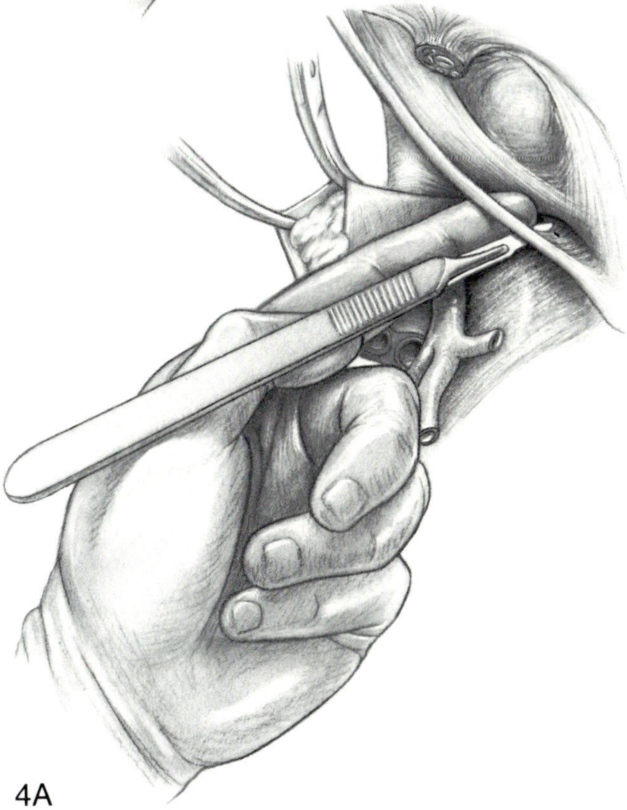

4A

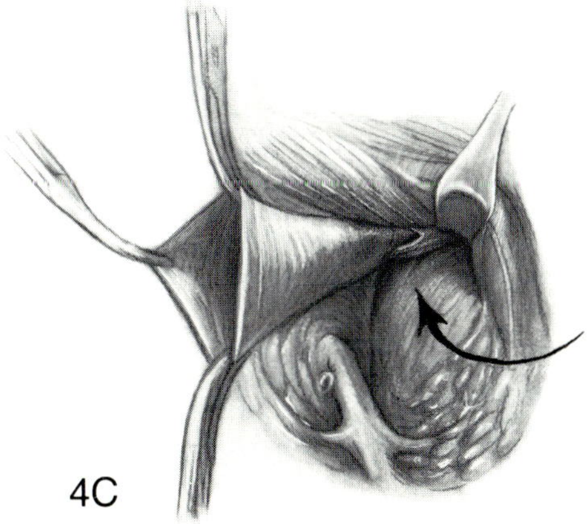

4C

FEMORAL ("LOW") APPROACH TO REPAIR OF A FEMORAL HERNIA *Continued*

5 The empty sac of the femoral hernia is shown in relation to the surrounding structures.

6 Downward and outward traction on the hernial sac is applied to show the relationship of its medial wall to the prevesical fat and urinary bladder. The surgeon must always be aware of this anatomic relationship in order to avoid injury to the bladder whenever the sac of a femoral hernia is dissected from below.

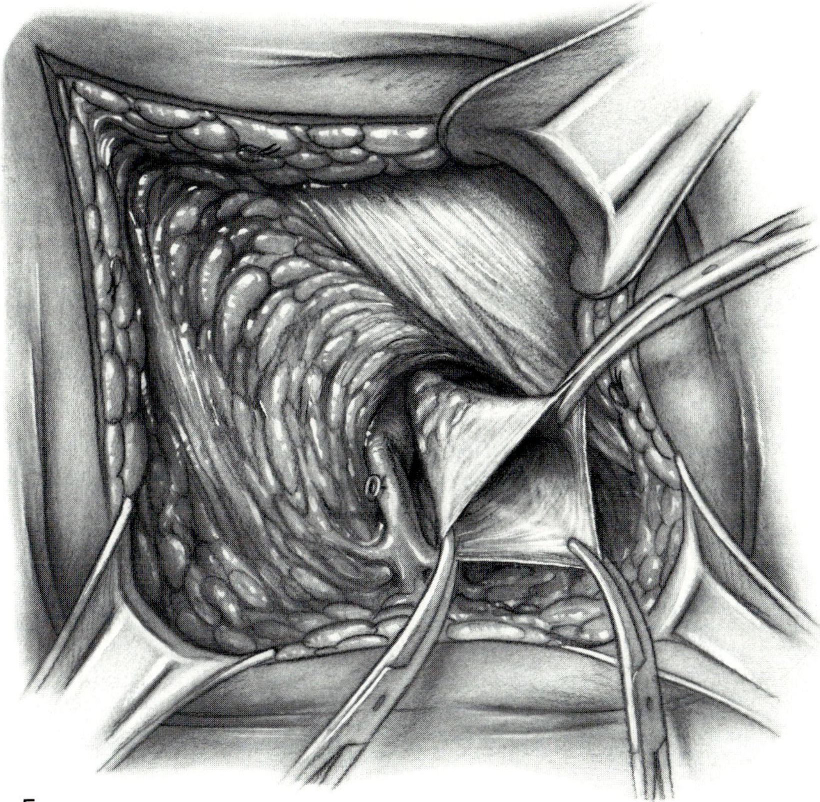

5

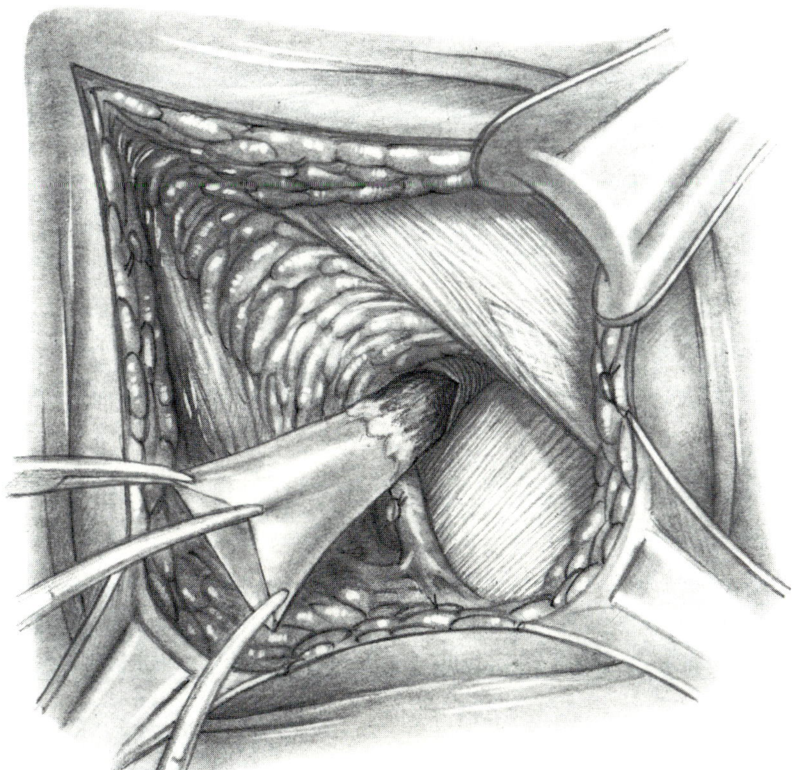

6

FEMORAL ("LOW") APPROACH TO REPAIR OF A FEMORAL HERNIA *Continued*

7, 8 The neck of the sac is transfixed by the curved needle of a swaged-on suture of 3-0 silk **(7)**, which is tied medially. Its strands are then brought laterally around the neck of the sac, preparatory to being tied **(8)**.

9 The insertion of the transfixion suture of silk (3-0) is completed, and the redundant portion of the hernial sac is resected (*dashed line*) with scissors.

10 The ligated cuff of the neck of the sac has retracted from view, and the site of the femoral hernial orifice (Lytle), in relation to the adjacent structures, is visible. This orifice, in the lower portion of the femoral sheath, is approximately 1.5 cm below the femoral ring and lies in juxtaposition to the crescentic margin of Gimbernat's ligament.

10A, 10B, 10C The lower border of the external oblique aponeurosis is retracted up to expose the femoral hernial orifice **(10A)**. The lower angle of the opening in the femoral sheath is closed by the insertion of a crown suture of 3-0 silk **(10B)**. A similar suture was previously inserted and tied to close the upper angle. The closure of the femoral hernial orifice is completed by the insertion of two interrupted sutures of 3-0 silk between the respective angle sutures **(10C)**.

11 The insertion of the pursestring suture (3-0 silk) was advocated by Lytle for the closure of the femoral hernial orifice. This suture approximates Gimbernat's ligament to its normal attachment on the inner wall of the femoral sheath, with minimum tension and distortion.

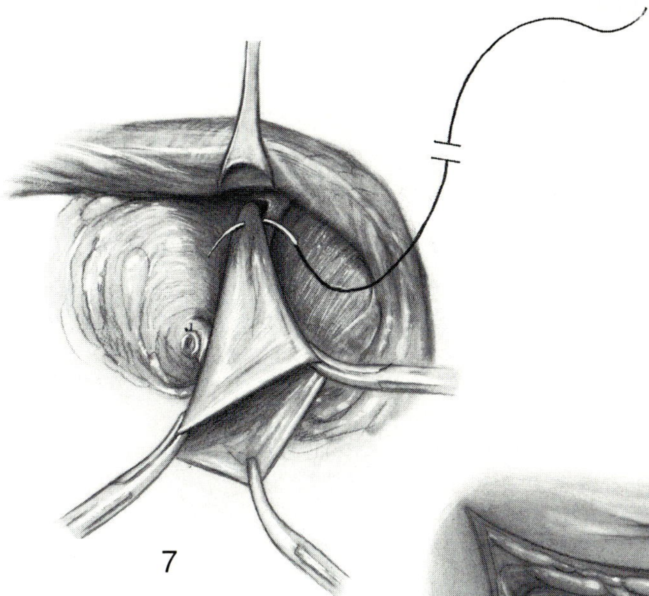

7

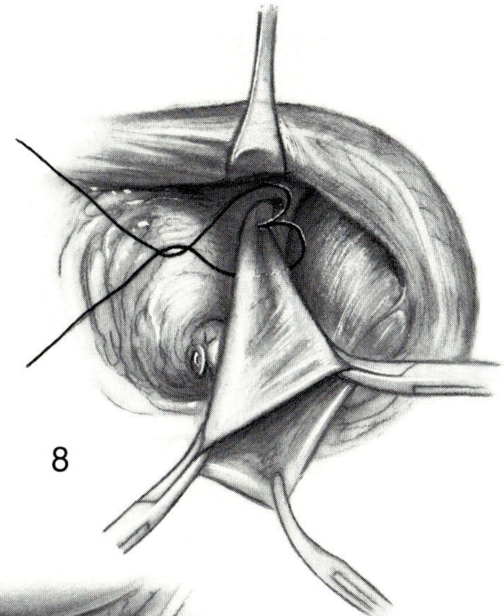

8

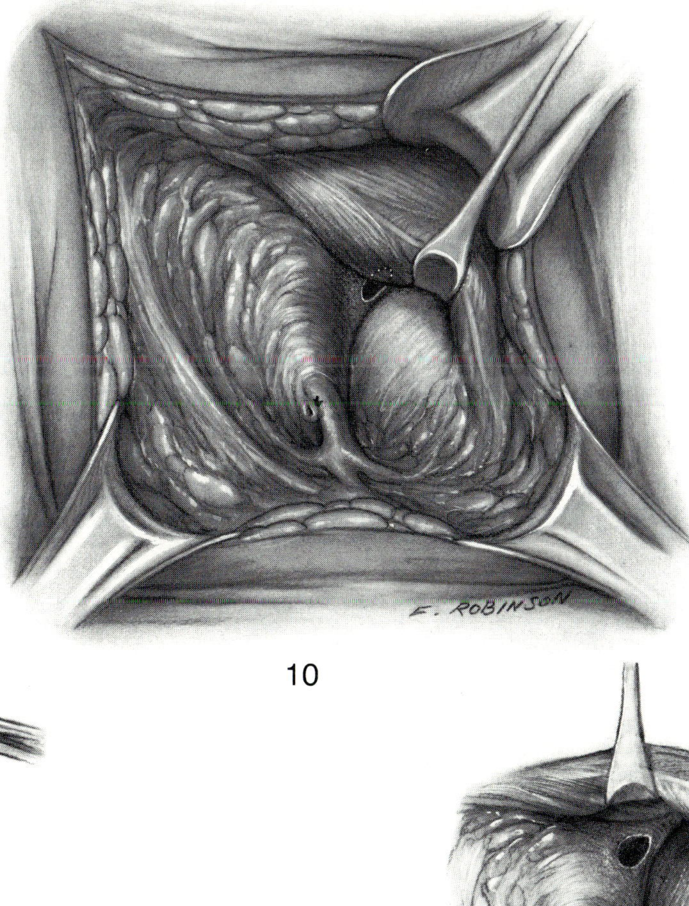

10

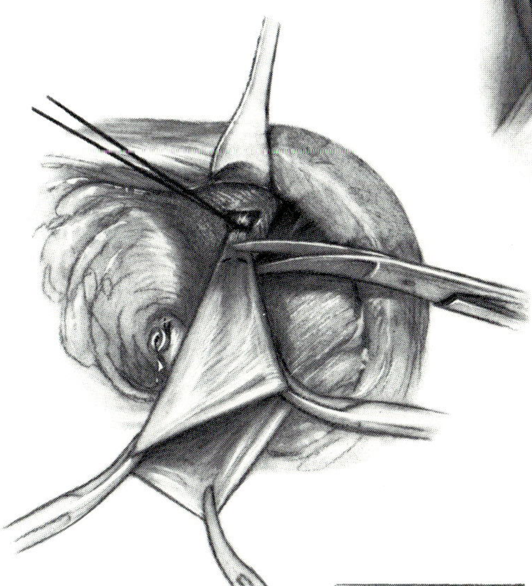

9

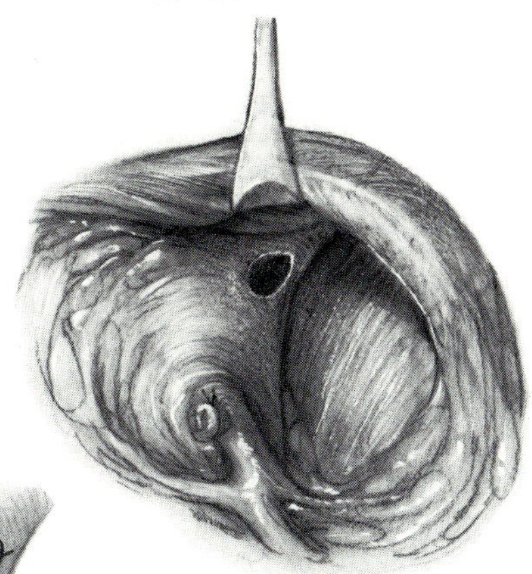

10A

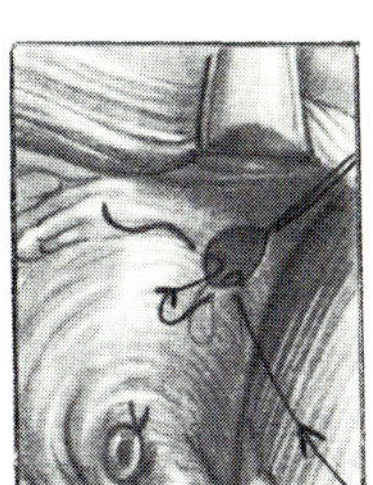

10B

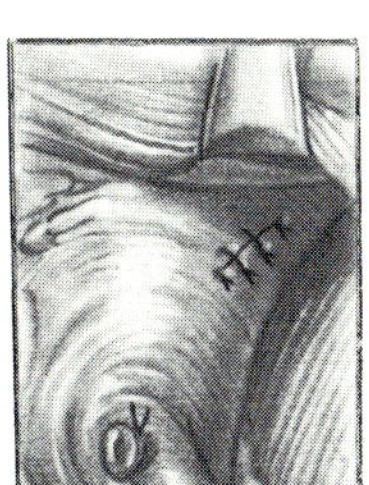

10C

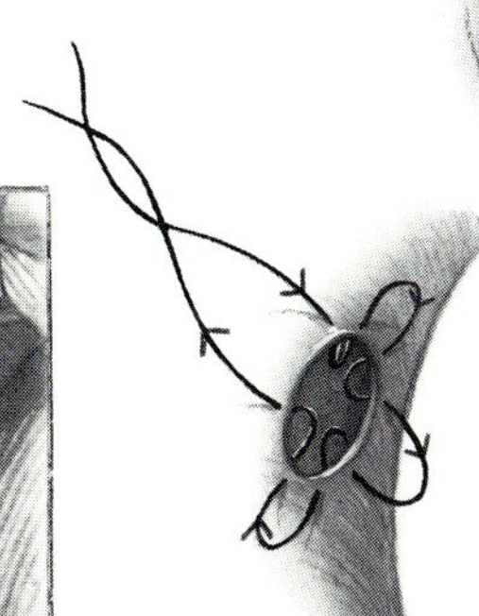

11

OPERATION 12

INGUINAL ("HIGH") APPROACH TO REPAIR OF A FEMORAL HERNIA

Plate XLVIII
Plate IL
Plate L

1 The right oblique inguinal incision is deepened through the subcutaneous tissue plane to expose the underlying aponeurosis of the external oblique muscle and the exit of the spermatic cord and ilioinguinal nerve through the external inguinal ring. The subjacent femoral hernia, unduly magnified by the artist, typically is turned up to overlie the inguinal ligament. This anatomic characteristic of a femoral hernia accounts for its frequent clinical misdiagnosis as an inguinal hernia.

A stab incision in the plane of the intercrural fibers is extended medially (*dashed line*) by simply pushing the firmly held blades of the scissors through the external ring. This technique is a safeguard against injury to the ilioinguinal nerve. Since this is a sensory nerve, a painful neuroma may occur if it is transected.

2 The superior and inferior leaflets of the external oblique aponeurosis and the underlying spermatic cord are retracted to expose their relationships to the neighboring structures. The incision in the fascia of the posterior inguinal wall is shown (*broken line*).

3 The superior and inferior segments of the posterior inguinal wall are retracted to expose the underlying preperitoneal fat and peritoneum. The *dashed line* indicates the site of incision for entry into the peritoneal cavity.

3A In this illustration, which complements **3**, the cremaster muscle, the spermatic cord, and the related soft tissues have been removed to expose the femoral hernia and its relationship to the surrounding structures. The opening in the medial wall of the femoral sheath (the femoral hernial orifice of Lytle) and its juxtaposition to the lateral crescentic margin of Gimbernat's ligament are visible. Partial transection of this ligament, as originally described by Gimbernat, releases the constriction of the bowel in the treatment of the acutely strangulated femoral hernia.

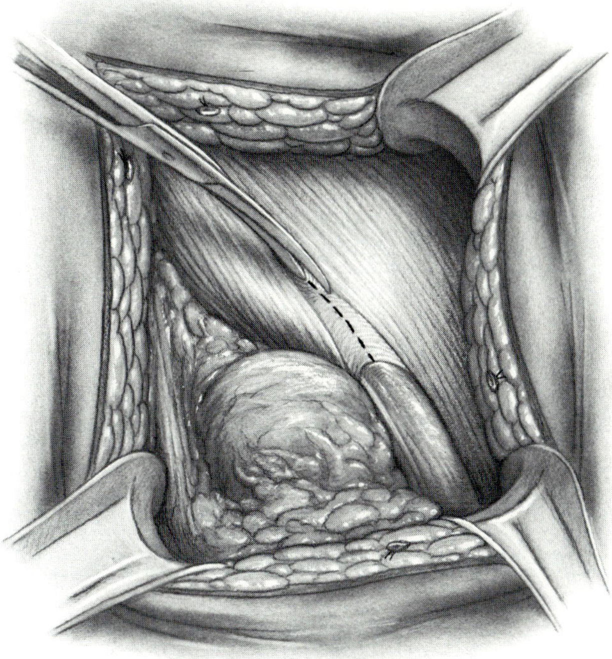

1

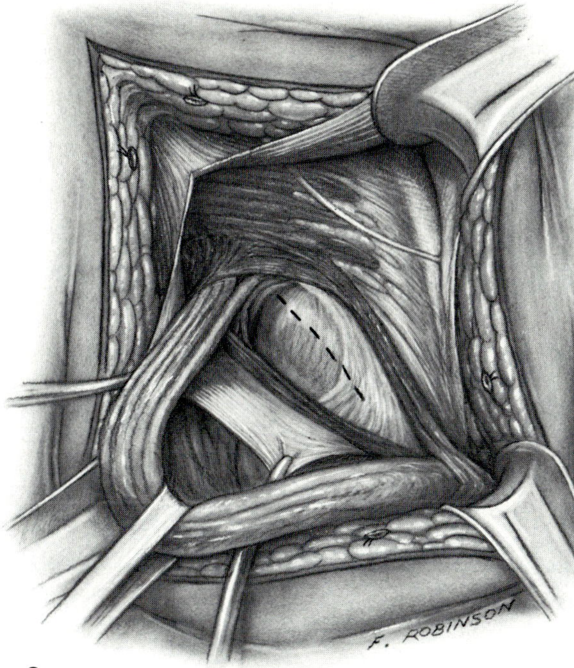

2

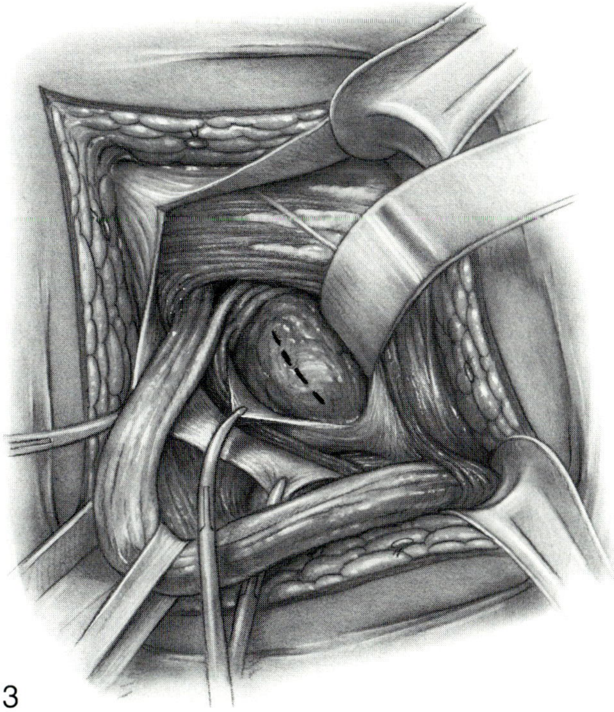

3

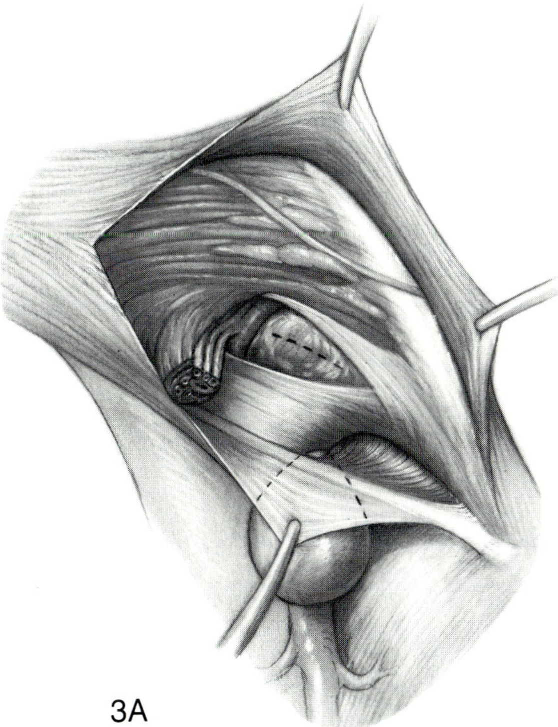

3A

4 The peritoneal cavity is entered. The bulging protrusion of an obstructed loop of small intestine is visible.

5 The tip of the left index finger is inserted medial to the peritoneum and its encased small bowel loop. With the handle of the scalpel held in the right hand (omitted from the illustration for visibility), a small cut is made (*dashed line*) with a No. 15 blade in the unyielding lateral crescentic margin of Gimbernat's ligament.

6, 6A The constriction of the neck of the sac of the femoral hernia is released, and the entrapped segment of small bowel is withdrawn into the wound. The narrow but irreversibly compromised white bands of constriction on the afferent and efferent limbs of the herniated bowel are evident **(6)**.

These ischemic bands are simply treated by inversion, using a series of encircling interrupted seromuscular sutures of 3-0 silk (Summers' stitch) as depicted in **6A**. However, when the circulation in the loop of bowel is irreversibly compromised (or in doubt), resection is mandatory.

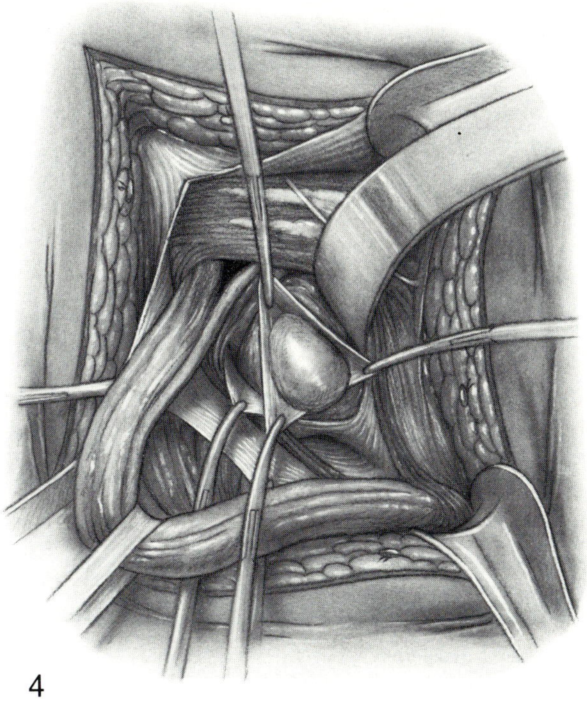

4

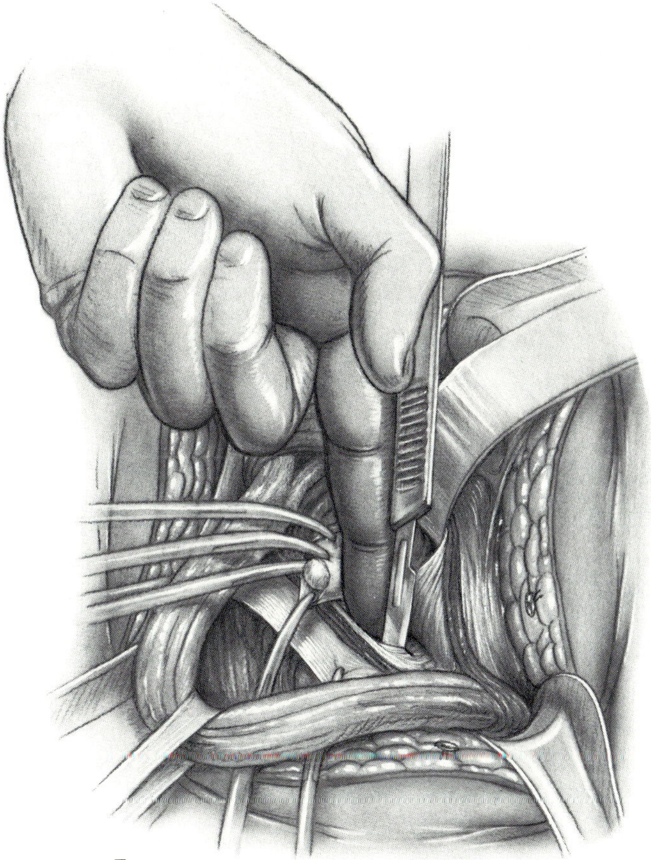

5

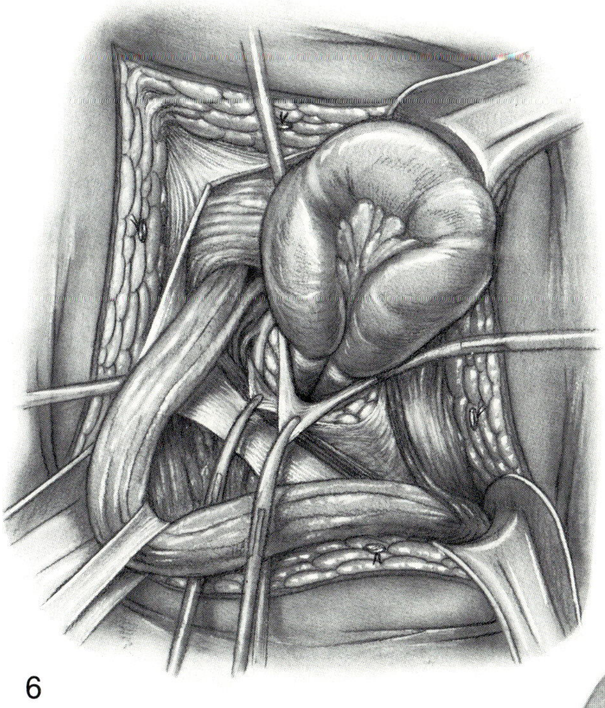

6

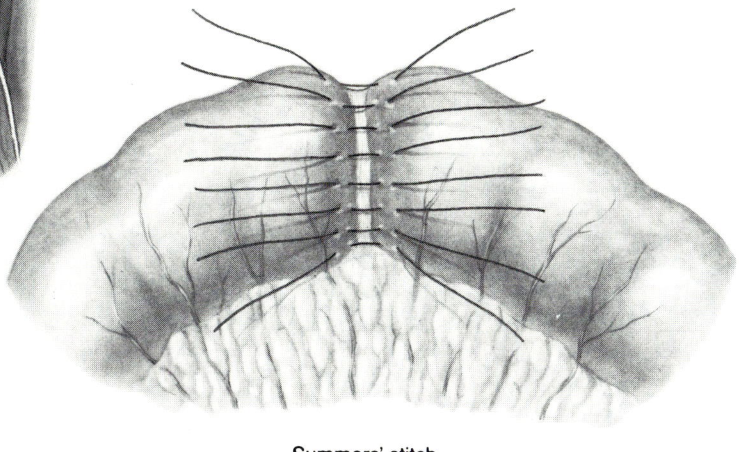

6A Summers' stitch

INGUINAL ("HIGH") APPROACH TO REPAIR OF A FEMORAL HERNIA *Continued*

7 A long curved clamp is inserted from the peritoneal cavity into the lumen of the femoral hernia sac. By digital counterpressure from below, a fold of the apex of the sac is grasped between the tips of the clamp preparatory to its retrograde inversion.

8, 9 The retrograde inversion of the sac is completed, and the level for transection of the sac is indicated by the *broken line* **(8)**. The transected cuff of the sac is oversewn with a continuous suture of 3-0 chromic catgut **(9)**, which is returned as an over-and-over (baseball) stitch to its starting point, where it will be tied (*inset*).

10, 10A The opening in the peritoneum is closed with interrupted sutures of 4-0 silk. Its relationships to the overlying large V-shaped defect in the fascia of the posterior inguinal wall and to the pyriform fossa, medially and subjacent, are evident. Downward traction is applied to the clamp on the inferior leaflet of the aponeurosis of the external oblique muscle to expose the incised crescentic margin of Gimbernat's ligament and its relationship to the femoral hernial defect in the medial wall of the femoral sheath **(10)**. Similarly, upward traction on the clamp shows the relationship of the hernial defect to the turn-in of the inguinal ligament and its continuation medially as the fascial part of Gimbernat's ligament **(10A)**.

Following the closure of the defect in the fascia of the posterior inguinal wall with interrupted sutures of 3-0 silk, the spermatic cord is repositioned onto the reconstructed floor. The overlying external oblique aponeurosis, subcutaneous fascia, and skin are then closed in layers to complete the operation.

This "high" approach may be complemented by the closure from below of the opening in the femoral sheath, at the site of the femoral hernial orifice.

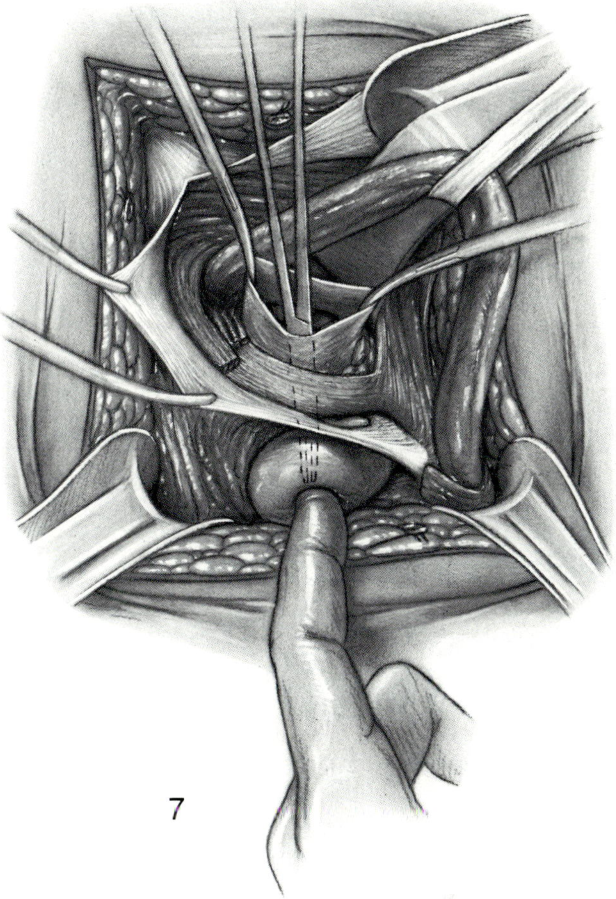

7

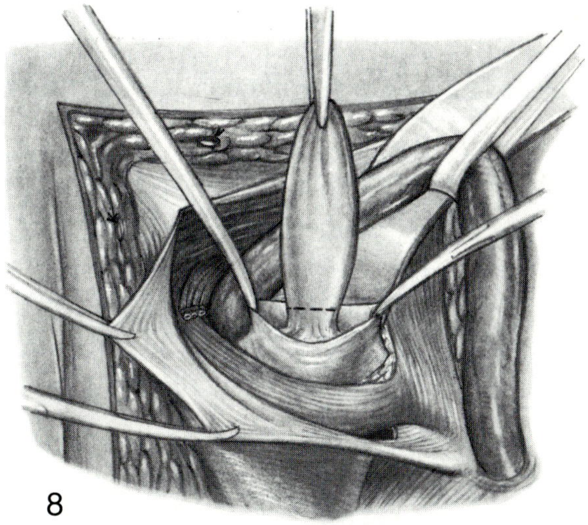

8

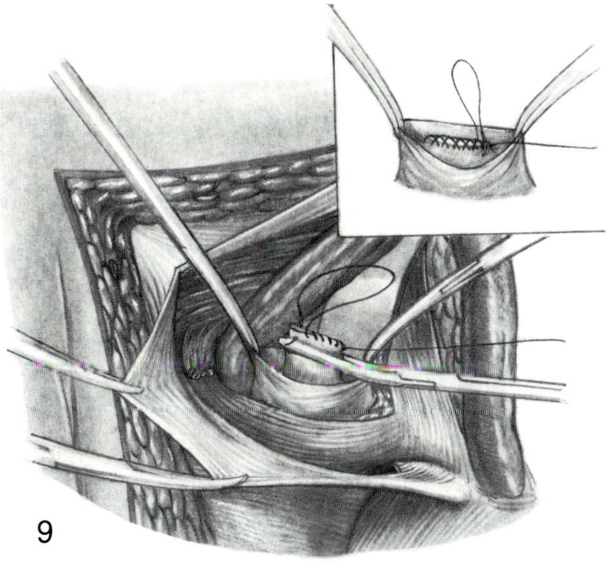

9

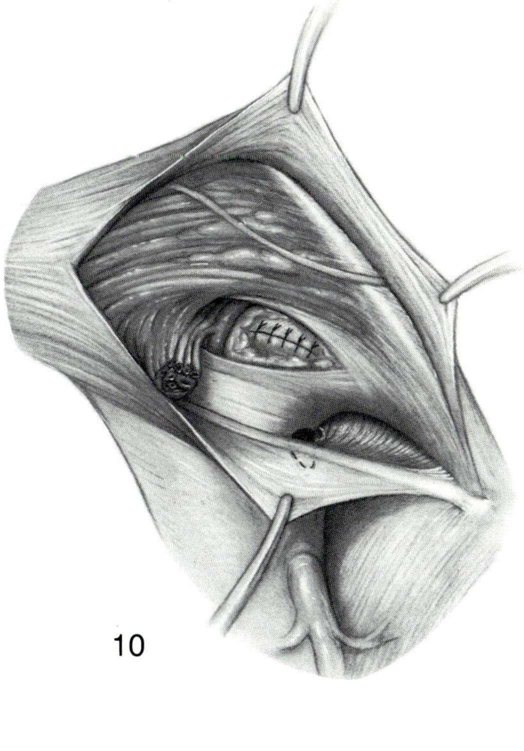

10

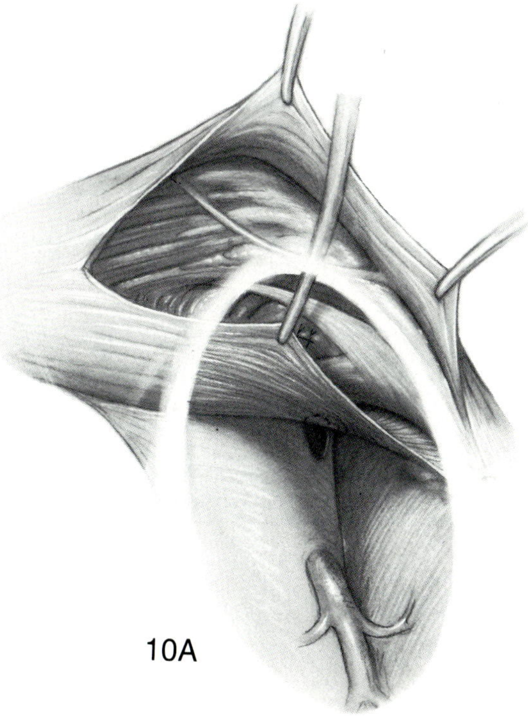

10A

INGUINAL APPROACH TO REPAIR OF A FEMORAL HERNIA: ANATOMIC SUPPLEMENT

Plate LI
Plate LII

1 This semidiagrammatic illustration shows the relationship of the lateral border of the fascial part of Gimbernat's ligament to the femoral sheath. The inferior leaflet of the external oblique aponeurosis and its subjacent inguinal ligament are transected and then retracted to expose the site of the femoral hernial orifice (indicated by the *black dot* at the lower part of the femoral canal). This orifice, as described by Lytle,[2] is 1.5 cm below the femoral ring.

In the intact anatomic state, the *black dots* superimposed on the center of the lateral crescentic border of Gimbernat's ligament and the lower part of the femoral canal represent the site of the femoral hernial orifice in the femoral sheath. Through this orifice a femoral hernia protrudes from the femoral canal. Accordingly, in the treatment of an incarcerated or strangulated femoral hernia, partial transection of the unyielding crescentic margin of Gimbernat's ligament is required to release the constriction at the neck of the sac.

2, 3 These magnified semidiagrammatic illustrations of superior **(2)** and oblique end-on **(3)** views of Gimbernat's ligament show its relationship to the surrounding structures—the inferior segment of the fascia of the posterior inguinal wall (iliopubic tract), the iliopectineal line (Cooper's ligament), the inguinal ligament, and the pectineus fascia.

In each of these views it can be seen that Gimbernat's ligament, as it ascends to insert into Cooper's ligament, is intimately fused to the pectineus fascia immediately below its site of origin from Cooper's ligament. Also demonstrated are the separate anatomic planes of the inferior segment of the fascia of the posterior inguinal wall (superior plane) and Gimbernat's ligament (inferior plane), enroute to their conjoint line of insertion into Cooper's ligament.

Gimbernat's ligament is shown in relation to Cooper's ligament and the inguinal ligament; its concavity has been exaggerated for emphasis. The lower part of the lateral crescentic border of the fascial part of Gimbernat's ligament (*black dot* in **1**) represents the level of its constant anatomic relationship to the site of the femoral hernial orifice in the lower portion of the femoral sheath, where it forms the sheath's medial boundary.

However, Condon[1] and McVay[3] share the opinion that it is the lateral extension of the inferior segment of the fascia of the posterior inguinal wall, and not Gimbernat's ligament, that forms the medial boundary of the femoral sheath. Furthermore, McVay[3] had observed in femoral hernias an attrition of the insertion of the fascia of the posterior inguinal wall into Cooper's ligament. Accordingly, he believed that as a femoral hernia enlarges, it abuts against the unyielding crescentic margin of Gimbernat's ligament, giving the false impression that this ligament forms the medial boundary of the femoral sheath. This concept, however, is not supported by the illustrations presented here. (See the discussion of this question in Section I.)

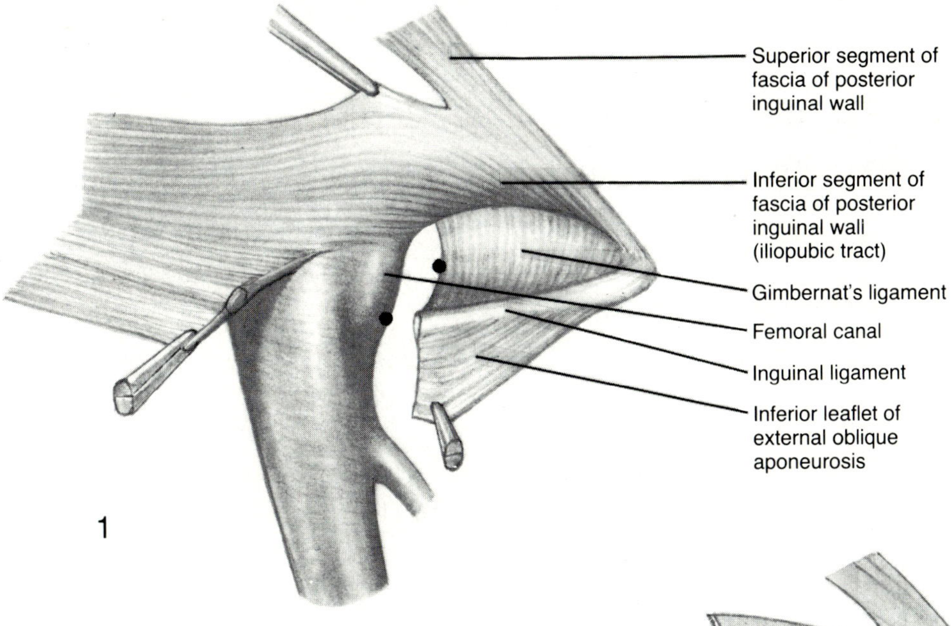

1

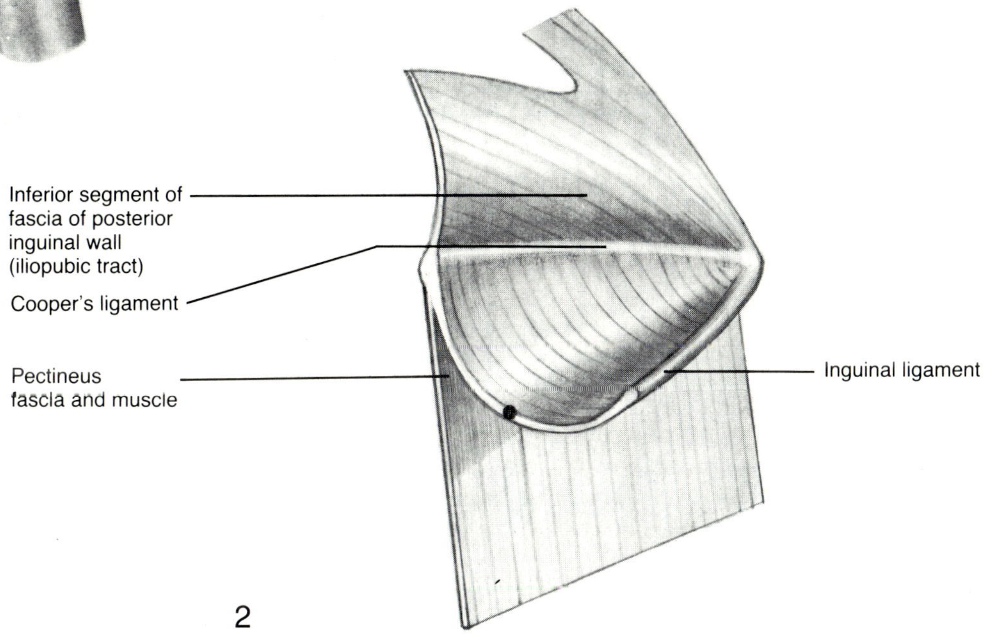

2

OBLIQUE MEDIOLATERAL VIEW

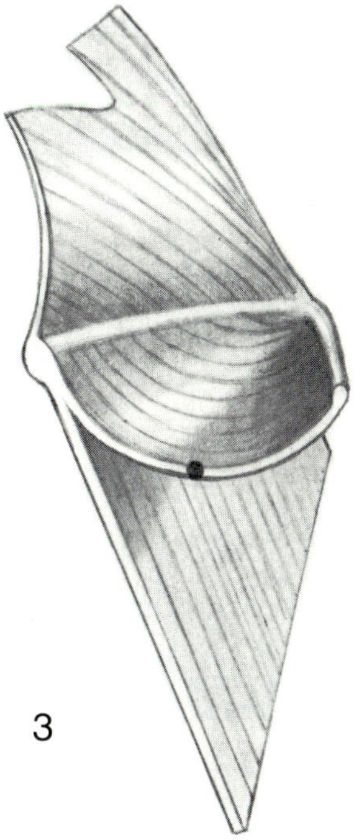

3

ON-END MEDIOLATERAL VIEW

INGUINAL APPROACH TO REPAIR OF A FEMORAL HERNIA: ANATOMIC SUPPLEMENT *Continued*

These illustrations of the surgical anatomy of a femoral hernia repair complement the semidiagrammatic views in Plate LI. For clarity of exposure, the cremaster muscle and cord structures have been deleted, with the exception of their transected ends laterally.

4 The femoral hernia is shown in relation to the surrounding structures. The *dashed line* overlying the external oblique aponeurosis and inguinal ligament indicates the site of transection to reveal the underlying surgical anatomy.

5 The transected ends of the inguinal ligament are retracted to show the protrusion of the hernia through the femoral hernial orifice in the femoral sheath. The lateral crescentic margin of Gimbernat's ligament forms the medial border of the femoral sheath at the site of the femoral hernial orifice. Furthermore, this unyielding border is the cause of the constriction of the neck of the sac in the incarcerated or strangulated femoral hernia. Therefore, the site of obstruction in such hernias is 1.5 cm *below* and not *at* the level of the femoral ring, as is commonly but mistakenly believed.

For purposes of illustration, the constriction of the neck of the sac is presented as if the inguinal ligament were intact and Gimbernat's ligament were not displaced. The *black dots* superimposed on the center of the concave lateral margin of Gimbernat's ligament and the medial wall of the neck of the sac, respectively, indicate the site of obstruction, as implied but not visible in **4.**

6 The hernial sac has been inverted in a retrograde manner, its redundant portion resected, and the incision in the peritoneum closed. The site of the hernial protrusion in the femoral sheath (the femoral hernial orifice) and its regional anatomic relationships—in particular to the V-shaped cut in the lateral crescentic margin of Gimbernat's ligament that is required to release the constriction of the neck of the hernial sac—are clearly depicted. Also visible are the separate anatomic planes of the inferior segment of the fascia of the posterior inguinal wall (superior plane) and the fascial part of Gimbernat's ligament (inferior plane) as they course to their conjoint line of insertion into the iliopectineal line (Cooper's ligament).

A single-layer closure of the defect in the fascia of the posterior inguinal wall, on which the spermatic cord is placed, and a serial-layer closure of the overlying structures complete the operation. When feasible, a complementary closure from below of the defect in the femoral sheath may be done. Even if this step is omitted, however, the possibility of a recurrence of the femoral hernia is remote, owing to the obliterative postoperative fibrosing tissue reaction around the femoral hernial orifice.

REFERENCES

1. Condon RE: The anatomy of the inguinal region and its relationship to groin hernias. In Nyhus LM and Harkins H (eds): *Hernia.* Philadelphia: JB Lippincott, 1964, pp 34–35.
2. Lytle WJ: Femoral hernia. Ann R Coll Surg Engl *21*:244–262, 1957.
3. McVay CB: *Hernia.* Springfield: Charles C Thomas, 1954.

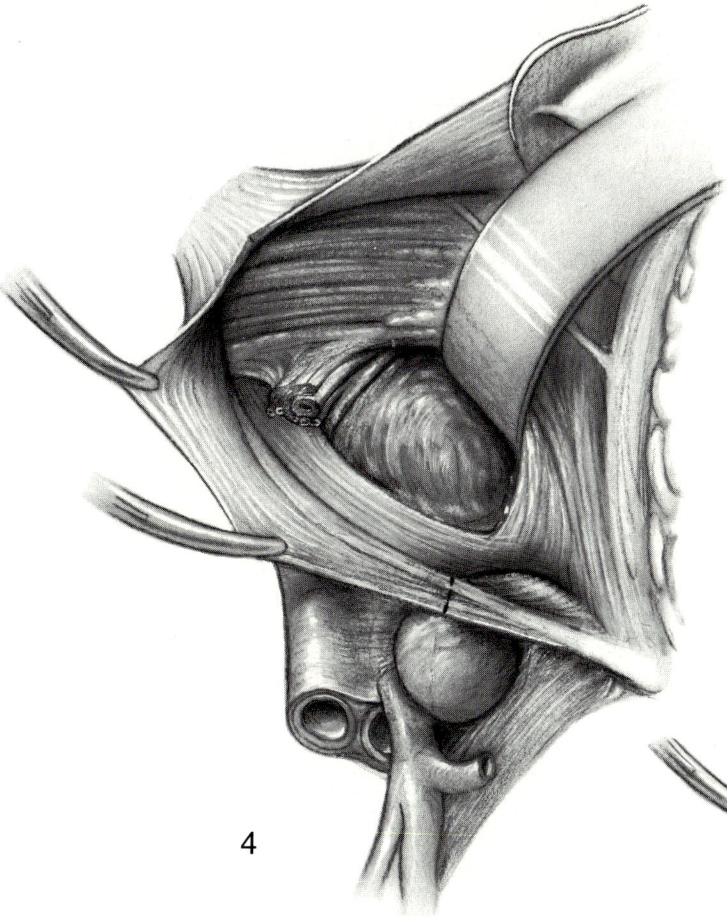

4

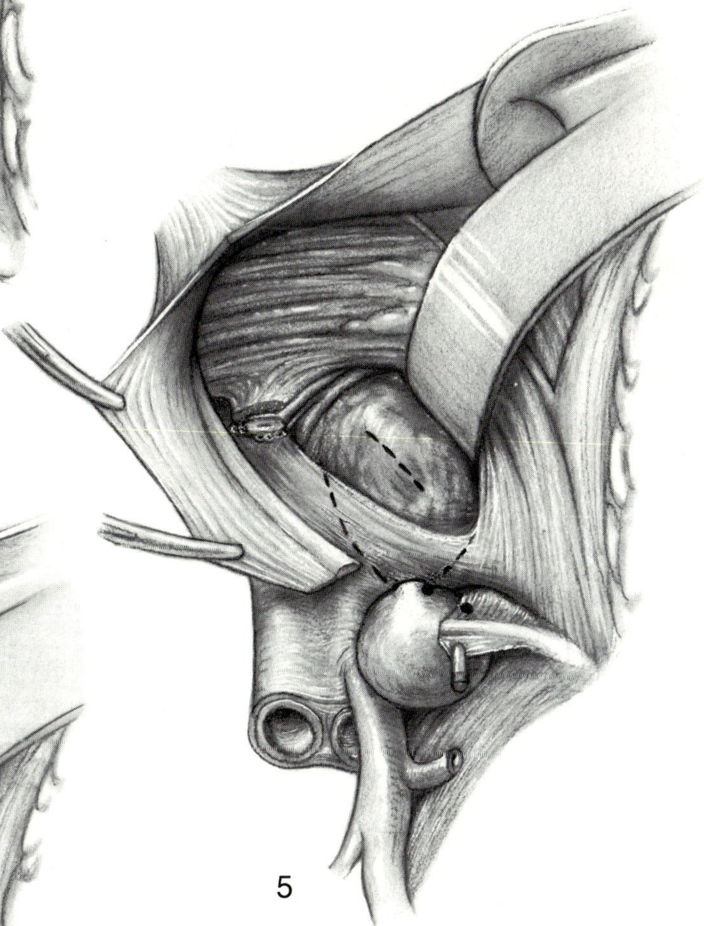

5

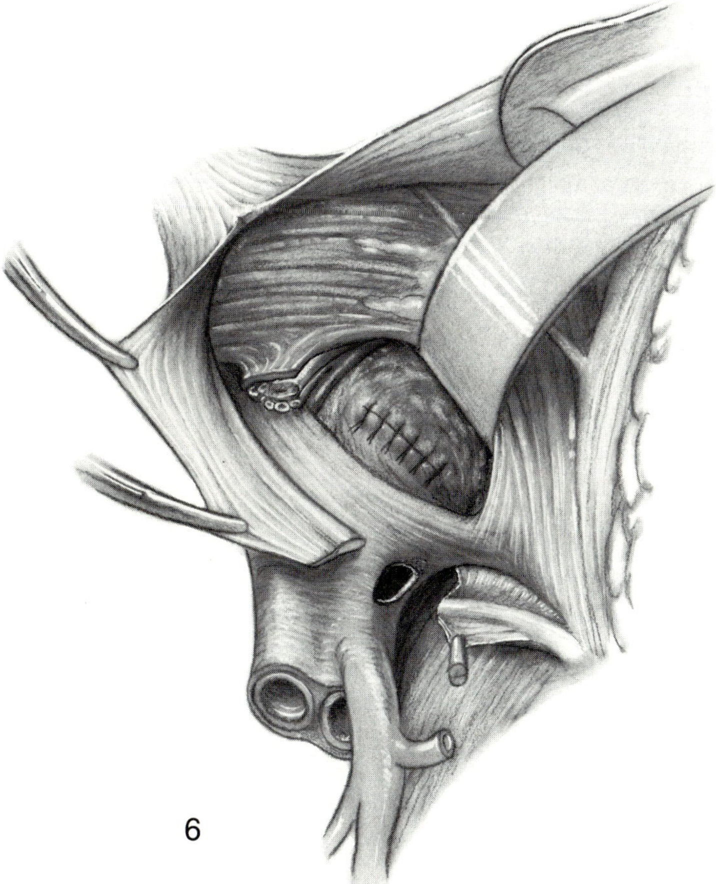

6

OPERATION 13

PREPERITONEAL (POSTERIOR) APPROACH IN THE TREATMENT OF GROIN HERNIAS

Technique of Lloyd M. Nyhus, M.D.

Plate LIII
Plate LIV
Plate LV
Plate LVI

PREPERITONEAL ANATOMY

1 In this illustration of the normal preperitoneal anatomy, the acute angle of convergence of the vas deferens medially and the spermatic vessels laterally, in relation to the internal ring, is clearly depicted. The vas deferens, however, is disproportionately large relative to the internal spermatic vessels. The origin of the obturator artery and vein from the inferior (deep) epigastric vessels is visible, as is the passage of the obturator vessels and nerve through the obturator foramen.

In the illustrated technique of the preperitoneal repair of groin hernias that follows, the artist has erred in the views (**5** through **11**) pertaining to the site of suspension of the spermatic cord with rubber tissue tape. As shown in Plate LIII, the acute angle of convergence of the vas deferens and the internal spermatic vessels to form the spermatic cord lies in immediate proximity to the internal ring. Thus, to depict the component parts of the cord suspended together at a site relatively remote from their normal angle of convergence is anatomically incorrect. However, these parts of the cord can be encompassed by a suspension tape, close to their entrance into the internal ring.

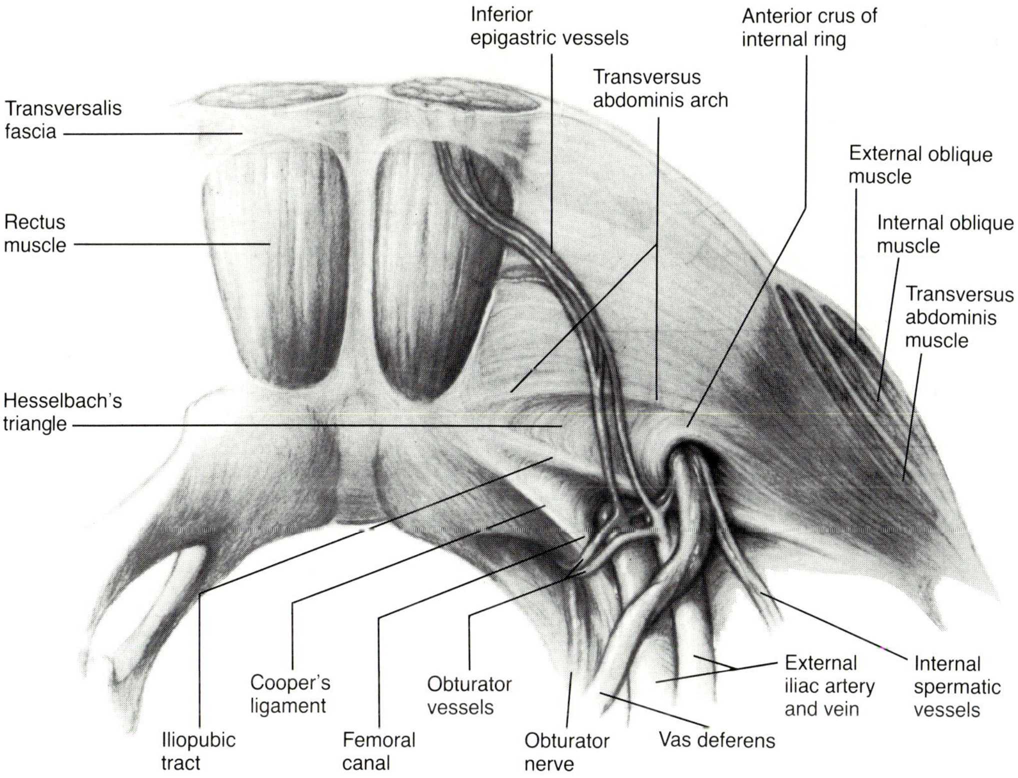
Inferior epigastric vessels
Anterior crus of internal ring
Transversus abdominis arch
Transversalis fascia
External oblique muscle
Rectus muscle
Internal oblique muscle
Transversus abdominis muscle
Hesselbach's triangle
Cooper's ligament
Obturator vessels
External iliac artery and vein
Internal spermatic vessels
Iliopubic tract
Femoral canal
Obturator nerve
Vas deferens

1

PREPERITONEAL (POSTERIOR) APPROACH IN THE TREATMENT OF GROIN HERNIAS
Continued

REPAIR OF A DIRECT INGUINAL HERNIA

The artist, Frank Robinson, was commissioned to visit Nyhus in order to illustrate his use of the posterior or preperitoneal approach in the treatment of groin hernias. The techniques for the repair of direct and indirect inguinal and femoral hernias are presented here.

2 The right transverse skin incision (*dashed line*) is made two fingerbreadths cephalad to the superior border of the pubis. This measurement can be made by the surgeon from either side of the operating table.

3 The skin and subcutaneous tissue layers are retracted to expose the incision in the aponeurosis of the external oblique muscle. This incision extends from its anterior component in the rectus sheath medially into the muscle layer of its site of origin laterally.

4 The incision is deepened through the underlying anterior lamella of the internal oblique muscle to uncover the rectus muscle and the subjacent inferior epigastric vessels deep to its lateral border. The incision is extended laterally and deepened through the external and internal oblique muscles and the transversus abdominis muscle to expose the transversalis (endoabdominal) fascia, beneath which lobulated segments of the preperitoneal fat can be seen. The endoabdominal fascia is cut to enter the preperitoneal space. After combined blunt and sharp tissue dissection, the posterior inguinal wall is exposed.

5 The direct hernial protrusion through Hesselbach's triangle is depicted. The spermatic cord, in proximity to the internal ring, is encircled by rubber tissue tape and retracted upward.

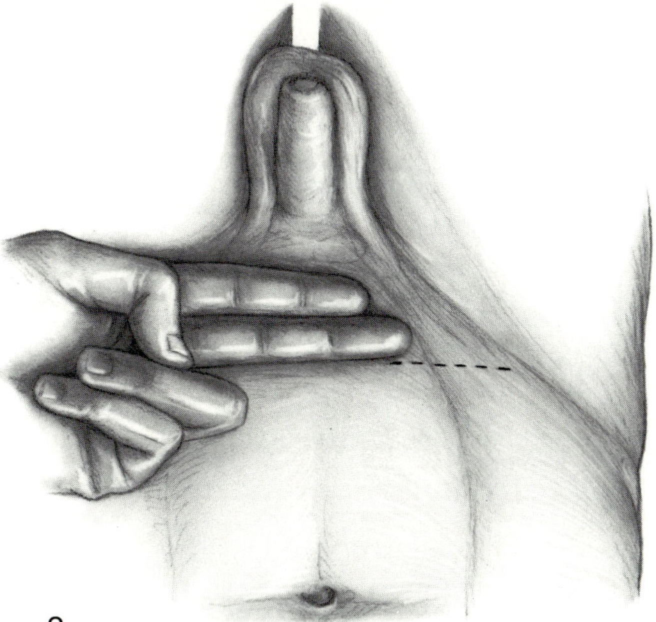

2

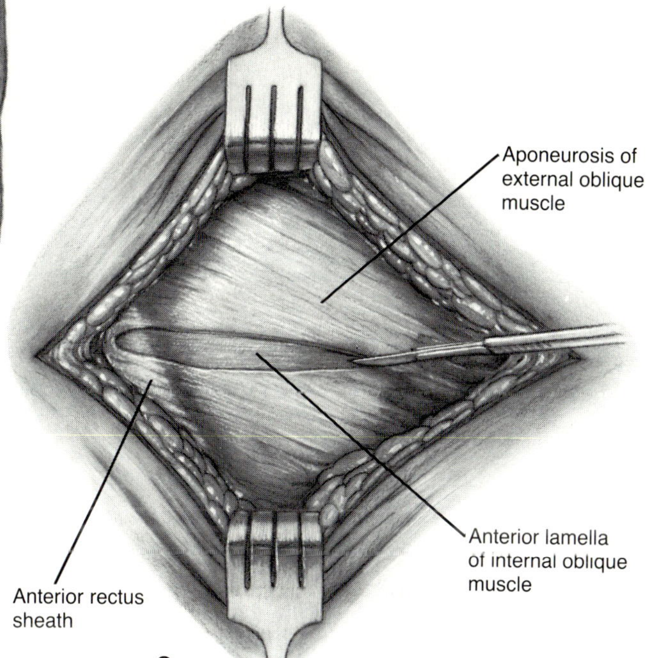
Aponeurosis of
external oblique
muscle
Anterior lamella
of internal oblique
muscle
Anterior rectus
sheath

3

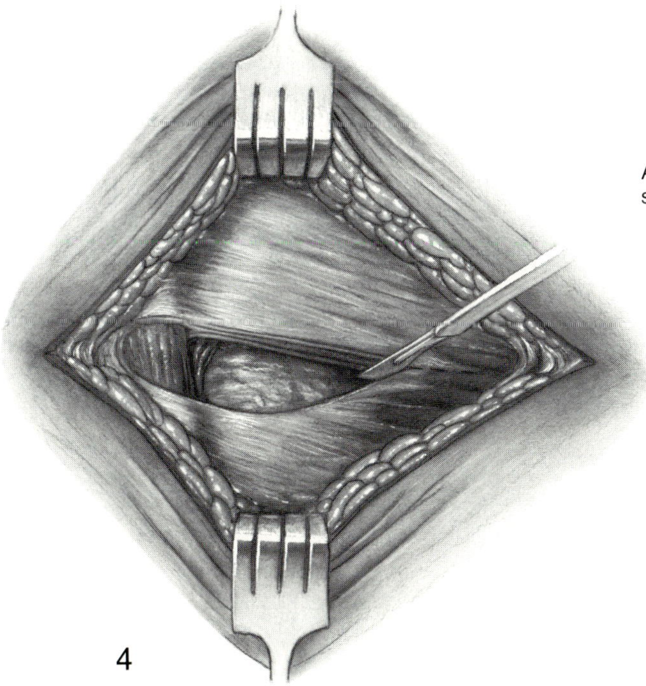

4

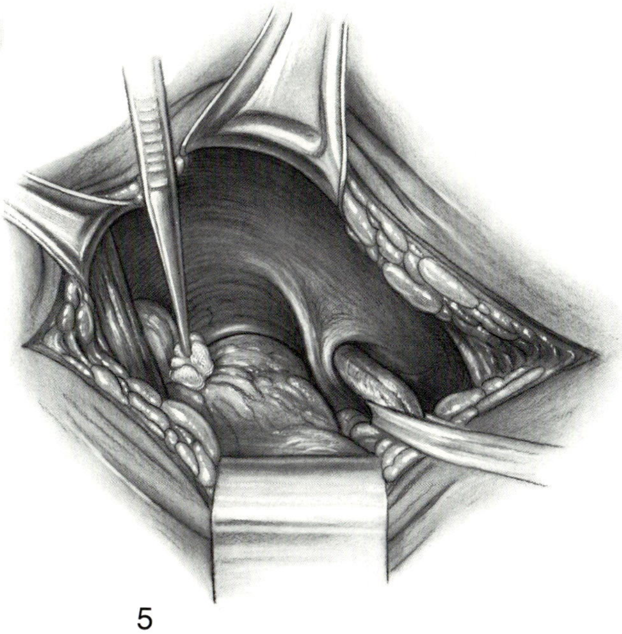

5

PREPERITONEAL (POSTERIOR) APPROACH IN THE TREATMENT OF GROIN HERNIAS

Continued

6 The "nipple" or apex of the herniated peritoneal sac is reduced and, later, may be inverted with interrupted 3-0 sutures of silk or chromic catgut. During the reduction of the sac, the line of transection of the adherent layer of transversalis (endoabdominal) fascia, which preceded the herniation of the peritoneum, may be seen. This line is especially well delineated in the reduction of a femoral hernia.

7 The closure of the medial angle of the hernial defect is initiated by the insertion of an interrupted and untied suture of 1-0 Prolene that includes the arch of the transversus abdominis muscle above and the iliopubic tract below.

8 For technical expediency, additional sutures of 1-0 Prolene are inserted before being tied. Another suture is inserted lateral to the cord for closure of the internal ring whenever there is any question of its laxity. The obturator vessels may be seen crossing over the external iliac vein and Cooper's ligament en route to their passage through the obturator foramen.

9 The sutures are tied and cut to complete the repair of the direct inguinal hernia and to effect a snug closure of the internal ring around the cord. The repair of all direct hernias should include a complementary relaxing incision to release the tension on the suture line.

To complete the operation, the abdominal wound is simply closed in layers in the reverse order to which it was opened.

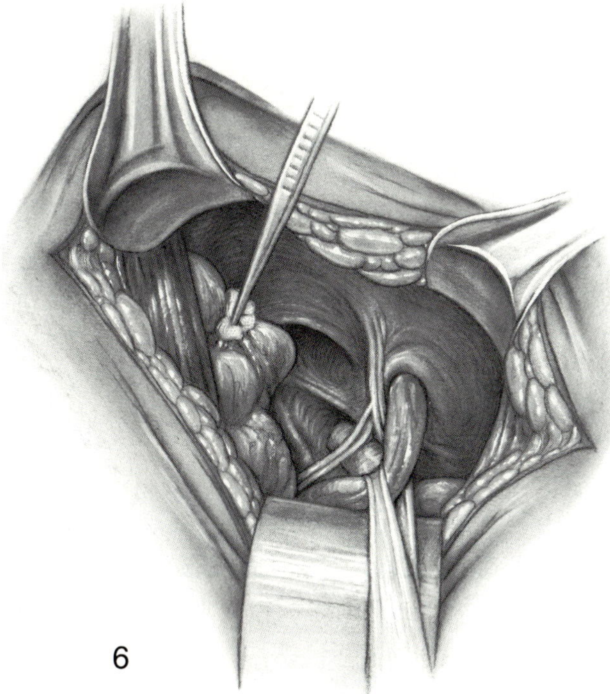

6

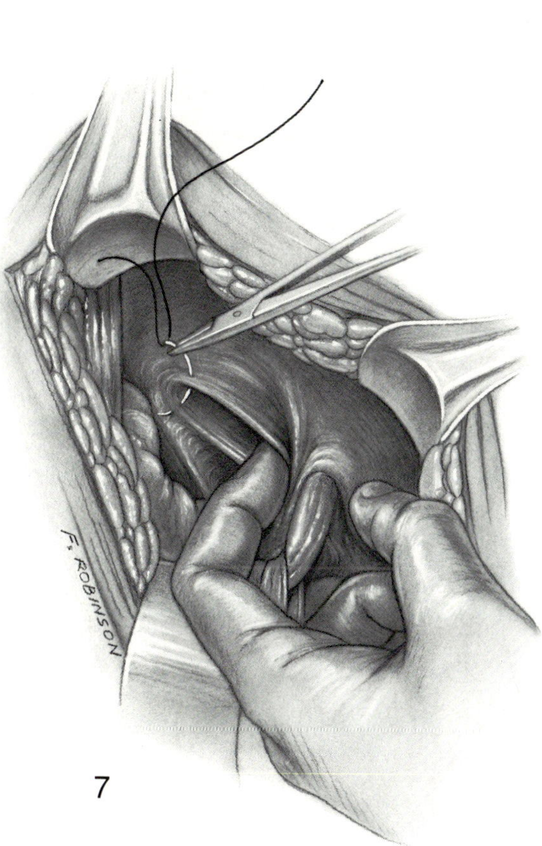

7

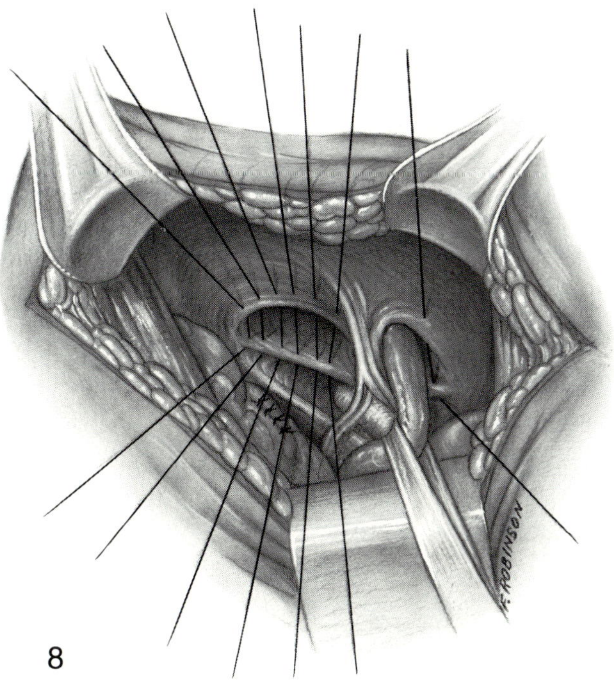

8

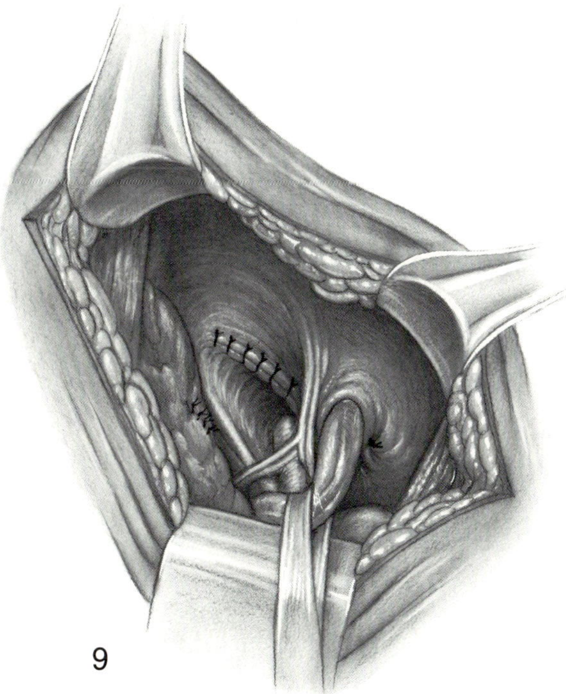

9

PREPERITONEAL (POSTERIOR) APPROACH IN THE TREATMENT OF GROIN HERNIAS
Continued

REPAIR OF INDIRECT INGUINAL AND FEMORAL HERNIAS

10 In the preperitoneal repair of an indirect groin hernia, the peritoneal sac is opened, the redundant sac is excised, and the peritoneum is closed with either a pursestring suture or interrupted sutures of 3-0 silk.

The hernial defect is repaired using two sutures of 1-0 Prolene medially and one or more laterally, depending upon the size of the hernial defect. Frequently, one suture laterally suffices.

11 The preperitoneal approach is ideal for the elective repair of unilateral or bilateral femoral hernias. Also, it is particularly effective in the treatment of an acutely incarcerated hernia or in a strangulated hernia when resection of a gangrenous segment of bowel is mandated. In the uncomplicated type, the hernia is simply reduced, the redundant sac is excised, and the peritoneum is closed with either a pursestring suture or interrupted sutures of 3-0 silk.

The hernial defect is repaired using interrupted sutures of 1-0 Prolene, which approximate the iliopubic tract to Cooper's ligament. Caution must be observed, however, to avoid encroaching on the femoral vein.

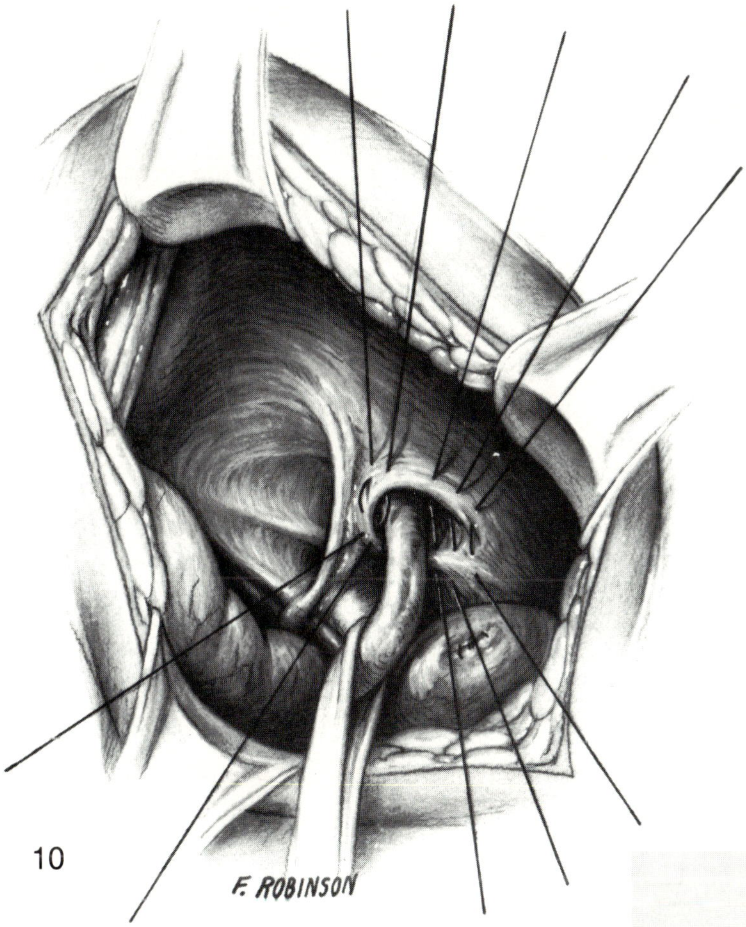

10

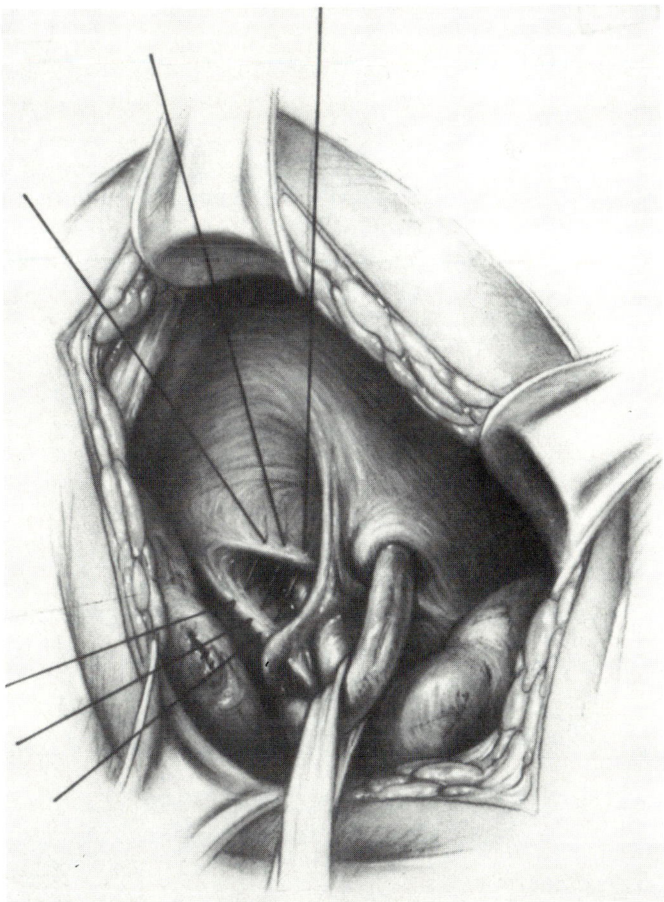

11

PREPERITONEAL (POSTERIOR) APPROACH IN THE TREATMENT OF GROIN HERNIAS
Continued

REPAIR OF A FEMORAL HERNIA

DISCUSSION

William P. Mikkelsen, M.D.

In 1949 I began using the suprapubic, preperitoneal approach for the repair of femoral hernias. My interest in its use was stimulated by the report of Musgrove and McCready[1] (in which credit to Henry[2] was given) on this method of approach. Further inquiry disclosed that primary credit belongs to Cheatle,[3] who in 1920 was the first to describe the basic principles of this procedure.

During the four-year period between 1949 and 1953, 113 patients with femoral hernias were operated on at the Los Angeles County Hospital utilizing this approach.[4] In the 34 years subsequent to this report, the preperitoneal approach has remained the method of choice in the surgical treatment of femoral hernias. The advantages of this approach include: (1) it provides superior exposure, especially if bowel resection is required; (2) the opposite side may be routinely explored and bilateral repair is easily accomplished; (3) injury to the external iliac vein and urinary bladder is minimized; and (4) an anomalous obturator artery or associated obturator hernia can be readily seen.

The only time the preperitoneal approach is not used is when a femoral hernia has been mistaken for an inguinal hernia. This error in diagnosis should be rare if strict precautions are taken to determine the exact anatomic location of the hernial protrusion. This can be done by placing the tip of one index finger on the pubic tubercle and the other on the anterosuperior iliac spine. A true femoral hernia will be found inferior to a line visualized between these two anatomic landmarks. Also, the femoral arterial pulsation will be immediately lateral to the hernial protrusion.

In performing the operation, either a vertical midline lower abdominal incision or a Pfannenstiel incision may be used. The vertical midline incision is easier and more quickly made, but for cosmetic reasons the Pfannenstiel incision is preferred in the younger female patient. The first time this approach is used, the invariable tendency is to explore too deeply or too far posteriorly. Actually, the femoral ring is quite superficial. The rectus muscle is elevated and displaced laterally with a small right-angle or Richardson retractor. The depth of the exploration should be limited to the superior pubic ramus, over which Cooper's ligament resides; this can be readily identified by digital palpation.

Even in obese patients the area to be dissected, the femoral ring, is easily exposed. Its boundaries, distinct and constant, are anteriorly, the inguinal ligament; posteriorly, Cooper's ligament; laterally, the external iliac vein; and medially, the lacunar or

Gimbernat's ligament. When the femoral ring is fully exposed, the hernial protrusion of the peritoneum into the femoral canal is visible. By careful dissection with the index finger, the funiculus is encircled and gently separated from the external iliac vein. Traction is then applied superiorly in an effort to extract the hernial sac from the femoral canal. This extraction can be facilitated by combining the traction with "stick sponge" counterpressure on the edges of the femoral ring. More often, however, an incision in the lacunar ligament with a scalpel is required. This is easily accomplished by first inserting a grooved director between the outside medial wall of the hernial sac and the lateral crescentic margin of Gimbernat's ligament. A scalpel with a No. 15 blade is then inserted in the groove of the director, and the ligament is cut.

In using this technique, one must always be aware that the obturator artery, when aberrant, courses along the lateral crescentic margin of Gimbernat's ligament and is thereby subject to severance and bleeding. This occurrence should be rare, however, since an aberrant artery is easily seen with this approach.

In the large incarcerated or strangulated femoral hernia, the incision in Gimbernat's ligament may prove inadequate to permit reduction. When this occurs, the inguinal ligament is transected and then reconstructed when the repair of the hernia is completed. Surgical repair of a transected Gimbernat's ligament is not required.

After the sac is liberated, it is immediately opened. If necessary, the opening can be extended superiorly as far as necessary and can even be converted into a routine lower abdominal laparotomy incision. In such circumstances the resection of the bowel, if required, is readily done. The actual hernioplasty is accomplished by suturing a fold of the fused transversalis fascia and aponeurosis of the transversus muscle to Cooper's ligament. This provides a strong repair without tension and completely obliterates the femoral ring. Nyhus prefers to suture the iliopubic tract to Cooper's ligament, as depicted in **11.** Most frequently, however, I find the iliopubic tract to be a "will-o'-the-wisp," and McVay[5] referred to it as "an illusion."

The lattice-like repair of Kinnear,[6] in which floss silk or floss nylon is interwoven between the inguinal ligament and Cooper's ligament, is not advocated. The technique in which the inguinal ligament is sutured to Cooper's ligament causes excessive tension on the suture line and may even compromise the lumina of the external iliac vein and artery. Furthermore, elevating a flap of pectineus fascia and attaching it to the inguinal ligament is most cumbersome. Accordingly, neither of these two techniques is recommended.

PREPERITONEAL (POSTERIOR) APPROACH IN THE TREATMENT OF GROIN HERNIAS

Continued

Complications of the preperitoneal approach are rare. In fact, this approach eliminates the potential complications of the infra- and suprainguinal approaches for the repair of femoral hernias. Hematomas are uncommon, and hernial recurrences are rare. Personally, I have never seen a recurrent femoral hernia that previously had been repaired by the suprapubic, preperitoneal approach.

Although the preperitoneal approach is ideal for the repair of femoral hernias, it is generally unsuitable for the repair of inguinal hernias. Admittedly, in the repair of small indirect inguinal hernias—especially in the young adult—the reduction, ligation, and excision of the hernial sac are easily done. However, these can also be accomplished easily by the inguinal route.

Use of the preperitoneal approach in the repair of direct and large indirect inguinal hernias is associated with an unacceptably high failure rate. In fact, the early recurrence of the hernia in a significant number of these cases led me to abandon this approach early on. This decision later received credence when McVay[5] stated, "Available reports . . . have indicated a recurrence rate as high as 35 per cent . . . of direct hernias . . . with only a 3 or 4 year follow-up." This statement echoed the views expressed by Henry in a letter to Nyhus 24 years ago: "An attempt to enlist the extraperitoneal method for work on inguinal hernia was met on three occasions with the rebuff of rapid recurrence, in two patients within 10 days of operation." He concluded, "I have long relinquished the extraperitoneal approach for inguinal hernia as discouraging and unsatisfactory."[7]

REFERENCES

1. Musgrove JE and McCready FJ: The Henry approach to femoral hernia. Surgery *26*:608, 1949.
2. Henry AK: Operation for femoral hernia by a midline extraperitoneal approach. Lancet *1*:531, 1936.
3. Cheatle GL: An operation for the radical cure of inguinal and femoral hernia. Br Med *2*:68, 1920.
4. Mikkelsen WP and Berne CJ: Femoral hernioplasty: Suprapubic extraperitoneal (Cheatle-Henry) approach. Surgery *35*:743, 1954.
5. McVay CB: Preperitoneal hernioplasty. Surg Gynecol Obstet *123*:349–350, 1966.
6. Kinnear N: The femoral hernia: The Henry operation. In Nyhus LM and Harkins HN (eds): *Hernia*. Philadelphia: JB Lippincott, 1964, pp 307–309.
7. Nyhus LM and Harkins HN (eds): *Hernia*. Philadelphia: JB Lippincott, 1964, p 306.

SUMMATION

Lloyd M. Nyhus, M.D.

POSTERIOR ILIOPUBIC TRACT REPAIR (PREPERITONEAL APPROACH)

In the 1980's the operative treatment of groin hernias continues to be based on an accurate knowledge of anatomy. Understanding of the endoabdominal (transversalis) fascia and its analogues (iliopubic tract, anterior femoral sheath) is a key to our knowledge of the etiology, development, diagnosis, and cure of these common problems.

The employment of the posterior approach to the transversalis-transversus layer has been periodically advocated during the past 112 years. During this interval the technique has been useful in the repair of three major types of hernias: the recurrent inguinal hernia (recent), the primary femoral hernia, and incarcerated hernias of all types.[1] Table 1 summarizes the relation of the posterior iliopubic tract repair to other methods in the operative care of specific groin defects. An operation should be carefully selected for an individual problem, not performed automatically. One should note the variety of operations suggested for a given anatomic defect.

Table 1. TYPES OF GROIN HERNIAS AND THE PROCEDURE OF CHOICE FOR EACH

Hernia	Repair*
Small indirect inguinal	Transversalis fascial repair of internal ring
Large indirect inguinal	Iliopubic tract repair of posterior inguinal wall, or Cooper's ligament–McVay repair
Small direct inguinal	Iliopubic tract repair of posterior inguinal wall
Large direct inguinal	Cooper's ligament repair of posterior inguinal wall, or iliopubic tract repair with Marlex mesh buttress by the posterior approach
Pantaloon (combined direct-indirect)	Iliopubic tract repair of posterior inguinal wall plus transversalis fascial closure of internal ring
Femoral	Preperitoneal approach and iliopubic tract repair
Sliding indirect inguinal	Preperitoneal approach and iliopubic tract repair, or iliopubic tract repair (anterior approach), or Cooper's ligament repair
Strangulated indirect and femoral	Preperitoneal approach, intestinal resection and anastomosis, iliopubic tract repair
Recurrent	Preperitoneal approach and iliopubic tract repair with Marlex mesh buttress
Massive (loss of right of domain)	Ten-day pneumoperitoneum, and iliopubic tract repair of posterior inguinal wall with Marlex mesh buttress or Cooper's ligament–McVay repair

*Excision of the hernial sac and high ligation are performed for all defects except direct hernias.

It is not surprising that surgeons who are unfamiliar with the posterior approach should sometimes encounter difficulty in achieving effortless exposure of the proper tissue planes. For this reason, it is imperative for anyone interested in this procedure to first observe an experienced surgeon perform the preperitoneal approach to the repair. In this operation there is no substitute for experience in defining the sometimes subtle transversalis fascial layer.

Anatomic Considerations

I am concerned about Mikkelsen's comment regarding the posterior approach. The anterior limit of the femoral canal is the iliopubic tract (anterior femoral sheath), *not* the inguinal ligament. The lacunar or Gimbernat's ligament cannot be seen from the posterior view. The medial boundary of the femoral canal, which must be cut to release an incarcerated femoral hernia, is made up of reflected fibers of the iliopubic tract. In my technique, the iliopubic tract— *not* the "aponeurosis of the transversus muscle," as stated by Mikkelsen—is sewn to Cooper's ligament in the closure of the femoral defect. These aponeurotic fibers of the transversus abdominis muscle are used for repair of the femoral defect in the Cooper's ligament—McVay technique from the anterior approach. Mikkelsen's comments regarding the use of the posterior approach for inguinal hernial repair apply to the old and outmoded Cheatle-Henry approach (vertical midline) and repair (use of inappropriate anatomic fascial structures). It is little wonder that Henry, Mikkelsen, and others obtained such poor results with the posterior approach. Greenburg[2] has demonstrated the exceptionally good results that can be obtained when the proper techniques for the posterior approach and repair are used.

Technical Considerations

The incision should be made transversely in a line passing just cephalad to the internal inguinal ring. After the anterior rectus sheath is incised, the rectus muscle is retracted toward the midline, and an incision is made in the transversalis fascial layer to permit access to the preperitoneal space. This space always has a variable amount of fat. The appearance of fatty tissue is the signal that the proper plane has been entered, and at this point the incision through the abdominal musculature is widened toward the anterosuperior iliac spine to pass about 2.0 cm above the internal ring. This accomplished, the posterior inguinal wall is bared of fatty and areolar tissue from the line of incision to the superior pubic ramus. A moist gauze sponge is useful for sweeping most of these tissues down toward the pelvis, and an assistant places gentle cephalad traction on the preperitoneal fat and peritoneum. A slight depression of the head of the operating table helps to maintain the exposure. If small portions of areolar tissue obscure the fascial plane of the posterior inguinal wall, they should be promptly removed; similarly, if the epigastric vessels are in the way, they can be ligated and divided.

Next, the herniated structures are identified and reduced. If there is an incarcerated hernia, it is prudent (and easy) to inspect all portions of incarcerated intestine for signs of ischemia or infarction. If there is any doubt, the surgeon can easily observe the tissues in question until the decision whether or not to resect has been made. The walls of the hernial defect can then be identified in preparation for the repair.

In the repair itself, permanent suture material (1-0 polypropylene) is used to approximate the margins of the defect. Sutures must approximate these fascial margins without excessive tension. The spermatic cord must also be examined to ensure that an additional oblique hernia is not present. A relaxing incision must be performed in every direct hernia repair.

Recurrent Inguinal Hernias

The posterior approach is strongly recommended for recurrent hernias. The opportunity to perform the operation in virgin tissue is a distinct advantage in this type of repair. The only difference in the repair is that a synthetic mesh buttress is sutured to the posterior wall to prevent further herniation. This step should be carried out for any recurrence of a groin hernia.

The routine use of synthetic mesh remains somewhat controversial, but the outstanding results achieved in many medical centers, including my own, cannot be denied. Of the several methods of inserting the mesh, the direct application of a shield-shaped piece to the posterior wall is recommended. Heavy polypropylene sutures are used to sew the mesh (Marlex) to the borders of the preperitoneal space, anchoring it posteriorly to Cooper's ligament, with care taken not to encroach on the femoral vein. The hernial defect is repaired with 1-0 polypropylene sutures before the mesh is inserted.

Again, relaxing incisions are always used in direct hernias treated by the posterior approach. Whether or not a relaxing incision is an unnecessary addition to mesh insertion remains controversial.

Complications

Complications following hernial repairs by the posterior approach are unusual. Fortunately, wound infections, either superficial or deep, are rare. The posterior or preperitoneal approach and iliopubic tract repair of groin hernias, when properly applied and performed, can be expected to serve knowledgeable surgeons and their patients well.

REFERENCES

1. Nyhus LM and Condon RE (eds): *Hernia,* 3rd ed. Philadelphia: JB Lippincott, 1988.
2. Greenburg AG: Revisiting the recurrent groin hernia. Am J Surg *154*:35–38, 1987.

OPERATION 14

REPAIR OF AN UMBILICAL HERNIA

Plate LVII
Plate LVIII
Plate LIX
Plate LX
Plate LXI
Plate LXII

1, 1A, 1B The elliptical incision (*broken lines*) for the removal of the umbilicus is indicated (**1**). When the umbilicus is preserved either a supra- (**1A**) or infraumbilical (**1B**) incision is used, depending upon the size of the hernia and its relationship to the umbilicus.

2 A sagittal view of the omentum incarcerated in the hernial sac shows its relationship to the structures of the anterior abdominal wall and the subjacent loops of small bowel.

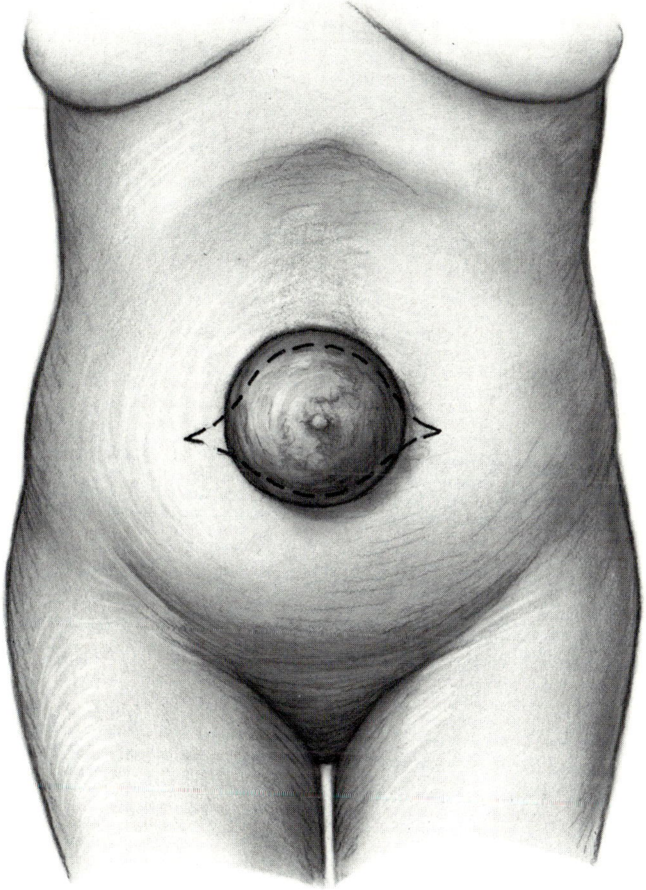

1

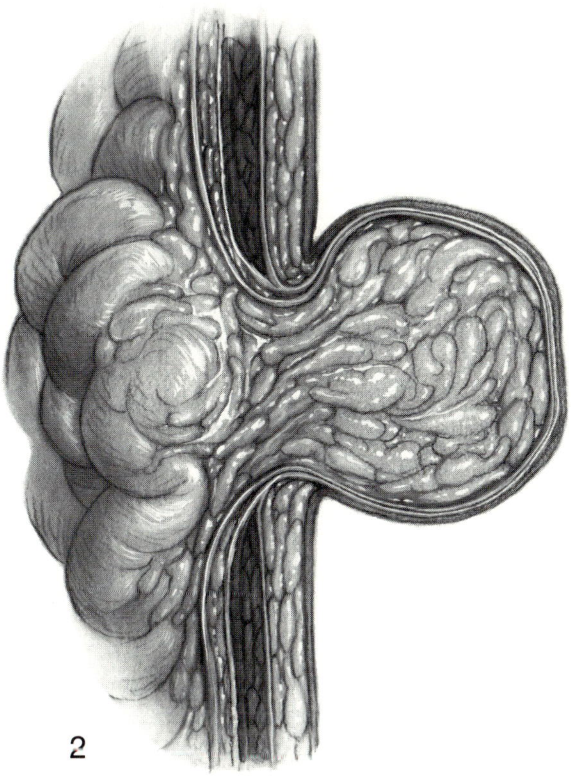

2

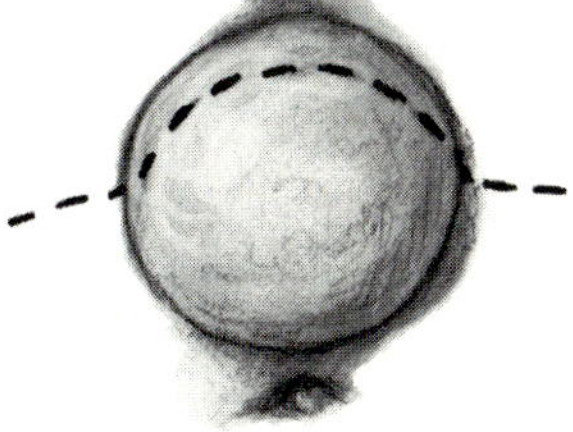

1A

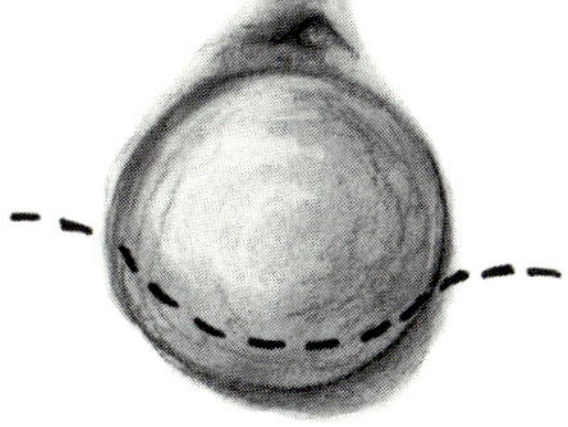

1B

REPAIR OF AN UMBILICAL HERNIA

Continued

3, 4 The lower part of the elliptical incision (**3**) is made first. This is done to avoid masking of the site of the lower incision by the flow of blood from the upper incision (**4**).

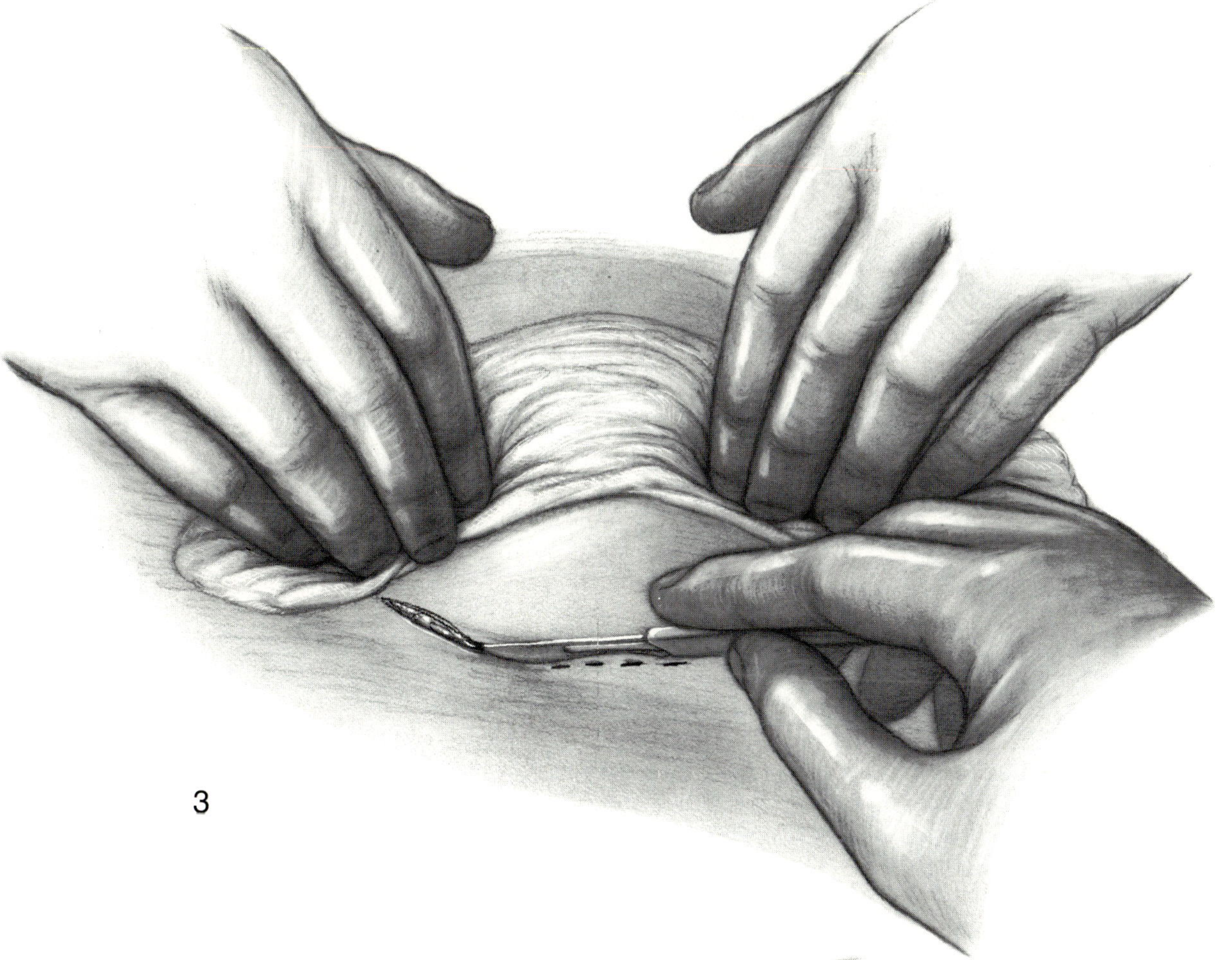

3

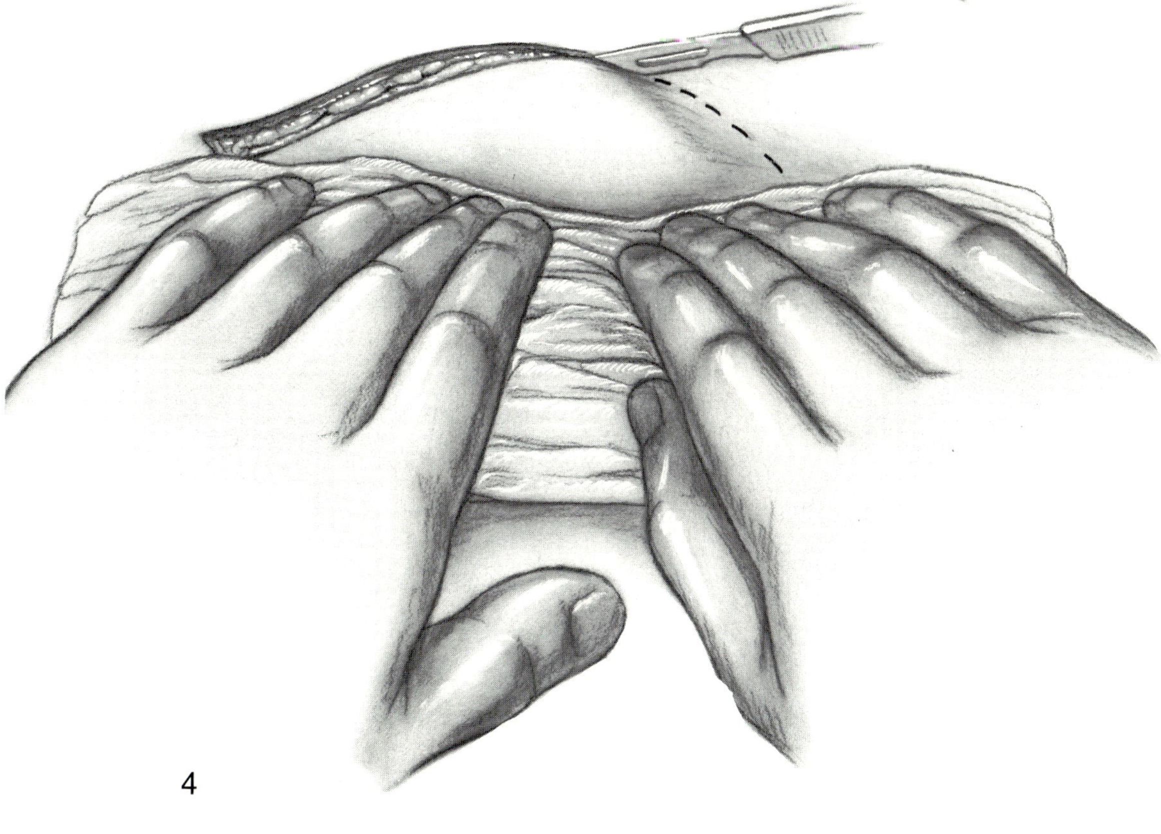

4

REPAIR OF AN UMBILICAL HERNIA
Continued

5 When the incision into the subcutaneous fatty tissue plane is completed, large clamps are applied to the incised skin margins of the herniated segment. A large, dry gauze "lap pad" is stuffed onto the island of skin and held secure by tying the handles of the clamps around it, using a length of gauze bandage. The cut strands of the tied gauze bandage are held in a clamp in one hand by the assistant, and the encased handles of the clamps are grasped in the other hand. While upward traction is maintained on the clamps, the surgeon exerts clamp countertraction serially as the scalpel dissection is continued to expose the underlying fascia of the anterior abdominal wall.

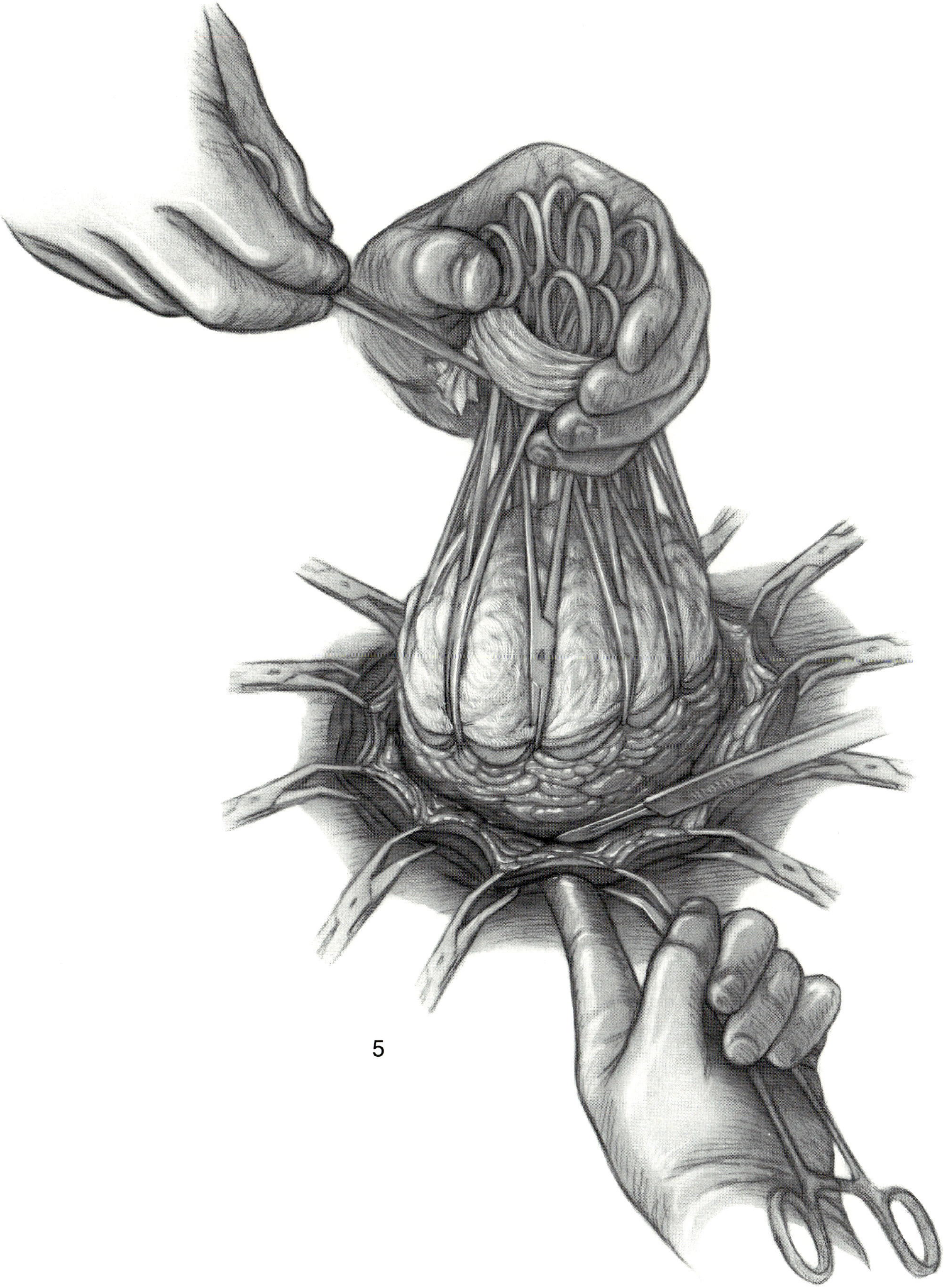

5

REPAIR OF AN UMBILICAL HERNIA

Continued

6, 6A, 6B The incision in the fascial layer is extended circumferentially (*broken lines*) by both scissors and scalpel dissection (**6**). Similarly, the opening in the underlying peritoneum, exposing part of the herniated segment of omentum, is extended circumferentially by scissors dissection, as indicated by the *broken line* (**6A**). The peritoneal cavity is entered, and the incarcerated segment of omentum within the hernial sac is detached from its intraperitoneal origin by serial clamping and severance of its wide pedicle attachment (**6B**).

The clamps are replaced serially with transfixion sutures of 3-0 silk. Simple ligatures are never used because of their propensity to slip off fatty tissue pedicles.

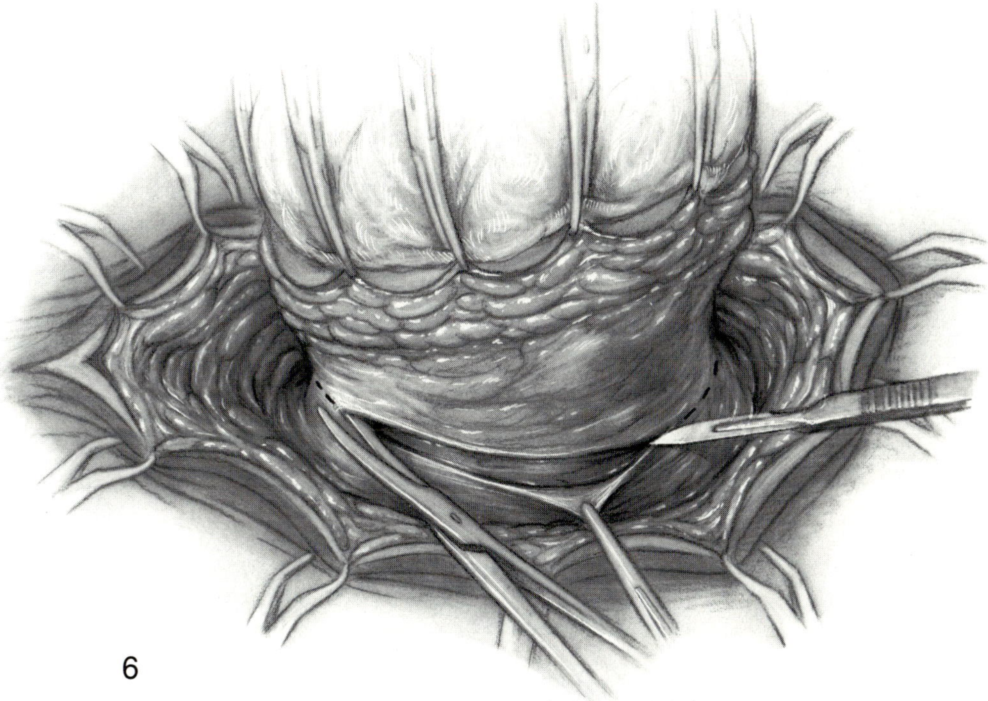

6

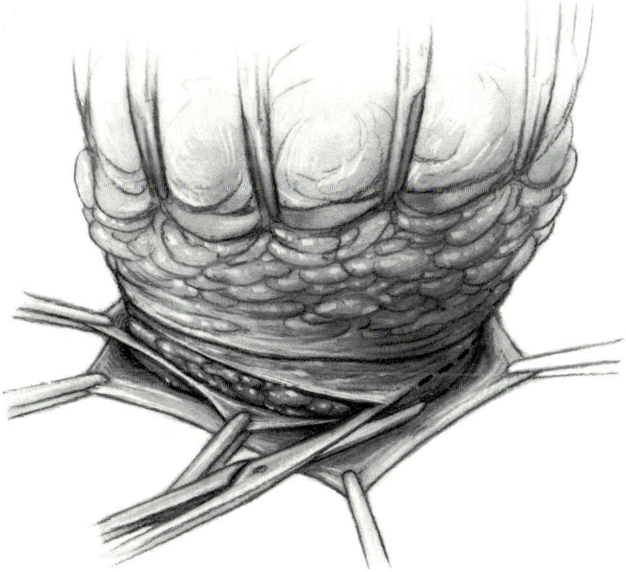

6A

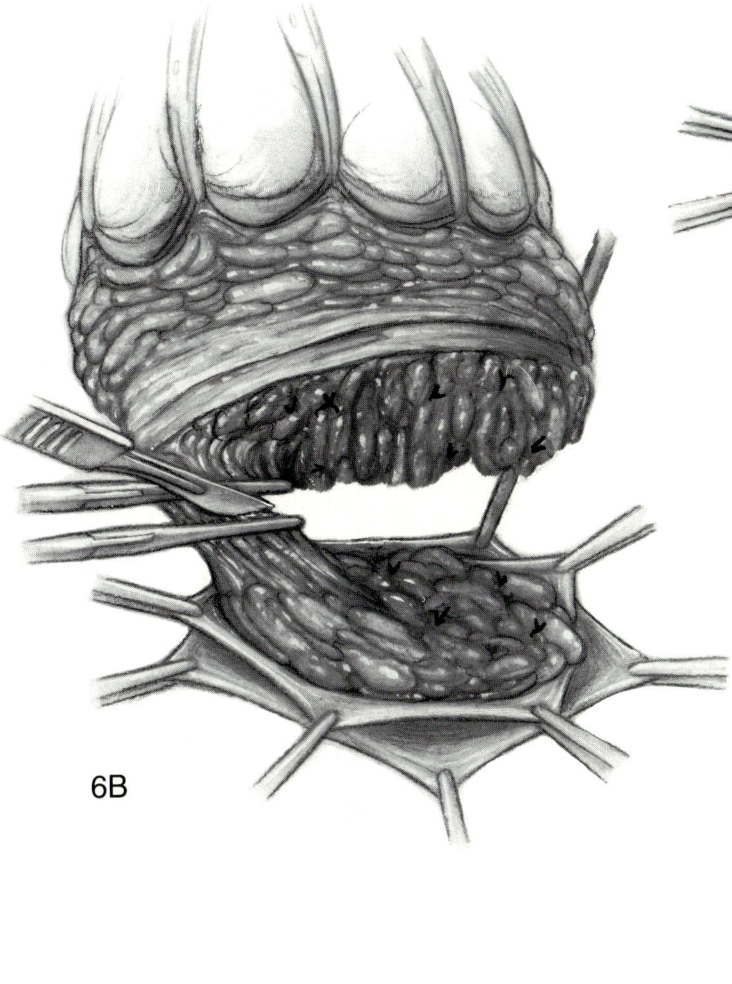

6B

REPAIR OF AN UMBILICAL HERNIA
Continued

7, 7A, 7B, 7C The peritoneum is closed with a continuous suture of 3-0 chromic catgut, and a crown suture of 3-0 silk, to close the fascia at its left lateral angle, is being inserted (**7**). A similar suture has been previously inserted and tied to close the right lateral angle. The insertion of the angle suture is completed (**7A**), and the fascial layer is being closed (**7B**) with a series of interrupted figure-of-eight mattress sutures of 3-0 silk to its completion (**7C**).

8, 8A, 8B, 8C, 8D A catheter for continuous suction is placed beneath each skin flap (**8**), and the skin is closed with interrupted sutures of 3-0 silk (**8A**). When the operation is completed, the well-like depression at the former site of the umbilicus is visible (**8B**).

Preservation of the umbilicus is commonly done. Placements of the suction catheters for the supraumbilical (**8C**) and infraumbilical (**8D**) incisions are shown.

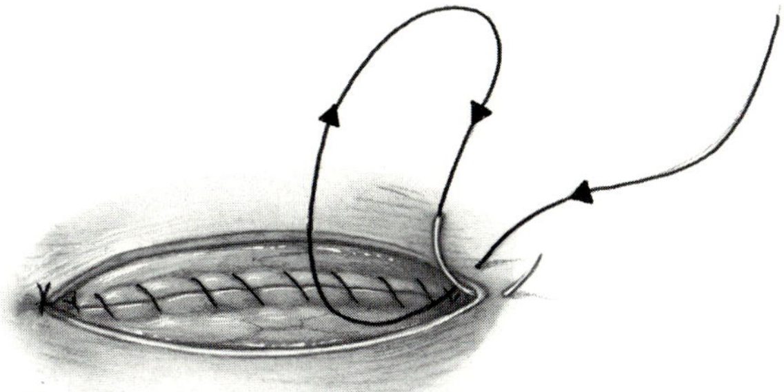
7

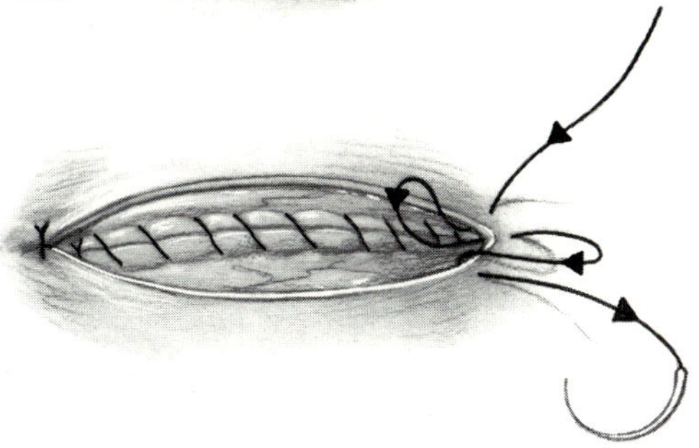
7A

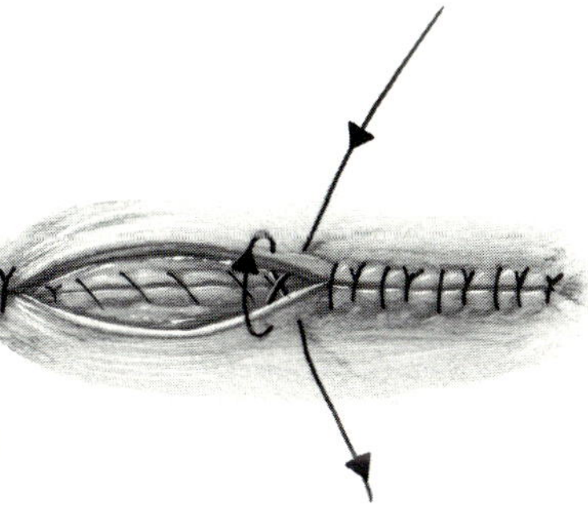
7B

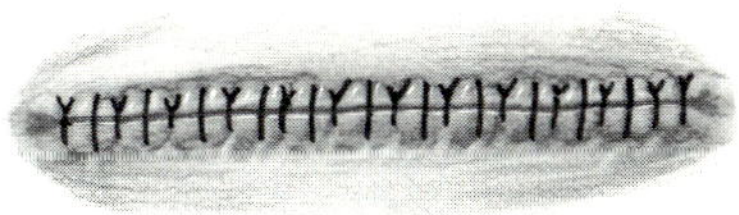
7C

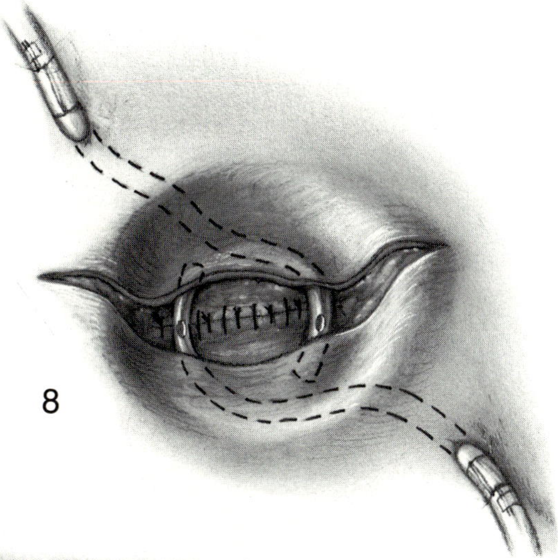
8

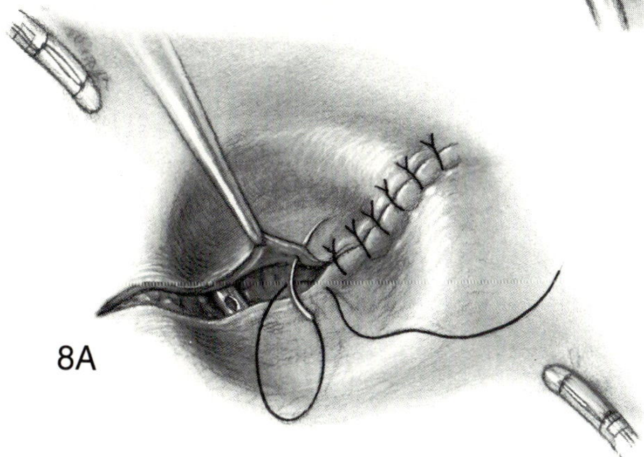
8A

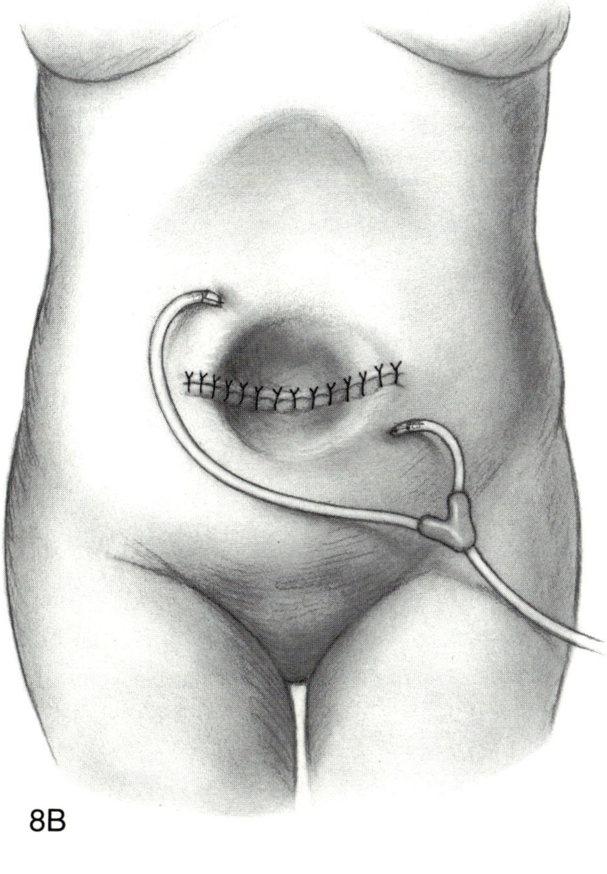
8B

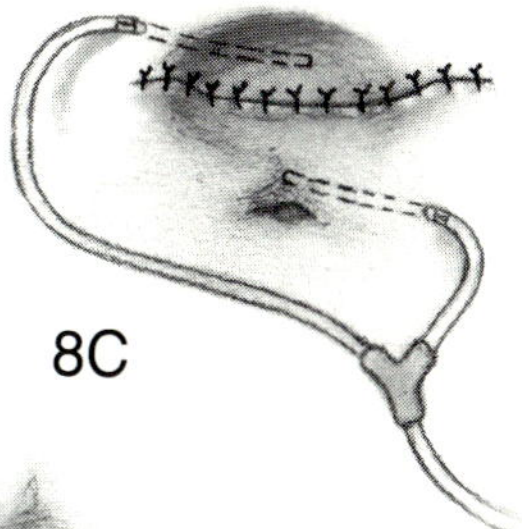
8C

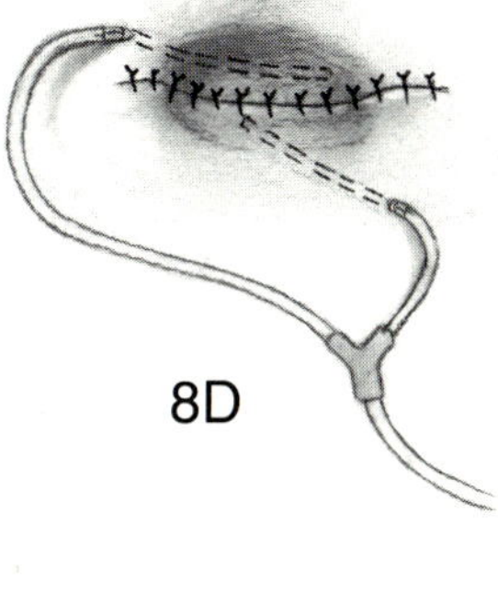
8D

REPAIR OF AN UMBILICAL HERNIA
Continued

9, 9A, 9B, 9C, 9D Enlarged schematic representations show the fixation of the suction catheters to the skin to prevent their accidental withdrawal.

The suture (3-0 silk) is first anchored to the skin (**9**) and then encircles the catheter just distal to its site of exit (**9A**). The first knot of the suture is tied, followed by the second knot (**9B**). The strands of the second knot are laid slack as its ends are tied around the catheter more distally (**9C**). They are then fixed to the catheter with strips of paper adhesive (**9D**).

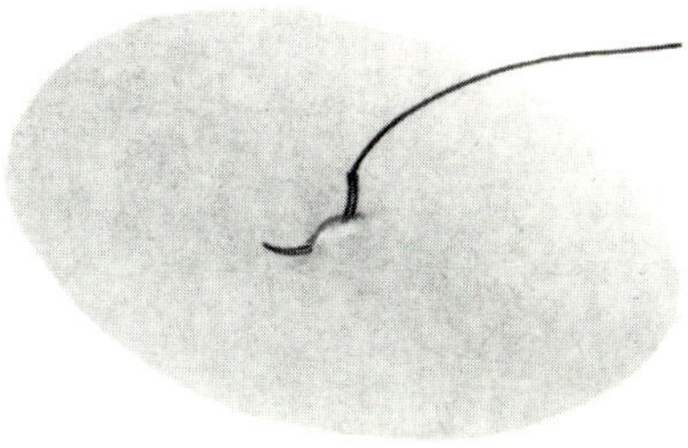

9

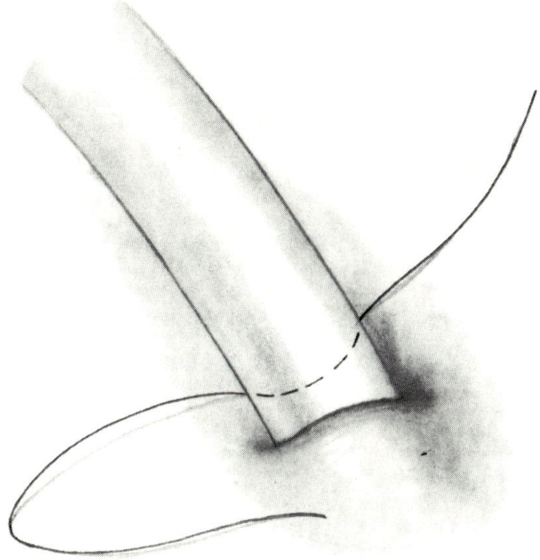

9A

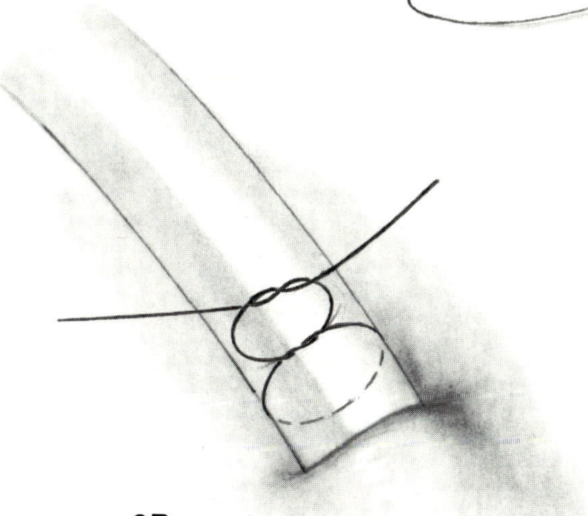

9B

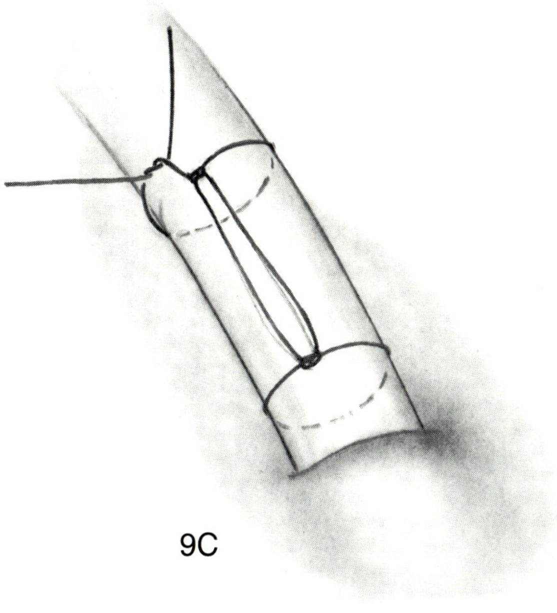

9C

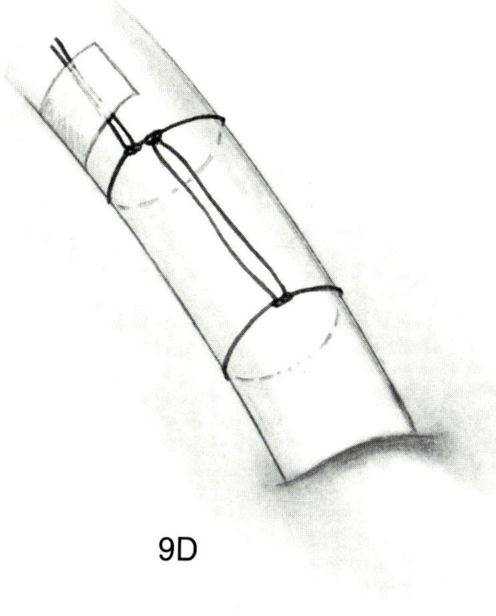

9D

OPERATION 15

REPAIR OF AN INCISIONAL HERNIA

Plate LXIII
Plate LXIV
Plate LXV
Plate LXVI
Plate LXVII
Plate LXVIII

1 The elliptical excision of a widened scar in a large incisional hernia is indicated by the *dotted outline.*

INTRODUCTION

The technique presented here for the repair of an incisional hernia has proved most effective. Previously, the standard practice was to dissect the peritoneum, muscle, and fascia and suture them separately in layers. However, the approximation of the fused margins of these tissues in a single-layer closure, as illustrated here, is now preferred.

Admittedly, in some patients the size of the hernia and the lack of adequate holding power of the tissues preclude a primary repair. In such instances the use of either autogenous tissue (fascia or skin*) or a plastic prosthesis is required. The preference is for a plastic prosthesis—specifically, polyethylene mesh (Marlex), as proposed by Usher.[1,2] (See Operation 16.)

Prosthetic meshes are frequently used when a primary repair would suffice. Their use varies in direct ratio to the particular interest and enthusiasm of the surgeon and in inverse ratio to the extent of tissue dissection. The more extensive the dissection and mobilization of the tissues, the greater is the incidence of primary repair.

Finally, emphasis should be placed on the value of lateral relaxing incisions on each side of the line of primary closure. When there is undue tension on the suture line, their use may prove to be the difference between success or failure of the operation.

*Although skin is mentioned for the sake of completeness, its use is not recommended.

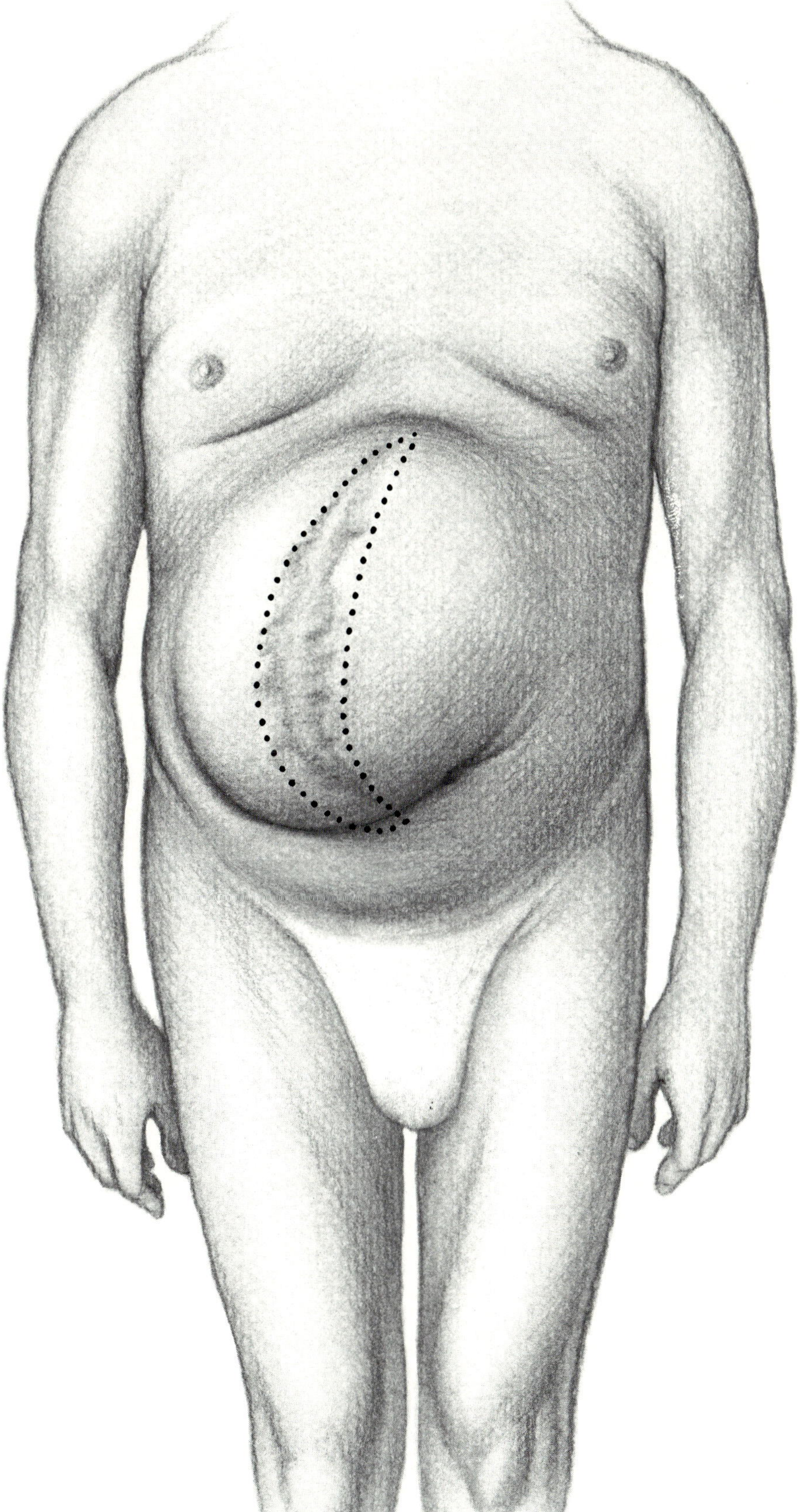
1

REPAIR OF AN INCISIONAL HERNIA
Continued

2, 3 The scar is excised by scalpel dissection. During this excision, one must be aware of the underlying intraperitoneal viscera; otherwise, the lumen of an adherent loop of bowel may be entered inadvertently.

4 The folded margin of a wet towel is attached to the skin edge with the first of a series of toothed clamps, which will be used subsequently for traction.

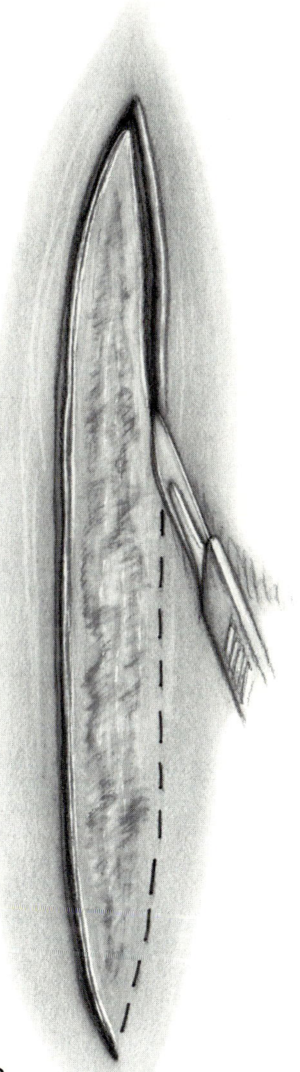

2

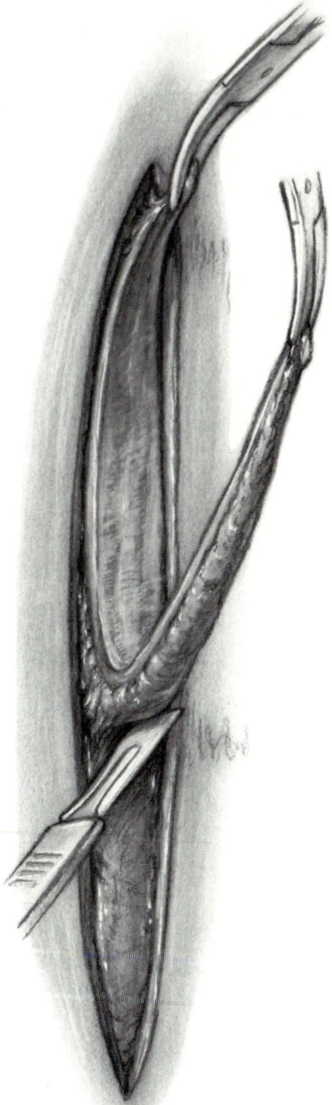

3

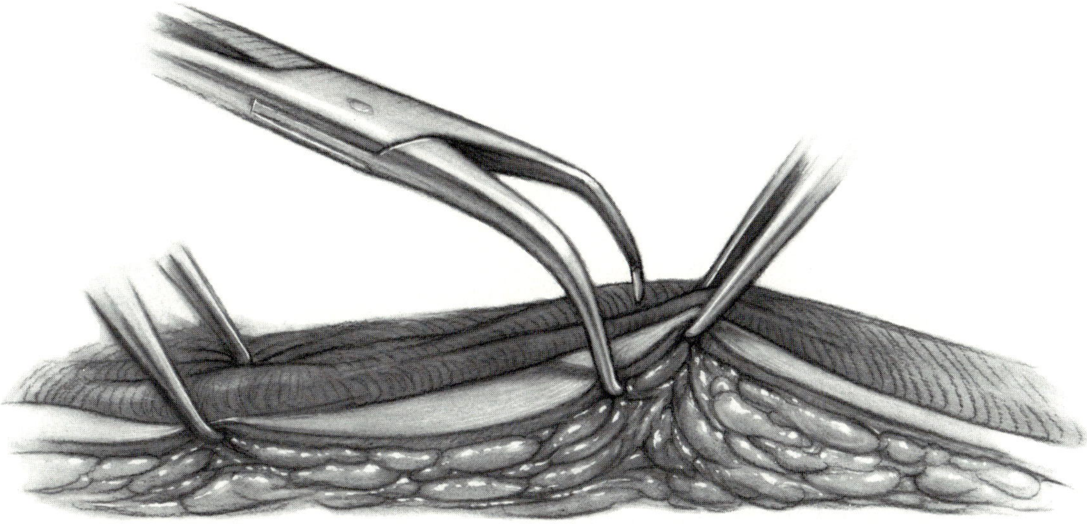

4

5 Upward traction is maintained on the clamps in sequence as the skin flap is mobilized by scalpel dissection in the subcutaneous tissue plane.

6 The opposite skin flap is similarly dissected to complete the mobilization of the skin flaps.

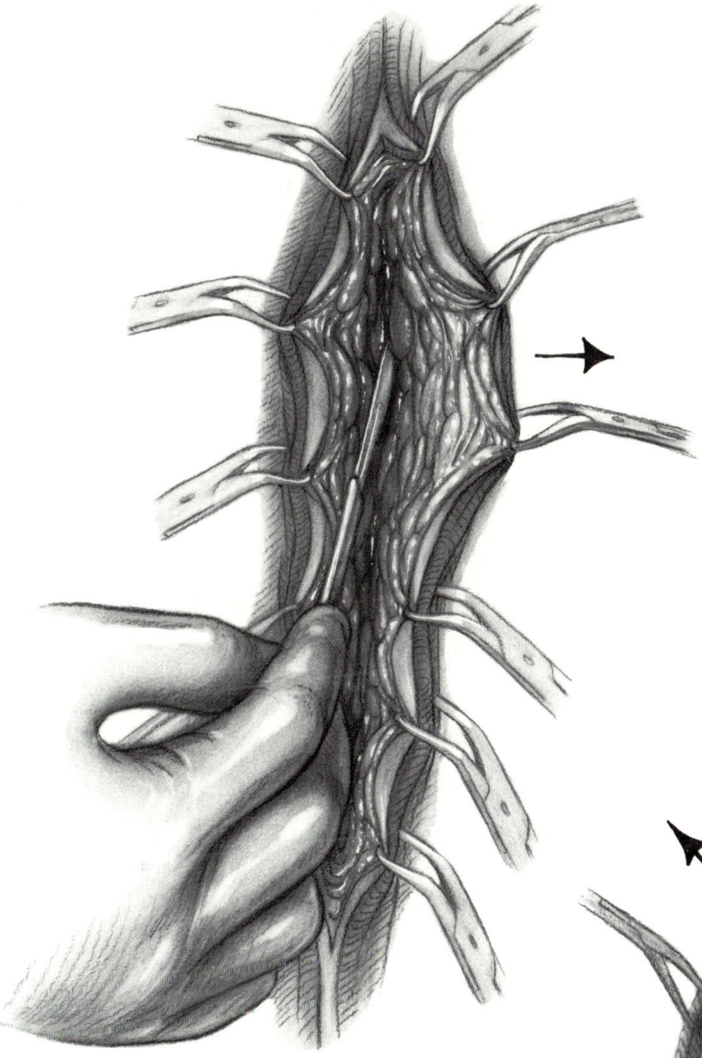

5

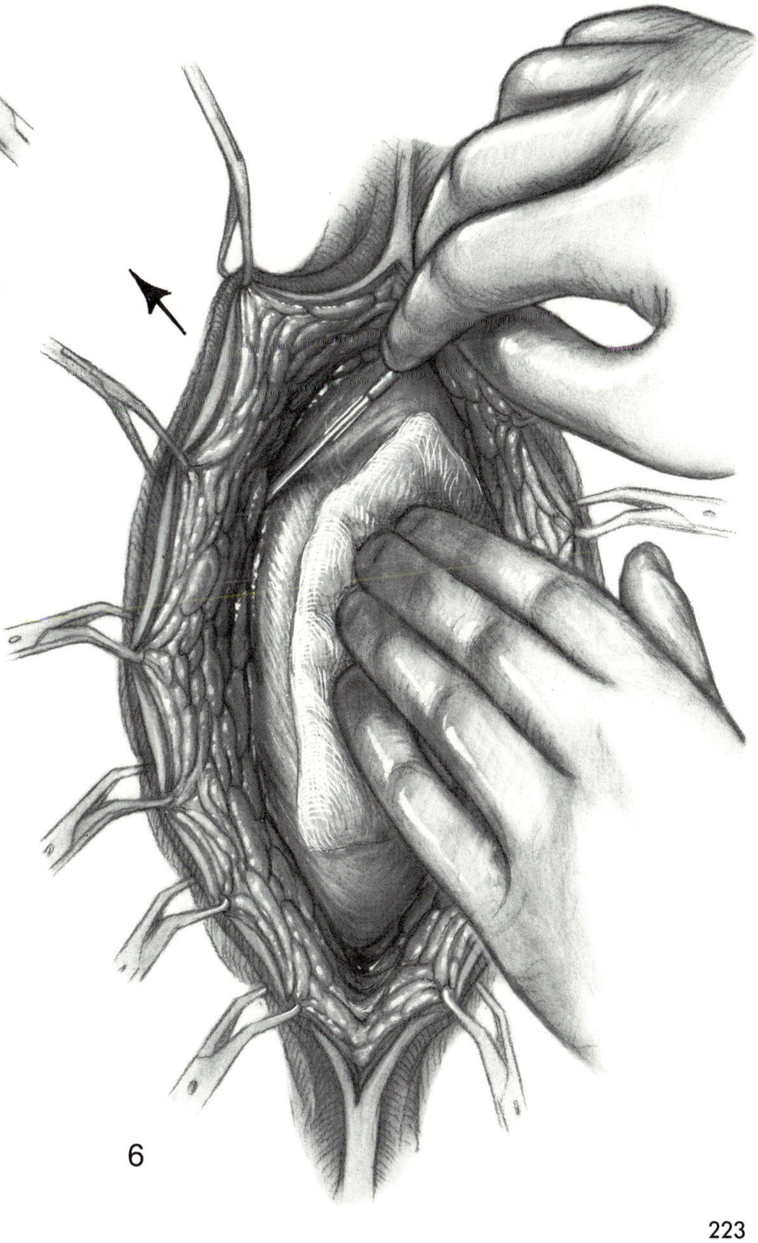

6

REPAIR OF AN INCISIONAL HERNIA
Continued

7 The "false" sac is incised, and the opening is enlarged caudad by severing the sac wall with a scalpel.

8 The peritoneal cavity is entered, and an adherent loop of the small intestine is freed from the undersurface of the sac by scissors dissection. This intimate adherence of the bowel to the sac is commonly found in large incisional hernias, and the possibility of its presence is considered a prime indication to open rather than enfold the sac.

9 The false sac, freed from the attachments of the underlying bowel, is severed with scissors in a cephalad direction, as indicated by the *broken line.*

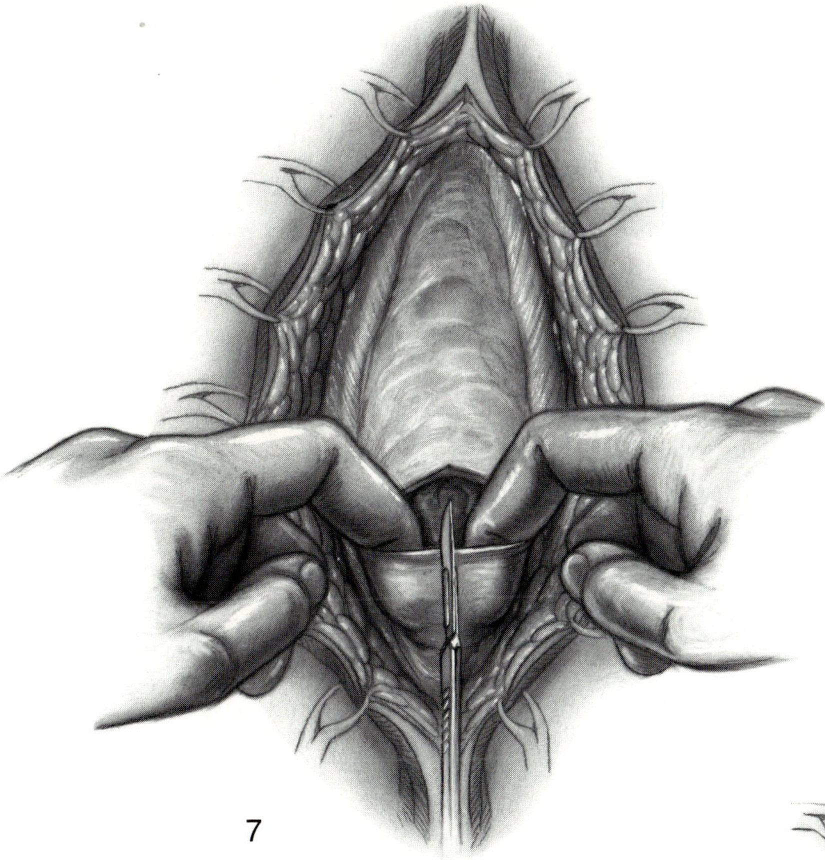

7

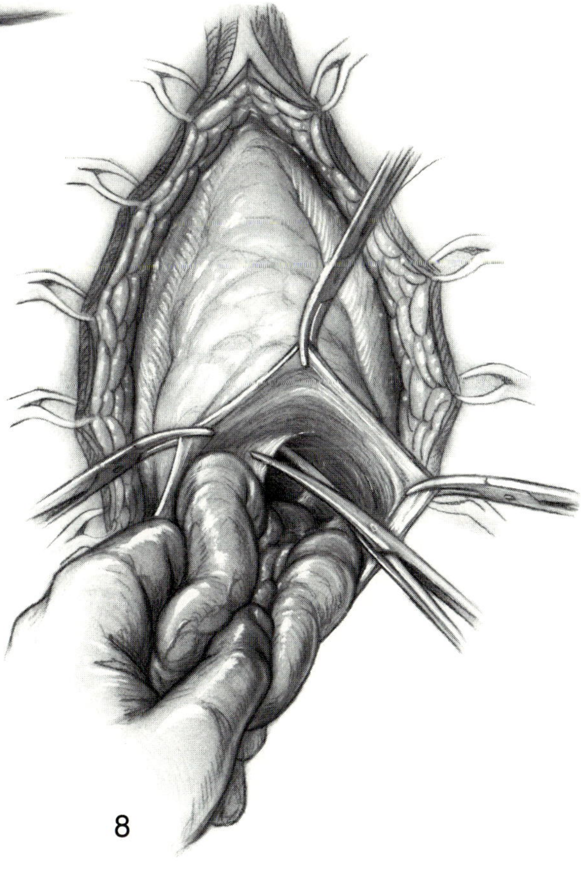

8

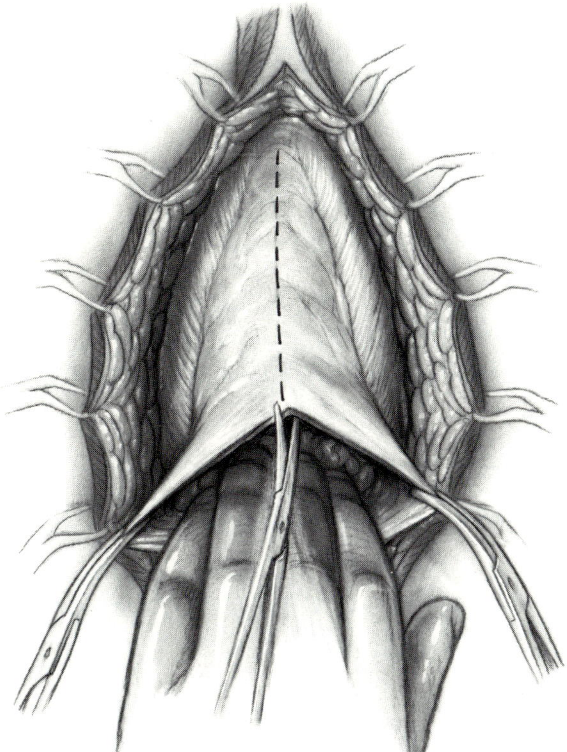

9

REPAIR OF AN INCISIONAL HERNIA

Continued

10 Clamp traction is maintained on the left lateral leaflet of the false sac as its caudad portion is severed by scalpel along the line of fusion with the normal structures that form the anterior abdominal wall.

11 The dissection of the false sac is continued with scissors to complete its excision (*broken line*) cephalad. The right lateral leaflet is subsequently excised in a similar manner.

12 The closure of the hernial defect is continued by the approximation of the fused margins of the anterior abdominal wall with interrupted far-and-near, near-and-far mattress sutures of 1-0 silk (the so-called pulley sutures). If required, lateral relaxing incisions in the fascia may be made. The inserted but untied crown suture in the caudad angle of the wound is visible. Similarly, a crown suture was previously inserted and tied to close the cephalad angle of the wound.

Previously, the tissues forming the fused margins of the wound—the peritoneum, rectus muscle, and fascia—were first separated and then closed separately in layers. However, experience has shown that approximating the fused margins of the wound in one layer provides greater holding power of the tissues and is less time consuming.

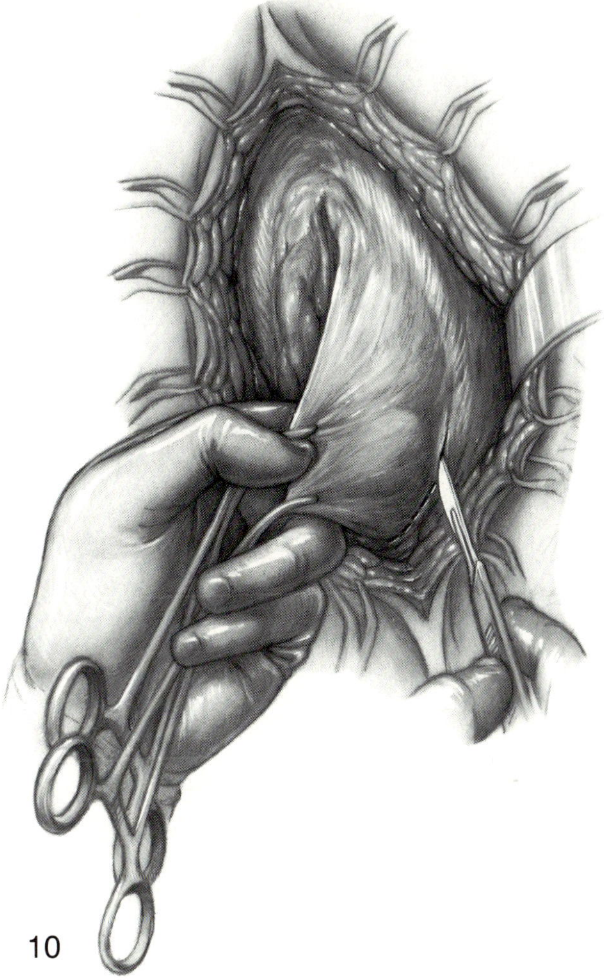

10

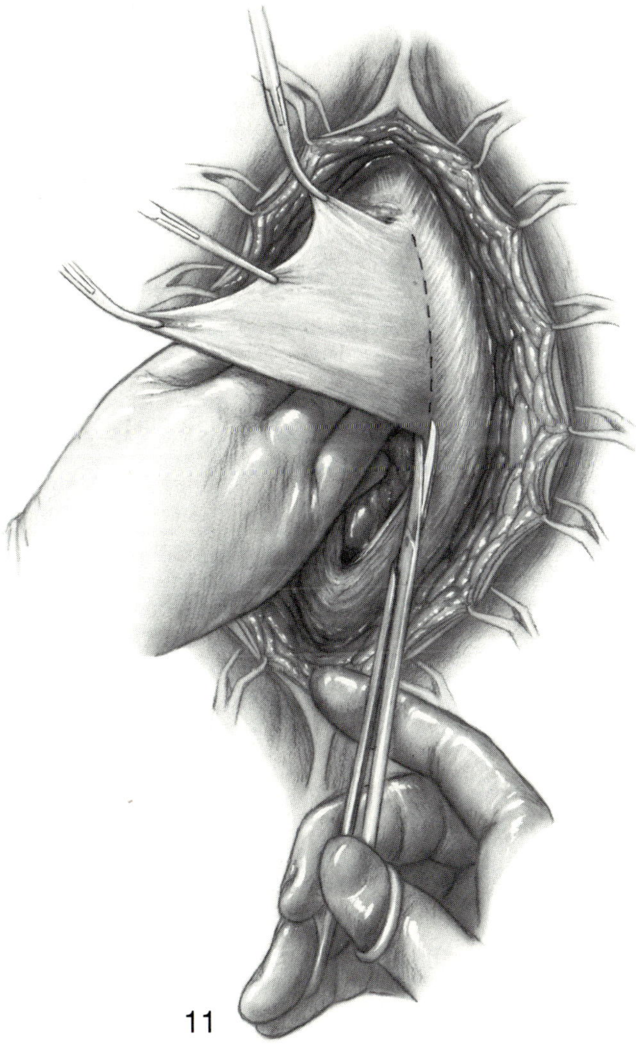

11

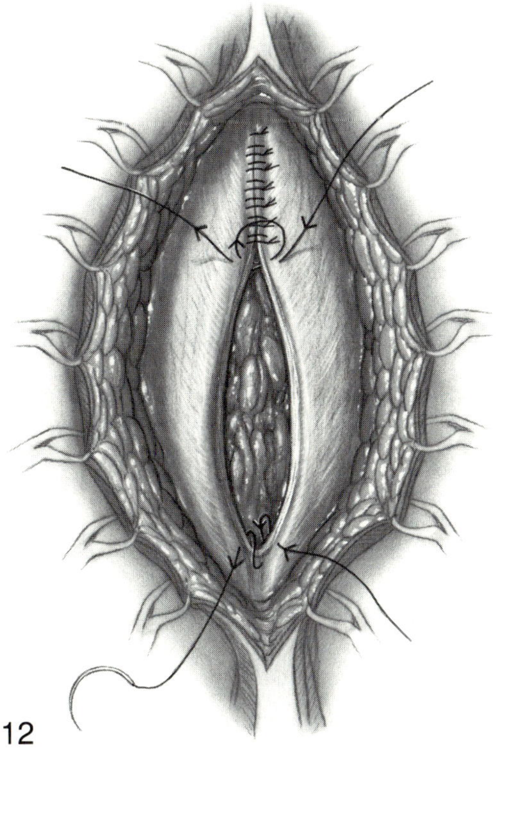

12

REPAIR OF AN INCISIONAL HERNIA
Continued

13 The closure of the hernial defect is completed, and perforated plastic tubes are inserted beneath the skin flaps for drainage. An alternate method for tube drainage is to direct one tube cephalad and the other caudad, with their corresponding exits at opposite poles.

14 The skin is closed with interrupted sutures of 3-0 silk threaded on straight (cambric) needles. The needles are inserted separately and then withdrawn individually, and the sutures are tied.

15 This illustration shows the completed closure of the wound. The tube drains are secured by silk sutures and exit through stab incisions.

REFERENCES

1. Usher FC: A new technique for repairing large abdominal wall defects. Arch Surg *82*:870–877, 1961.
2. Usher FC: The repair of incisional and inguinal hernias. Surg Gynecol Obstet *131*:525–530, 1970.

DISCUSSION

Joseph L. Ponka, M.D.

I am in complete agreement with Madden's technique in which the cicatrix from the previous operation is excised (**2, 3**). Since adherent bowel commonly is present just beneath the scar, caution must be observed in its excision to avoid injury to the bowel. Furthermore, any excess skin may be excised to effect a better cosmetic result.

Multiple rake retractors or small skin hooks may be used instead of towel clamps for upward traction on the skin flap (**5**) to facilitate its mobilization. The principle of tissue tension by traction and countertraction is demonstrated (**6**). The clamps are pulled up by an assistant for traction and the left hand of the surgeon exerts downward countertraction as the skin flap is being mobilized by scalpel dissection in the subcutaneous tissue plane.

Freeing the false sac of adherent intraperitoneal viscera and omentum must be carefully done, preferably by sharp dissection as illustrated (**8**). It is most important that the dissection of the false sac be extended laterally to expose the normal fascia of the anterior abdominal wall (**10, 11**).

I frequently use the same technique for excision of the false sac as the one depicted (**9–11**). However, there are occasions in the repair of large incisional hernias when extensive destruction of the abdominal wall has occurred. Since the implantation of a mesh prosthesis is required in these circumstances, a portion of the false sac may prove useful as a cover for the mesh.

The illustrations of the closure of the defect in the abdominal wall (**12, 13**) are excellent. The accurate approximation of normal anatomic structures is axiomatic. Frequently, however, I use figure-of-eight sutures in the closure of the abdominal wall.

The use of the plastic tubes for drainage of the wound (**13**) is commendable. Mechanical suction applied to these tubes evacuates air, blood, or serum, which otherwise could cause elevation of the skin flaps and provide a potential nidus for postoperative wound infection.

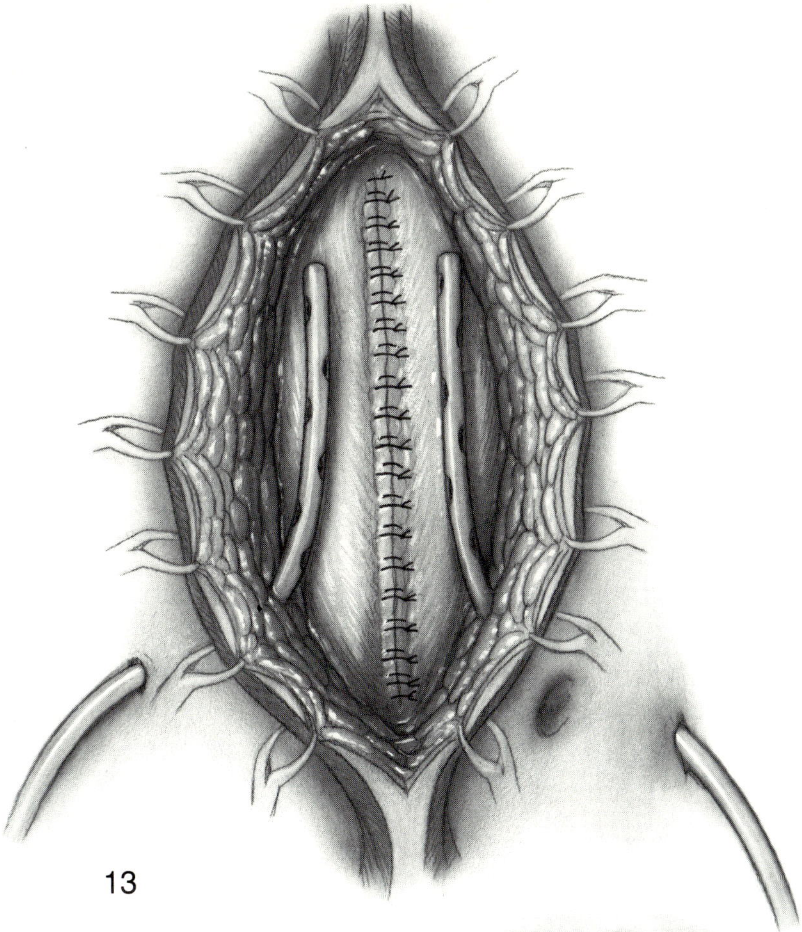

13

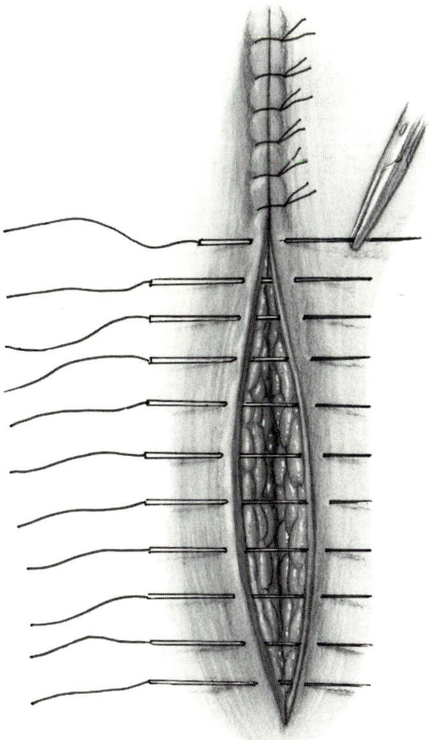

14

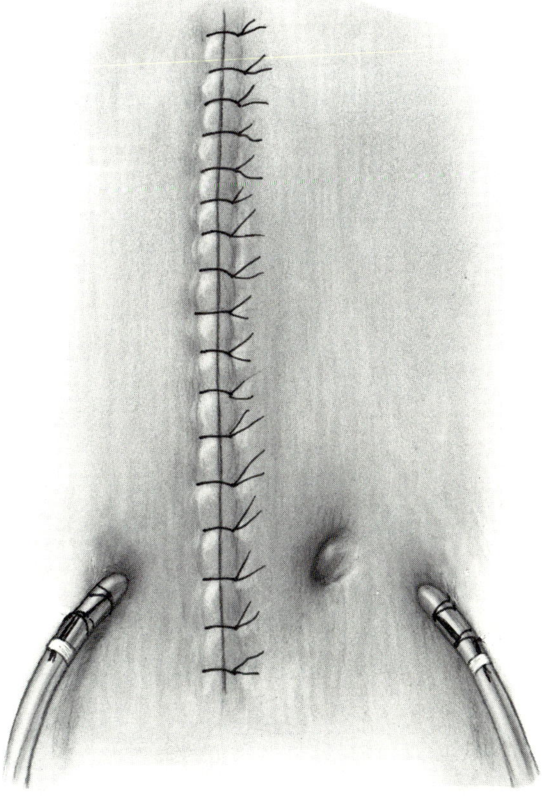

15

OPERATION 16

REPAIR OF AN INCISIONAL HERNIA WITH MARLEX MESH

Technique of Francis C. Usher, M.D.

Plate LXIX
Plate LXX

The technique illustrated here was witnessed by the artist, Frank Robinson, during his visits with Usher. The first two illustrations were done by Robinson. The remainder were executed by Grant Lashbrook from the finished sketches done previously by Robinson.

1 The false sac of the incisional hernia has been excised, and the fascial margins of the hernial ring are exposed. A 2-inch-wide rectangular strip of polypropylene mesh (Marlex) is sutured to the anterior fascial margin, using a continuous suture of polypropylene monofilament (1-0).

2 An assistant everts the fascial margin to facilitate the insertion of a similar continuous suture posteriorly, to form a mesh "cuff" over the edge of the hernial ring. In like manner, a second cuff of polypropylene mesh will cover the opposing hernial edge.

3, 3A Imbricating on-end vertical mattress sutures of polypropylene monofilament (1-0) are inserted 3/4-inch apart; each suture must pass through the anterior and posterior layers of the mesh. Four sutures have been inserted; the lower two are tied to imbricate the cuffed margins of the hernial ring at its lower angle (**3**). A diagrammatic representation of the insertion of the mattress suture is shown in **3A**.

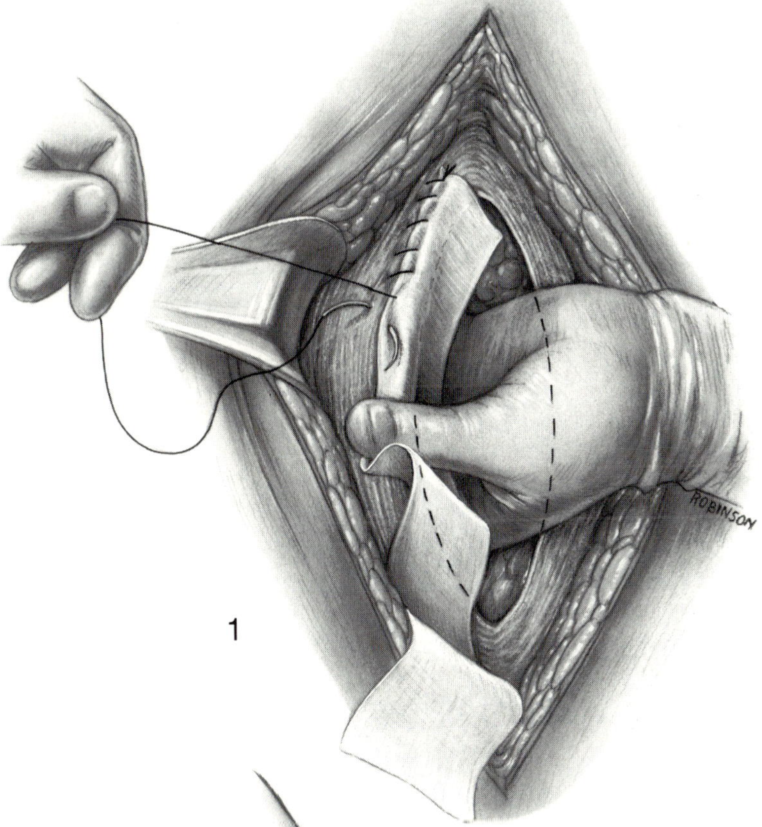

1

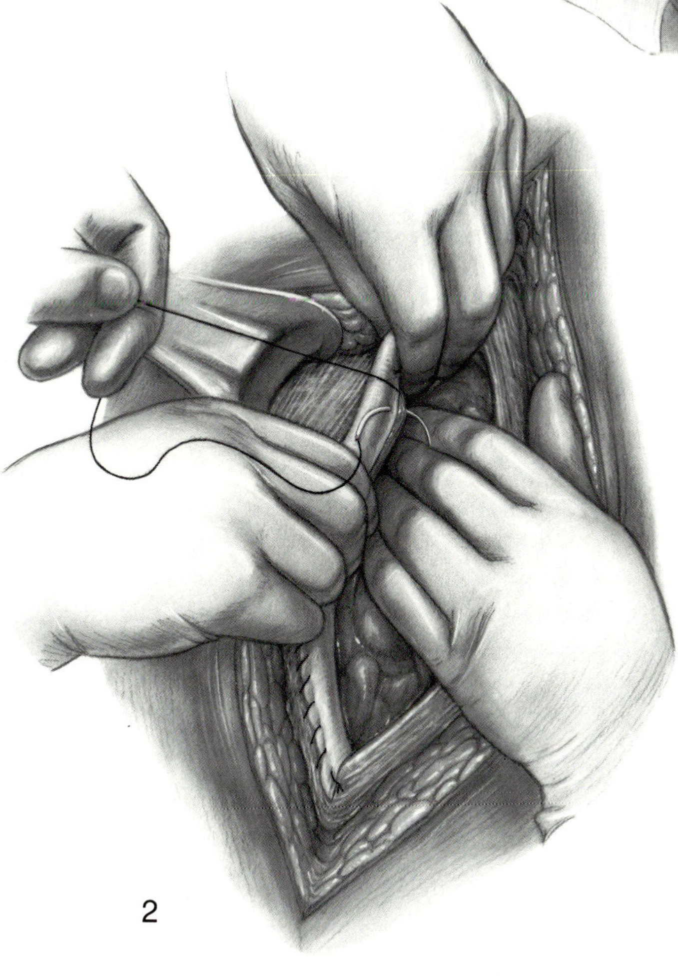

2

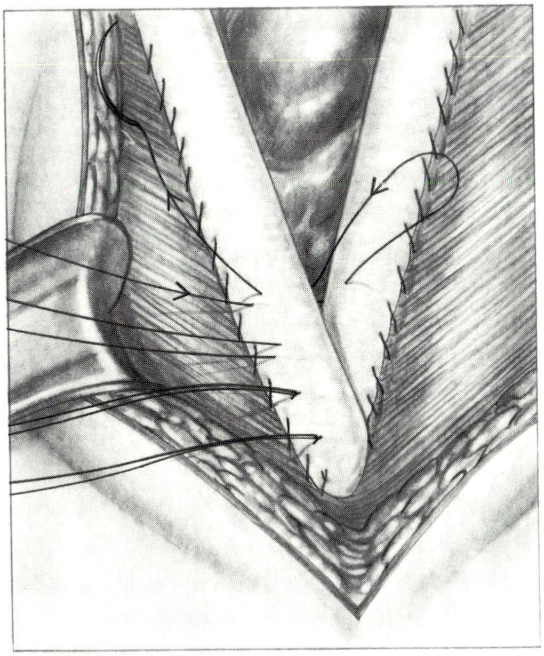

3

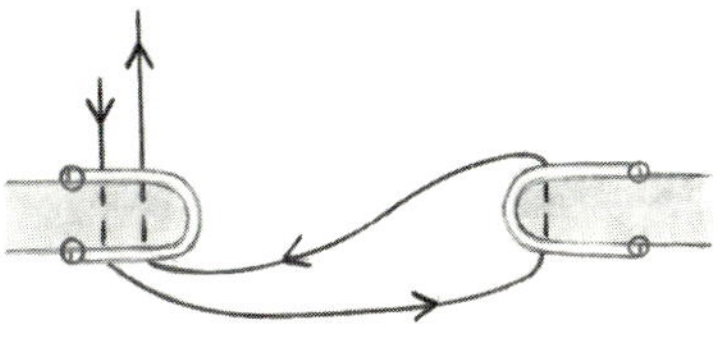

3A

REPAIR OF AN INCISIONAL HERNIA WITH MARLEX MESH *Continued*

4 For technical expediency, the succeeding mattress sutures are inserted before being tied. Simultaneous upward traction is maintained on the strands of these sutures by the assistant as they are tied in sequence to imbricate the opposing margins of the hernial ring.

The tissue reinforcement provided by the mesh cuff permits the closure of large incisional hernial defects, even under considerable tension, without the imbrication sutures cutting through.

5, 5A The imbrication closure of the hernial defect is completed, and interrupted sutures of polypropylene monofilament (1-0) are used to secure the edge of the mesh cuff of the overlying layer to the base of the underlying mesh cuff (**5**). The sutures are placed about 1 inch apart; for security of closure, they must pass through both mesh and fascia (**5A**).

6, 6A The repair of the incisional hernia is completed. Redundant subcutaneous fat and skin are excised from each side of the wound to eliminate dead space. Suction catheters are inserted as shown, and the subcutaneous fat and skin are closed with interrupted sutures of 3-0 chromic catgut and 3-0 silk, respectively (**6**). An alternative method for the placement of the suction catheters is depicted in **6A**.

In the repair of large incisional hernias, pulmonary ventilation frequently is compromised. Accordingly, in the immediate postoperative period precautionary measures must be taken to prevent pulmonary complications.

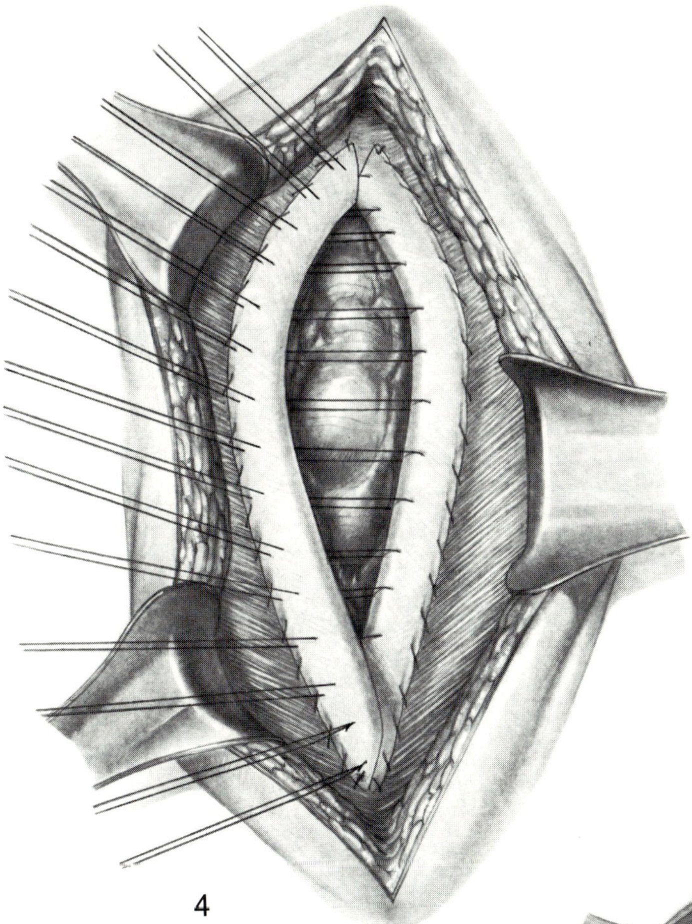

4

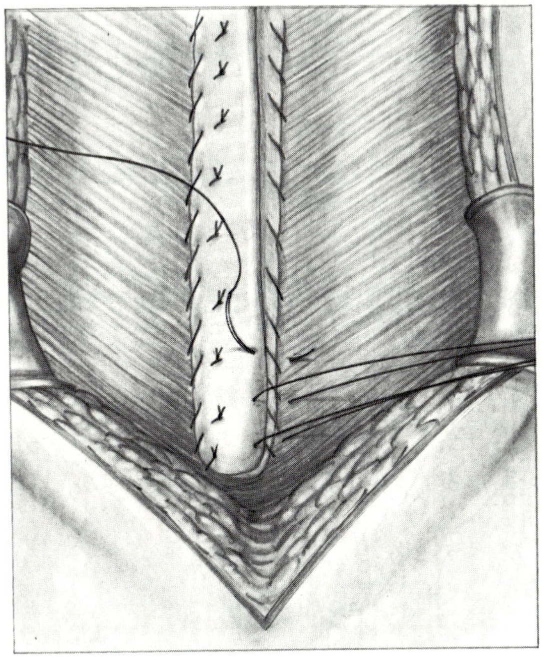

5

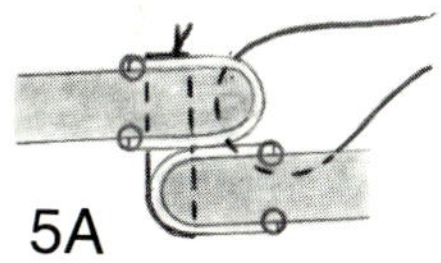

5A

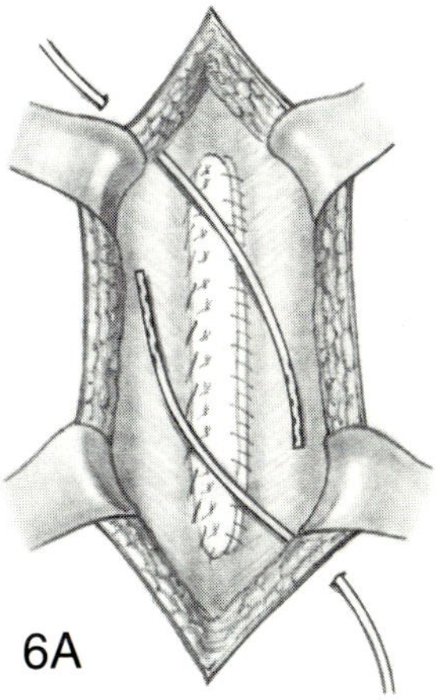

6A

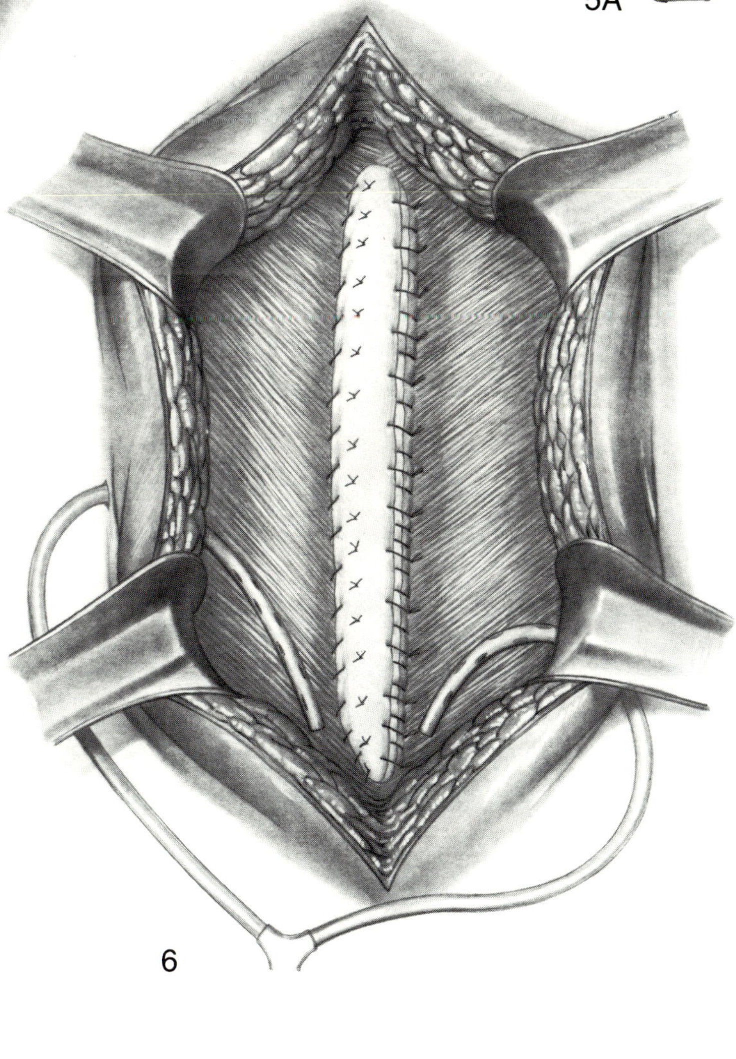

6

OPERATION 17

REPAIR OF LARGE INCISIONAL HERNIAS WITH INTERNAL MESH SUPPORTS

JOSEPH L. PONKA, M.D.

Plate LXXI
Plate LXXII
Plate LXXIII

In the surgical treatment of patients with large incisional hernias, the use of the patient's own tissues is preferred. However, an increasing number of these patients require the use of foreign body implants, either synthetic or metallic. The favored implant is polypropylene (Marlex) mesh.

In the use of mesh implants, certain basic requirements must be met to enhance the success of the implantation. The immediate essentials are the excision of the underlying scar tissue, careful hemostasis, and identification of the layers of the anterior abdominal wall. Next, an adequately sized sheet of mesh, selected to bridge completely the hernial defect, is sutured under slight tension.

Extraperitoneal implantation is advisable in order to avoid direct contact of the mesh with intestinal loops. Otherwise, the dense adhesions that form between the bowel and the mesh would make surgical dissection most difficult should a subsequent operation be required. If sufficient omentum is available to cover the exposed intestine, however, the mesh may be applied directly.

Chromic catgut or synthetic sutures have been used for the fixation of the mesh, which is covered whenever possible with a layer of muscle or fascia. Currently, catgut sutures alone are never used because they do not provide the long-term holding strength that is required. Should this coverage result in undue tissue tension, appropriate relaxing incisions may be made. However, if the uncovered area of mesh is small, it is simply covered by the overlying subcutaneous fatty tissue layer and skin. The use of a Hemovac suction apparatus with drainage tubes of 1/4-inch diameter is recommended to lessen hematoma or seroma formation postoperatively.

1, 2 The false hernial sac has been excised, and the layers of the abdominal wall are prepared for closure (**1**). The relationship of the layers of the anterior abdominal wall to the hernial defect is shown in cross-section (**2**).

3, 4 The mobilization of the layers of the anterior abdominal wall is completed (**3**), and the adjacent layers of the posterior rectus sheath and peritoneum are approximated with interrupted far-and-near, near-and-far (pulley) sutures of 2-0 chromic catgut.

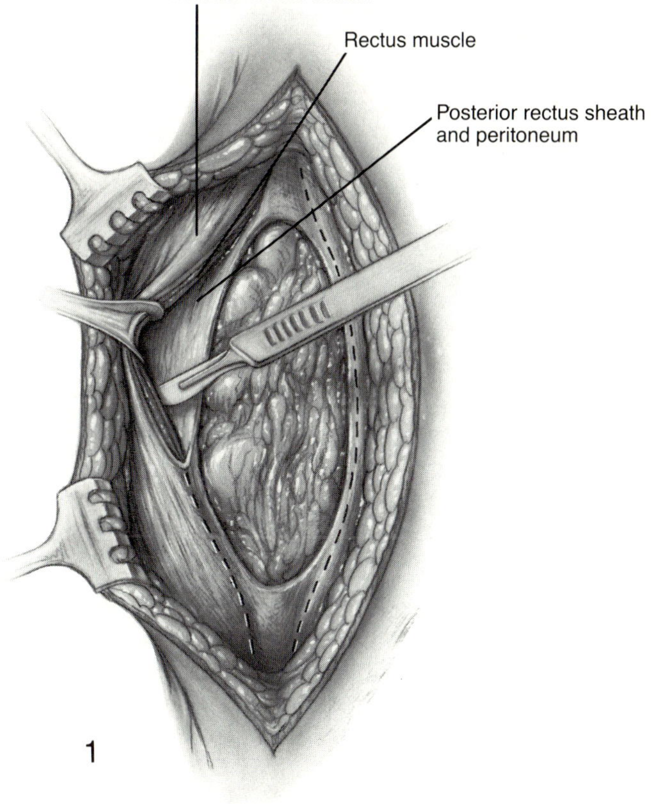
Anterior rectus sheath
Rectus muscle
Posterior rectus sheath
and peritoneum

1

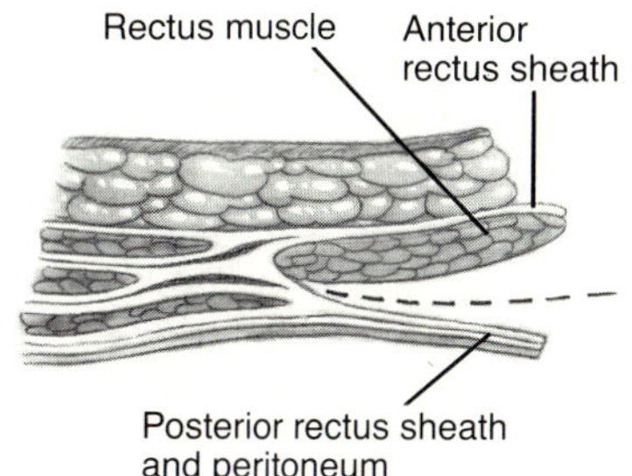
Rectus muscle
Anterior
rectus sheath
Posterior rectus sheath
and peritoneum

2

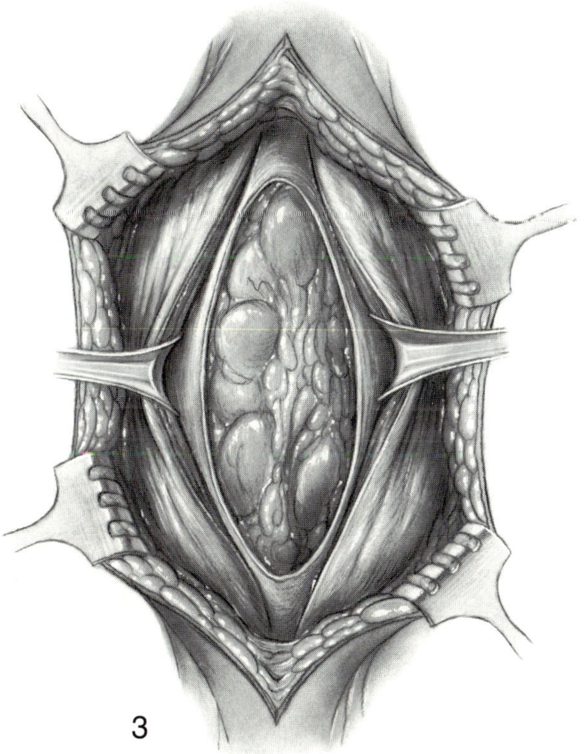

3

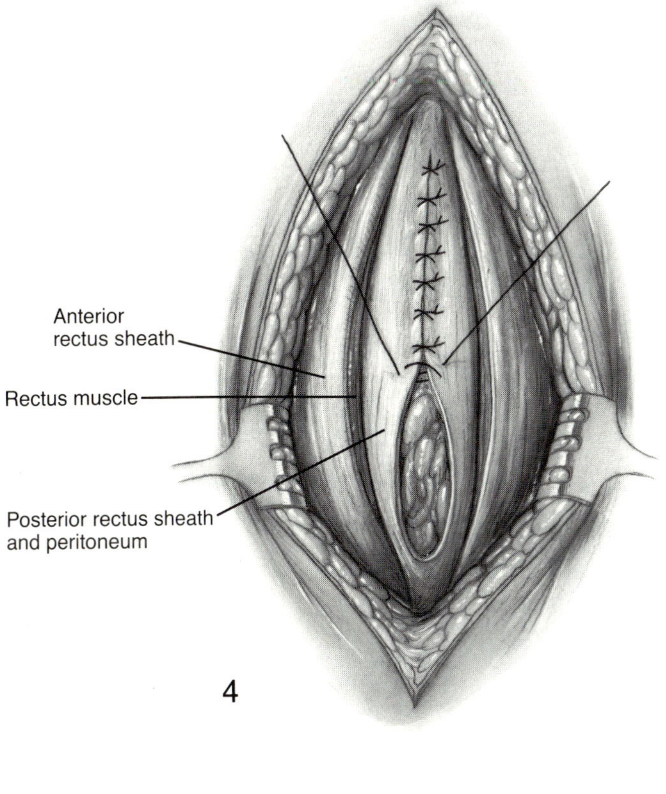
Anterior
rectus sheath
Rectus muscle
Posterior rectus sheath
and peritoneum

4

REPAIR OF LARGE INCISIONAL HERNIAS WITH INTERNAL MESH SUPPORTS *Continued*

5, 6, 7, 8, 9 The mesh is implanted beneath the musculofascial layer of the right side of the anterior abdominal wall, using interrupted mattress sutures of 1-0 chromic catgut (**5**). One of these sutures is shown in cross-section (**6**). The implantation of the mesh, which is under slight tension, is completed, and its relationship to the surrounding structures can be seen (**7**).

The margins of the musculofascial layer of the anterior abdominal wall are sutured together over the mesh implant with nonabsorbable 2-0 monofilament synthetic sutures, in conjunction with relaxing incisions in the fascia on each side (**8**).

To avoid tension on the line of closure over the mesh, a small segment is left exposed, which will be covered by the subcutaneous fat and skin (**9**). The use of multiple small relaxing incisions through the anterior rectus sheaths, as an alternative to the use of longitudinal incisions, is depicted.

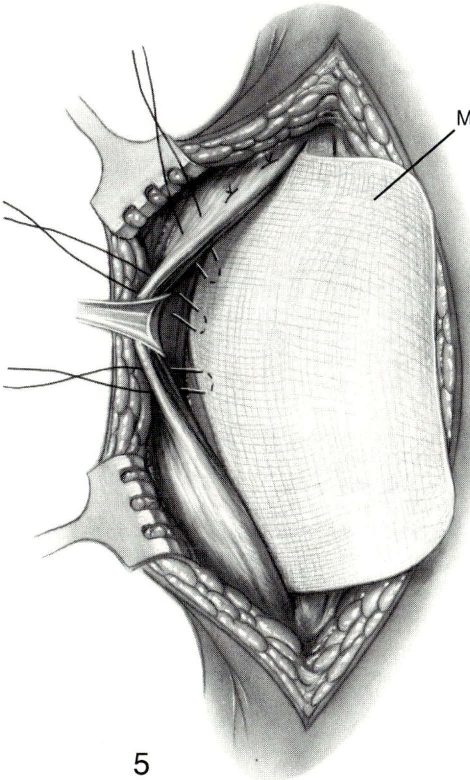

5

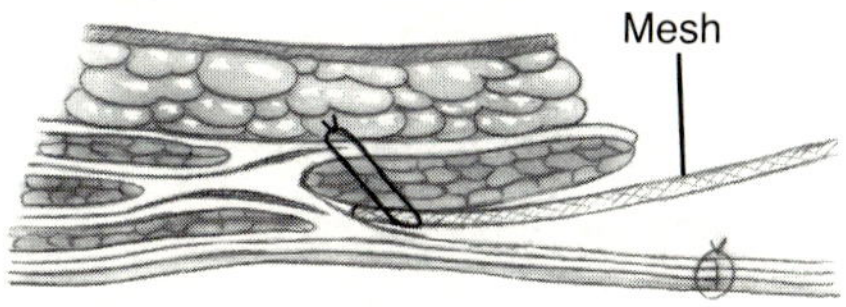

6

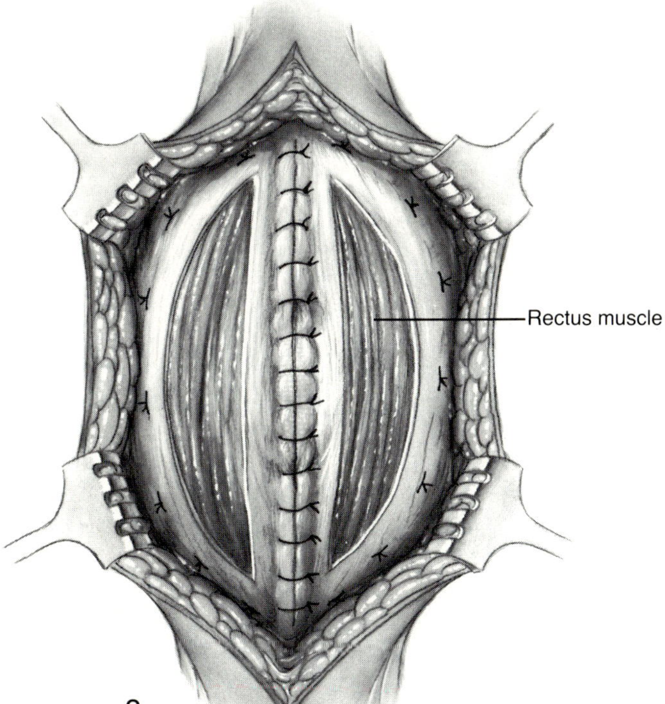

8

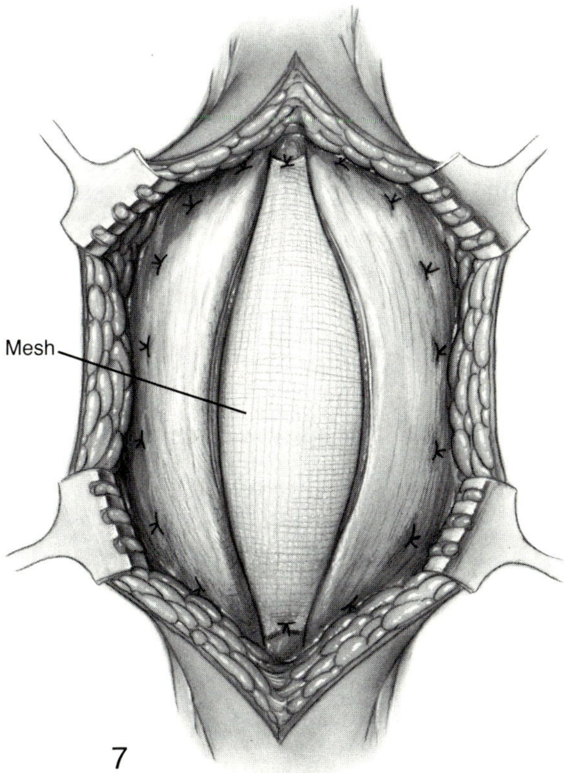

7

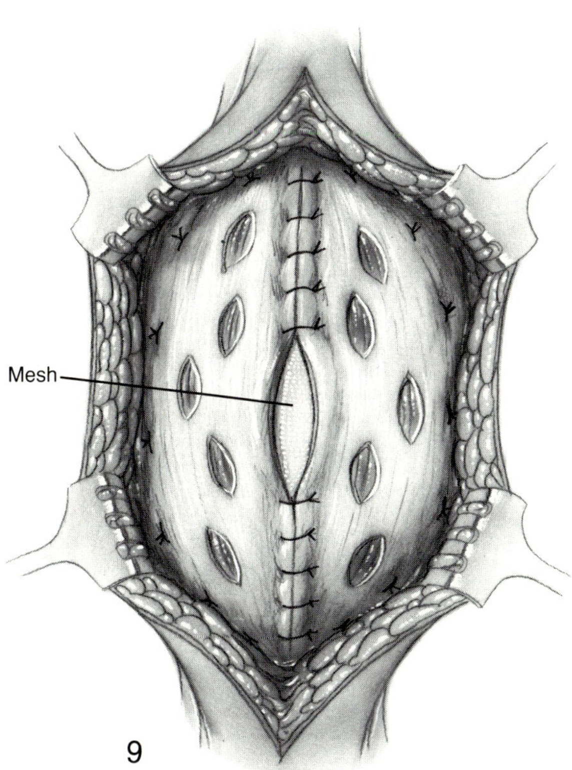

9

10 This preoperative sketch shows a patient with a huge, recurrent, infraumbilical midline incisional hernia. In a hernia of this type, a large sheet of Marlex mesh is placed deep and anterior to the peritoneum. Furthermore, since the bladder may protrude into the hernia, its recognition and replacement into its normal retropubic position are essential to the success of the operation.

10A A sheet of Marlex mesh is implanted in front of the peritoneum. It is attached cephalad to the lower middle and lateral portions of the anterior abdominal wall with 2-0 polypropylene monofilament sutures. Using the same type of sutures, the mesh is sutured caudad to the symphysis pubis and laterally, on each side, to Cooper's ligament.

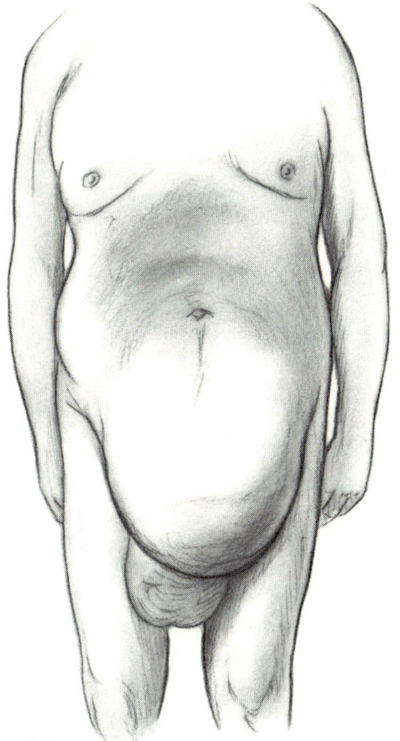

10

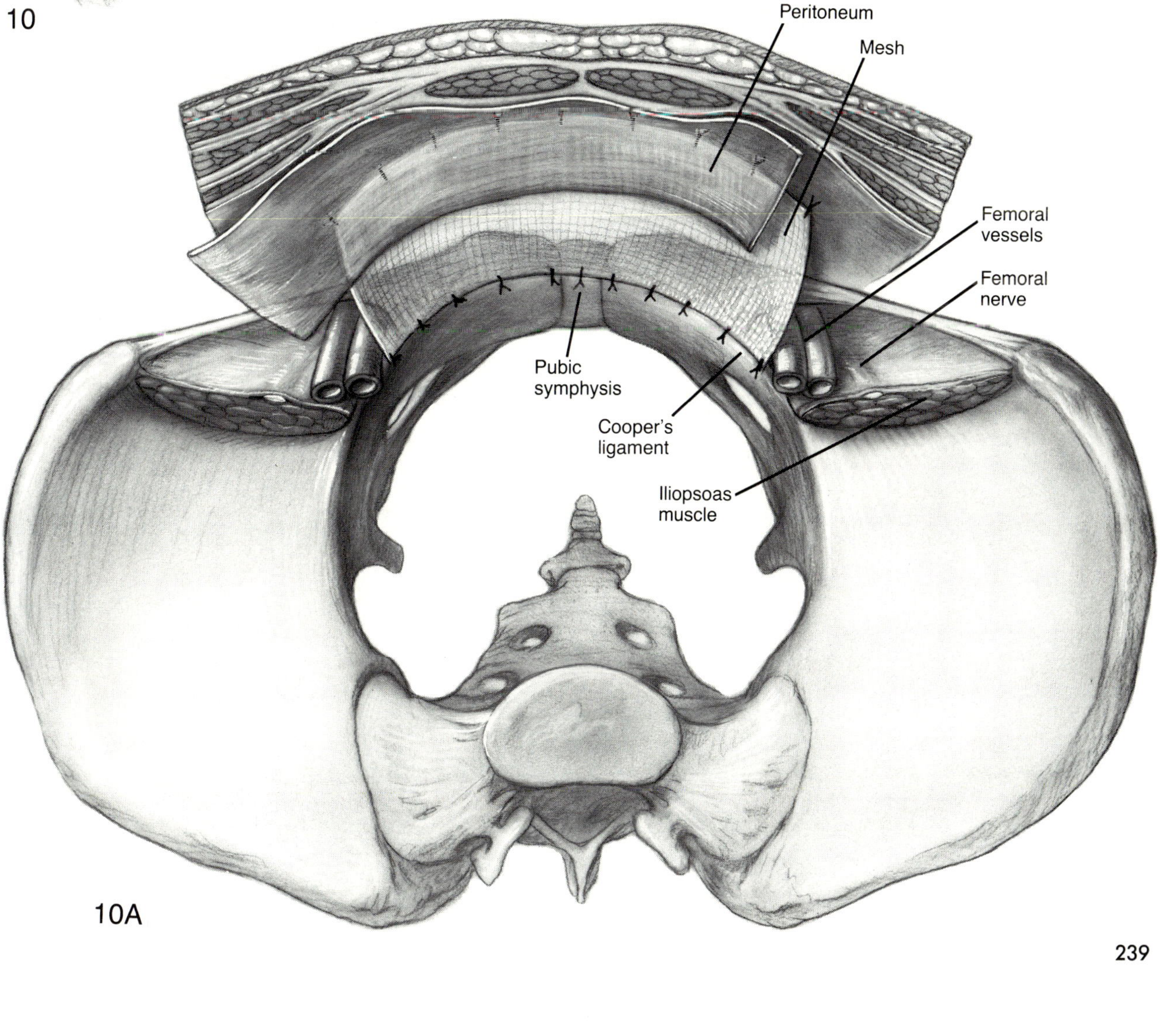
Peritoneum
Mesh
Femoral vessels
Femoral nerve
Pubic symphysis
Cooper's ligament
Iliopsoas muscle

10A

REPAIR OF LARGE INCISIONAL HERNIAS WITH INTERNAL MESH SUPPORTS *Continued*

11 This preoperative sketch depicts a woman with a large inguinofemoral recurrent hernia. In this type of hernia, the inguinal ligament and a portion of the anterior abdominal wall may be absent; not infrequently the hernia will extend into the upper part of the thigh. Therefore, the use of a large sheet of Marlex mesh is mandatory.

The incision for the repair of the hernia extends obliquely down from the anterior-superior iliac spine to the symphysis pubis, 2 or 3 cm superior to the inguinal ligament. The surgical dissection extends to the depths of the incision to expose the aponeurosis of the external oblique muscle, the rectus sheath, and the area of the upper part of the thigh. The femoral vessels and nerve are identified and kept in view throughout the duration of the tissue dissection.

When the dissection of the false sac is completed, it is opened and freed of any incarcerated omentum or loops of bowel. The neck of the sac is then closed, and its redundant portion is excised.

11A A cut-away view of the completed implantation of the Marlex mesh shows its relationship to the neighboring structures.

The mesh is placed deep to and in front of the peritoneum to cover an area that encompasses the anterior-superior iliac spine, the pubic tubercle, and the iliopectineal fascia (Cooper's ligament). Caudad it is sutured (2-0 polypropylene monofilament) to the anterosuperior iliac spine, the transversalis fascia, and the iliopectineal fascia (Cooper's ligament). Cephalad it is attached to the musculofascial structures of the lower and middle portions of the posterior abdominal wall and then laterally in continuity to the lamina of the posterior abdominal wall. In effect, suturing the mesh to the anterior-superior iliac spine and pubic tubercle serves as a replacement for the transversalis fascia and inguinal ligament.

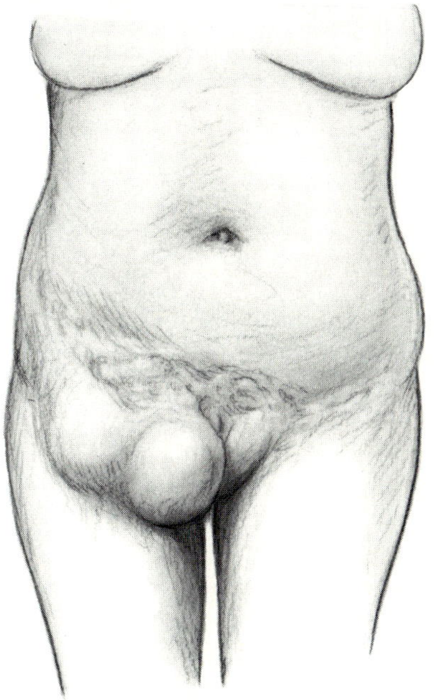

11

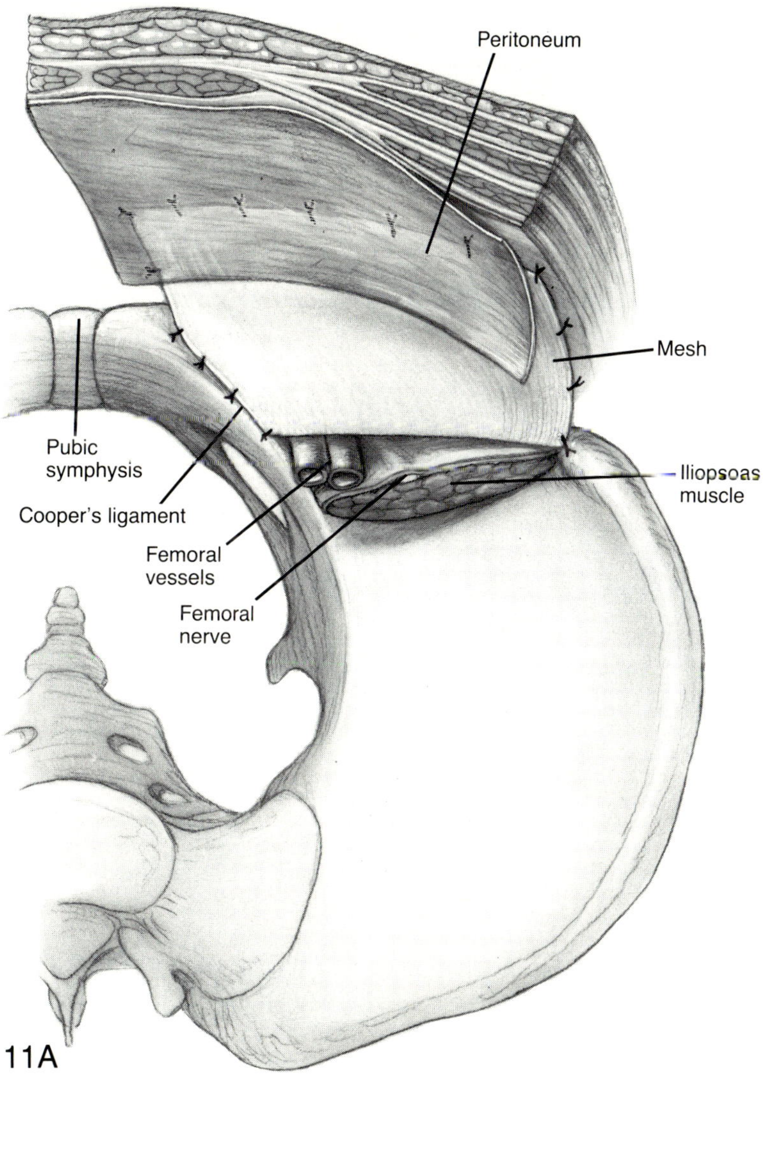
Peritoneum
Mesh
Pubic symphysis
Cooper's ligament
Iliopsoas muscle
Femoral vessels
Femoral nerve

11A

OPERATION 18

REPAIR OF RECURRENT GROIN HERNIAS BY THE INSERTION OF GIANT MESH PROSTHESES THROUGH THE MIDLINE PREPERITONEAL APPROACH (GPMPA)

R.E. STOPPA
C.R. WARLAUMONT

Plate LXXIV
Plate LXXV
Plate LXXVI
Plate LXXVII
Plate LXXVIII

We agree with the opinion that primary and recurrent groin hernias result from disruption or relaxation of the fascia of the posterior inguinal wall. The surgical cure of these hernias must restore the normal protective function of this fascia. Among the techniques proposed for this restoration, we would like to stress the technical advantages in the use of mesh prostheses in the treatment of recurrent hernias, particularly in patients who have had multiple recurrent hernias. It is also ideal in patients with recurrent hernias associated with contralateral groin hernias or lower incisional defects.

In our combined surgical experience of more than 20 years, we have treated such patients with the use of large Dacron mesh prostheses. These prostheses cover the groin areas on each side and are inserted between the peritoneum and posterior abdominal wall through a low midline preperitoneal abdominal incision. This original technique of the senior author (R.E.S.) is considered the "absolute weapon" against a further recurrence of the hernia. It is easy to perform and requires neither extensive surgical experience nor exceptional technical skills.

ANATOMY

In discussing the anatomy pertaining to our technique, we would like to stress structures that are seen through the posterior rather than the anterior route.

1. In support of the previous anatomic studies of Fruchaud, we emphasize the anatomic fact that all groin hernias protrude through the "musculopectineal hole" (**1**). This hole is seen perfectly through the posterior approach, after removing the peritoneum and preperitoneal fat. It is bounded medially by the lateral border of the rectus muscle, superiorly by the so-called conjoined tendon (falx inguinalis), and inferiorly by Cooper's ligament (pectineal ligament). These structures form a solid frame within which the sole tight layer resisting the intraabdominal pressure is the drum-like transversalis fascia, which has been damaged to some extent by previous operations in the repair of recurrent hernias. The insertion of a prosthetic mesh instantly and definitively tightens the musculopectineal hole.

2. The transversalis fascia is the reinforced inguinal part of the endoabdominal fascial layer, which at this level envelops the peritoneum. In the groin, it adheres intimately to the posterior surface of the transversus abdominis muscle, the lower margin of the inguinal ligament, and laterally to the iliac fascia. Below the inguinal ligament it forms the true femoral sheath (**2**).

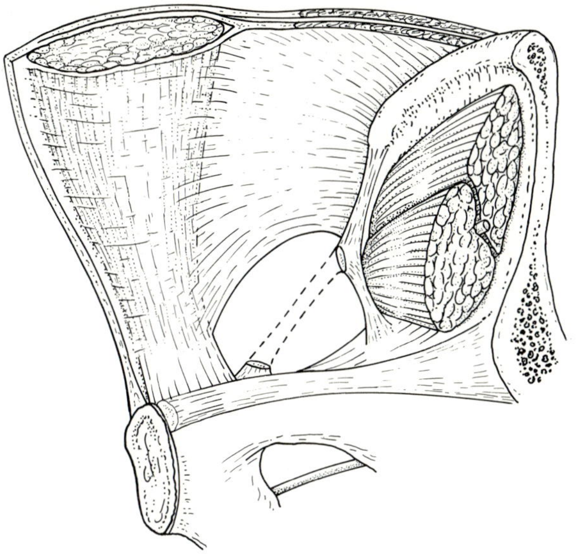

1 Schematic drawing of the right musculopectineal hole, from a posteromedial point of view (after Fruchaud). All groin hernias cross the wall through this hole and can be repaired by the use of the giant prosthesis. The iliopubic tract in relation to the musculopectineal hole is shown in dotted outline.

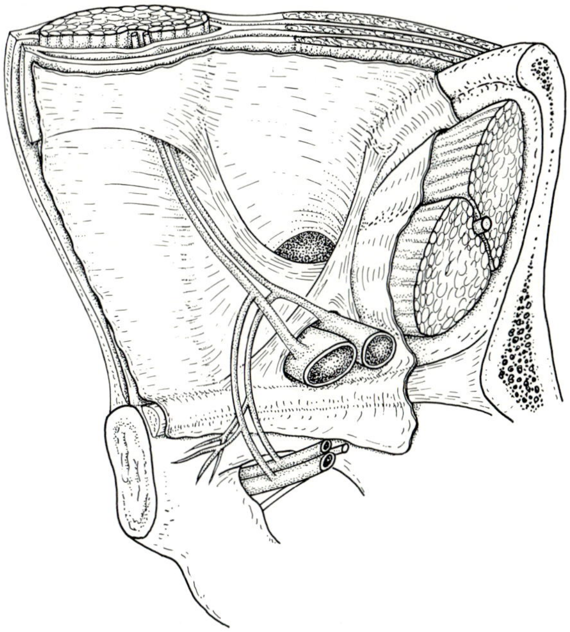

2 Schematic posterior view of the transversalis fascia in the right inguinal area. This is the deep inguinal layer that will be reinforced or replaced by the giant prosthesis.

3. The preperitoneal cleavage space, an areolar adipose layer of variable thickness, separates the transversalis fascia from the peritoneum, except above the arcuate line of Douglas, where it is absent. It penetrates forward and down between the bladder and the pubis into what is called Retzius' space (retropubic space) and laterally invests Bogros' space (retroinguinal space) in continuity with the iliac fascia. These spaces are useful surgical guides to the deep hernial defects of the groin and a perfect site for the placement of the giant bilateral groin prostheses that are frequently used (**3, 3A**).

4. The advantages of the subumbilical midline incision are striking when repairing recurrent hernias. Surgical dissection proceeds in the cleavage planes of the retroparietal spaces from the normal toward the abnormal surgical anatomy, with fast and direct exposure of the musculopectineal hole and hernial orifices. Therefore, there is no risk of injury to the surrounding structures—nerves, spermatic cord, and femoral vessels. The angle between the inferior epigastric vessels and the iliac vessels (*dashed lines* in **4**) marks clearly the site of the retroparietal convergence of the components of the cord (the vas deferens and the internal spermatic vessels). The hernial sac (or sacs) can be easily identified and reduced either by manual retraction or, when they are adherent to the neck of the hernial orifice, by combined scalpel and scissors dissection.

OTHER PRINCIPLES

Dacron polyester mesh has been used for more than 20 years. It is nonexpansive, supple, resistant, biologically well tolerated, and evokes a fibroblastic response for rapid fixation within the surrounding tissues. Marlex or Prolene (polypropylene) meshes are not used because they are less supple.

The excellent tissue tolerance for Dacron mesh permits the implantation of large pieces between the visceral sac and the endoabdominal fascia. Immediately following the implant, the inguinal hernial defect is corrected in keeping with Pascal's hydrostatic principle—the intraabdominal pressure rapidly fixes the position of the prosthesis, which is secondarily invested by the surrounding connective tissue. In other words, the intraabdominal force that was the cause of the herniation is now used to prevent its recurrence. This principle is considered the revolutionary basis of our method.

REPAIR OF RECURRENT GROIN HERNIAS BY THE INSERTION OF GIANT MESH PROSTHESES THROUGH THE MIDLINE PREPERITONEAL APPROACH (GPMPA)

Continued

The larger the prosthesis the more efficient is the repair, since there is no need for fixation of the mesh or for the use of sutures to close the hernial defect (or defects). The simplicity and effective clinical application of this technique have proved most gratifying to both patients and surgeons. Furthermore, this technique is particularly applicable in huge re-recurrent hernias, where the damage to the tissues overlying the hernial recurrence makes any attempts at an anterior repair difficult.

REPAIR OF A BILATERAL RECURRENT INGUINAL HERNIA: MIDLINE PREPERITONEAL APPROACH

Preparation

Because of the dire consequences of septic complications in the use of mesh prostheses, strict precautionary measures for the prevention of infection are mandatory. The skin of the operative area is carefully prepared with appropriate antiseptic solutions. In patients with enormous scrotal hernias and in those with ventilatory insufficiency, progressive pneumoperitoneum (Goni Moreno) may be required. General or spinal peridural anesthesia is preferred; conversely, local anesthesia is not used.

Useful surgical tools include mounted peanut swabs for cleavage of the retroparietal spaces; retractors for the abdominal wall; snares (rubber tissue tapes) for handling the cord; a sterile scale, straight scissors, and eight long curved Kelly forceps for measuring, cutting, and "no touch" handling of the mesh; small suction drains; and slowly absorbable synthetic sutures.

Procedure

Midline Preperitoneal Approach

The patient is placed in a mild Trendelenburg's position. The surgeon and nurse are positioned on the side of the larger defect; the assistant is on the opposite side. A sterile plastic adhesive is carefully placed on the skin, covering both sides of the lower abdominal wall. The layers of the abdominal wall are opened through a subumbilical midline incision extending from 2 cm above the pubis to 2 cm below the umbilicus (**5**). The subumbilical linea alba and the preperitoneal and prevesical fascia are cut with scissors.

Retroparietal Cleavage

The retroparietal cleavage is begun inferiorly in Retzius's space, using a mounted swab. The cleavage plane progresses laterally under the rectus abdominis muscle and posteriorly to the inferior epigastric vessels (**6**). The pedicle of the hernia, which is

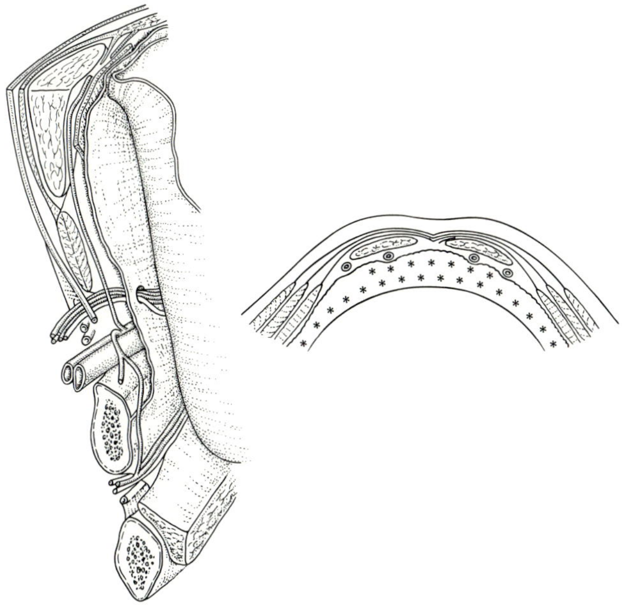

3, 3A Schematic cross-sections of the lower part of the abdomen showing the retroparietal cleavage spaces used for the placement of the giant prosthesis. 3 = sagittal representation; 3A = horizontal section.

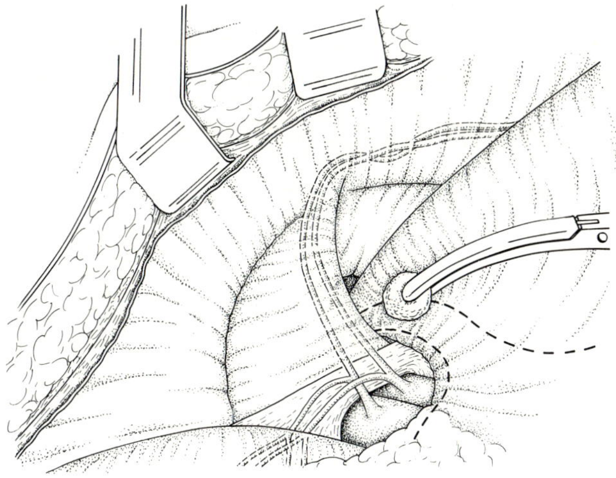

4 Schematic representation of the angle between the inferior epigastric vessels and the iliac vessels, as seen by the surgeon from the midline subumbilical approach. Also visible during the retroparietal cleavage is the angle of convergence of the internal spermatic vessels (*lateral dashed line*) and the vas deferens (*medial dashed line*), to form the spermatic cord at its passage through the deep inguinal orifice.

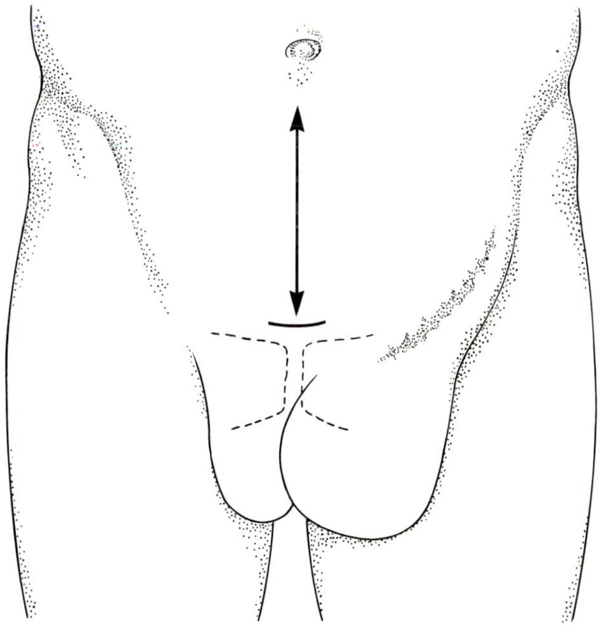

5 Schematic representation of the midline subumbilical incision for the insertion of a giant prosthesis.

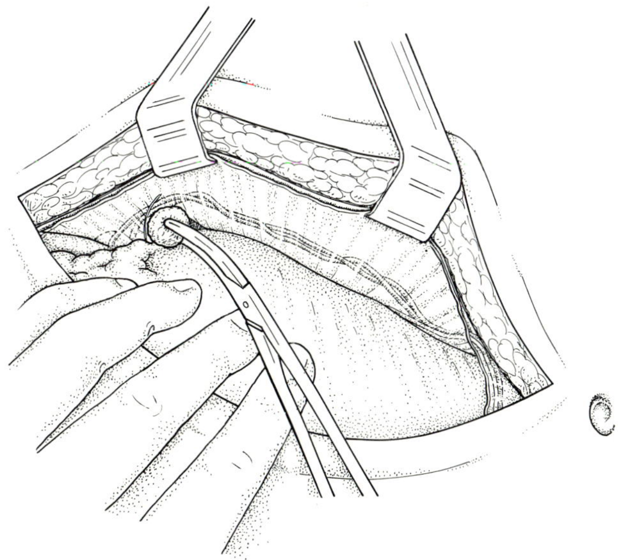

6 Schematic intraoperative view of the cleavage of the retroparietal Bogros' space (*right*), progressing posterolaterally to the inferior epigastric vessels. The linea arcuata of Douglas (*right inferior*), which is the superior limit of the retroparietal cleavage, may also be seen.

REPAIR OF RECURRENT GROIN HERNIAS BY THE INSERTION OF GIANT MESH PROSTHESES THROUGH THE MIDLINE PREPERITONEAL APPROACH (GPMPA)

Continued

rapidly isolated, is distinct from the spermatic cord in the direct inguinal (**7**) and femoral (**7A**) recurrences but is connected to it in the indirect inguinal recurrence (**8**). The hernial sac (or sacs) is treated according to the extent of the adhesion to its neck. Continuous moderate traction sometimes is sufficient to separate a small sac from the hernial defect. In other cases, both scalpel and scissors dissection are required to free the densely adherent sac of a re-recurrent hernia. The dissection frequently is aided by inserting the index finger into the lumen of the sac for traction. All clinically dubious or hidden defects are readily discovered and safely treated through this route. Furthermore, an accurate classification of the recurrent hernial defect may be made.

Treatment of the Sac (or Sacs)

No problem is encountered during this step of the operation. Small direct hernial sacs are simply reduced. Large indirect hernial sacs are easily resected, and the peritoneum is closed with absorbable sutures. Medium-sized indirect sacs may be treated by simple invagination and closure of the peritoneum infundibulum with a pursestring suture.

Parietalization of the Spermatic Cord Components

This step obviates the need to make an opening in the mesh for passage of the spermatic cord and simplifies the placement of the giant prosthesis. The spermatic cord is retracted forward and down with a rubber tissue tape (snare) as the peritoneum is retracted up by the surgeon's left hand. Beginning at the angle of their convergence, scissors and mounted swabs are used to separate the vas deferens and internal spermatic vessels from the peritoneal sac. Blunt dissection is continued posteriorly for a distance of 8 to 10 cm. When this dissection is completed, triangular areas of areolar tissue containing the vas deferens medially and the testicular vessels laterally can be seen (**9**). When the snare retracting the cord is removed, the funicular components, the vas deferens, and the testicular vessels appear parietalized.

The surgeon then changes sides and proceeds as previously described to perform the cleavage of the opposite side, which has the largest defect. Upon completion of the bilateral cleavage planes, one or more suction drains may be placed as desired.

Measurement of the Giant Prosthesis

The dimensions of the giant prosthesis are measured on the patient. The correct transverse dimension is 2 cm less than the distance between the two anterior-superior

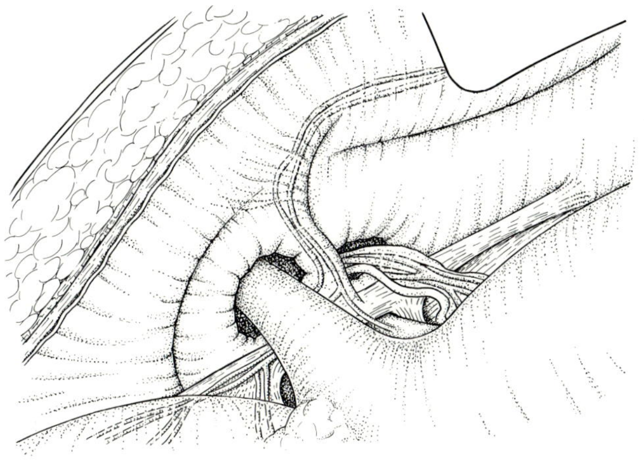

7 The pedicle of a right direct inguinal hernia, distinct from the cord, as seen in a schematic intraoperative view (opposite the surgeon).

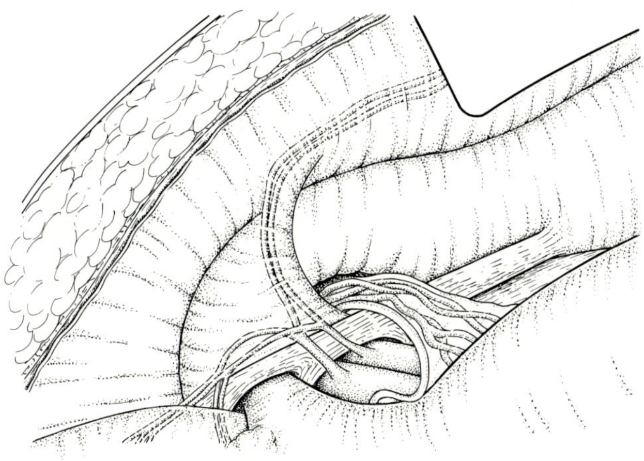

7A The pedicle of a right femoral hernia, also distinct from the cord, as seen from the posterior approach (schematic intraoperative view).

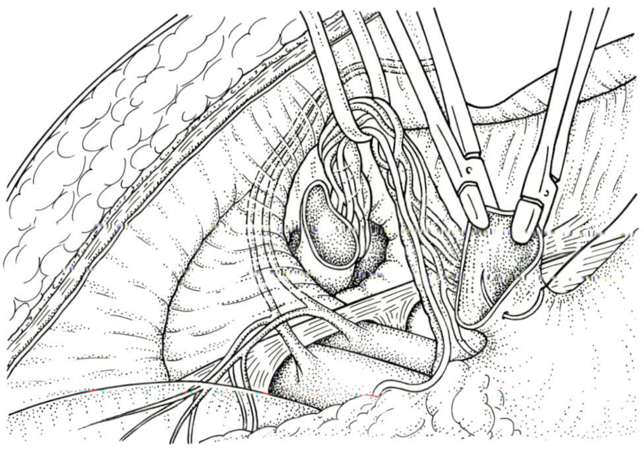

8 Schematic intraoperative view of the transected distal part of the sac of a right indirect inguinal hernia, previously connected to the cord. Its upper part is being closed; its open lower transected part will remain in situ in the scrotum.

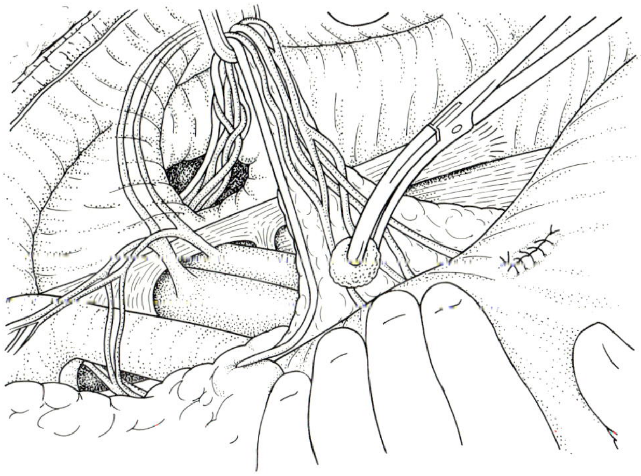

9 Schematic intraoperative view of the terminal step of the parietalization of the components of the right spermatic cord. The vas deferens is on the medial margin of the dissected triangular areolar sheet, and the internal spermatic vessels are on its lateral margin.

iliac spines; the correct vertical dimension is equal to the distance between the umbilicus and the pubis. The mean dimensions are 23 cm and 15 cm, respectively. The Dacron mesh is then cut to the correct measurement in a chevron shape, using a "no touch" technique. This shape corresponds cephalad with the arcuate line of Douglas; caudad, it overlaps the two musculopectineal holes (**10**).

Placement of the Giant Prosthesis

First, the corners and the middle of each margin of the prosthesis are grasped with long curved Kelly clamps. The peritoneum is then displaced upward by the surgeon's left hand while the abdominal wall is retracted by the assistant to open the retroparietal cleavage space. Using the Kelly clamps, the mesh prosthesis is simply inserted into place. The middle of the inferior margin of the prosthesis is placed between the pubis and the bladder. A Kelly clamp is placed on the inferior lateral corner, followed in

REPAIR OF RECURRENT GROIN HERNIAS BY THE INSERTION OF GIANT MESH PROSTHESES THROUGH THE MIDLINE PREPERITONEAL APPROACH (GPMPA)

Continued

succession by clamps on the midlateral margin and upper lateral corner. Each clamp is pushed as far as possible under the abdominal wall, thereby unfolding the mesh and at the same time placing it at the limits of the subparietal cleavage space. This maneuver permits the prosthesis to envelop the visceral sac on the side of the larger parietal defect. When the Kelly clamps have been pushed into place, they are immobilized by the assistant. The surgeon then removes his left hand, permitting the visceral sac to resume its normal position as the retracted abdominal wall is simultaneously released (**11**).

The surgeon again changes sides and repeats the placement procedure to cover the smaller defect on the other side. The resultant full unfolding of the giant Dacron mesh prosthesis envelops the visceral sac widely and extends well beyond the limits of the bilateral inguinal hernial defects. It also serves to protect the midline subumbilical surgical wound. A single absorbable mattress suture is inserted cephalad to fix the middle of the upper margin of the mesh to the lower margin of Richet's umbilical fascia (**12**).

Drainage and Closure of the Wound

One or two suction drains are placed anterior to the prosthesis. In large scrotal hernias, a suction drain is routinely placed in the scrotal cul-de-sac (**13**). Closure of the midline incisional wound is then performed with 3-0 and 5-0 absorbable synthetic sutures, which approximate the musculoaponeurotic planes. The subcutaneous tissue and skin are closed with fine monofilament sutures of nylon.

Postoperative Care

Early ambulation is prescribed and causes minimal postoperative discomfort. Slow-action heparin is given during the ensuing three to four days. Prophylactic antibiotic therapy is used under the following circumstances: (1) if sepsis has previously occurred after the repair of a recurrent hernia; (2) in huge inguinoscrotal hernias; (3) when scrotal incisions have been made to facilitate the reduction of the hernial contents; and (4) in the rare circumstance when the duration of the operation has exceeded one hour. If suction drainage has been used, the antibiotics are discontinued on the second postoperative day, at which time the dressing also is removed for inspection of the wound. Generally, patients are discharged on the fourth or fifth day after the operation.

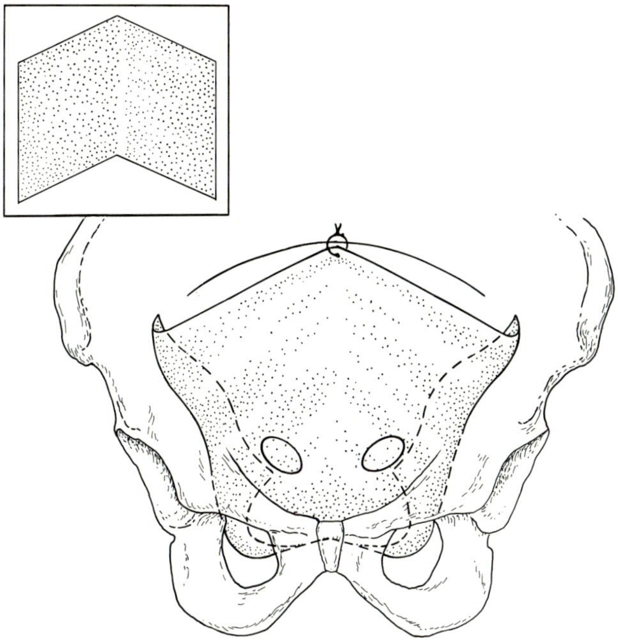

10 Schematic anterior view of the giant prosthesis in its correct position, showing the two overlapped musculopectineal holes. At the top is the linea arcuata of Douglas (*curved line*). The chevron shape of the measured prosthesis is shown in the inset.

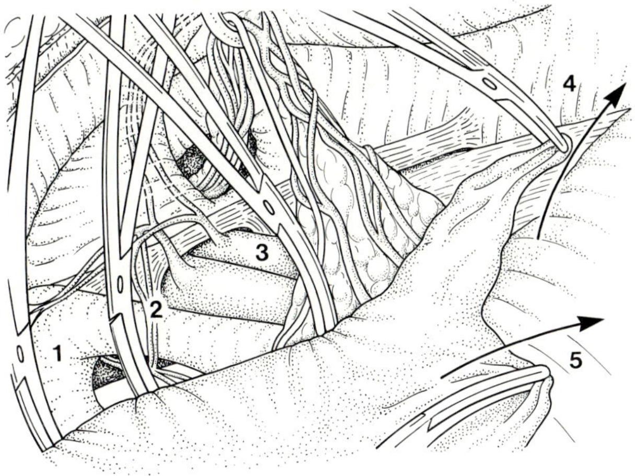

11 Schematic intraoperative representation of the placement of the giant prosthesis (*dotted gray area*) on the right side of the patient, using long curved Kelly clamps. The order of placement of the clamps is indicated by the numbers 1 to 5. The prosthesis is placed between the peritoneum and the parietalized components of the cord. *Arrows* indicate the direction for the placement of the No. 4 and 5 clamps, respectively, to achieve the placement of the mesh in its correct position on the right side of the patient.

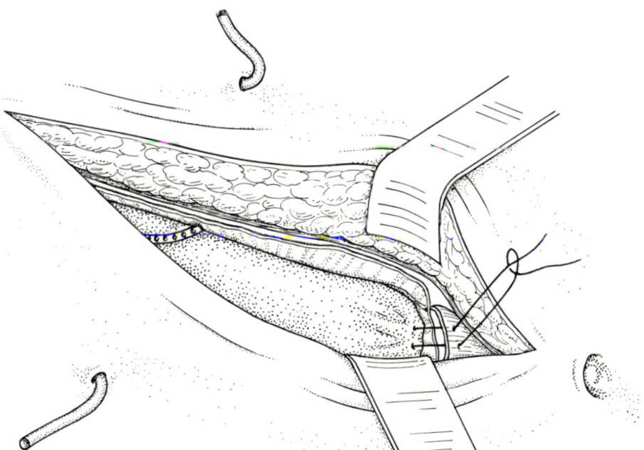

12 Schematic intraoperative view of the giant prosthesis correctly placed under both sides of the anterior wall, before closure of the midline incision. The single mattress suture for fixation of the mesh (*right*) on the inferior margin of Richet's umbilical fascia is being tied.

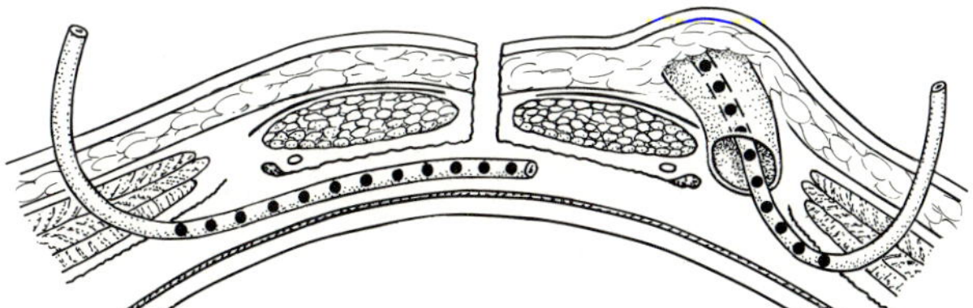

13 Schematic cross-section showing the position of the suction drains in front of the prosthesis (*left*) and into the lumen of the open transected distal end of the retained portion of the hernial sac within the scrotum (*right*).

Technical Variations

1. The Pfannenstiel incision, as proposed by Rignault, is of cosmetic interest only in the primary repair of a hernia with the use of a giant preperitoneal prosthesis. Furthermore, it is of no use in the repair of a recurrent hernia.

2. In the midline subumbilical preperitoneal approach, the contents of a huge scrotal hernia may be so adherent to the sac that its reduction may prove difficult. When this occurs, a separate incision is recommended to facilitate reduction (**14**).

REPAIR OF RECURRENT GROIN HERNIAS BY THE INSERTION OF GIANT MESH PROSTHESES THROUGH THE MIDLINE PREPERITONEAL APPROACH (GPMPA)

Continued

3. In huge hernias, the fundus of the sac may be left in the scrotum. Frequently, this is preferable as a prophylaxis for testicular atrophy. A hydrocele, incidentally, is not always prevented by suction drainage of the sac (**15**).

4. Most problems related to sliding recurrent hernias are simplified by the preperitoneal approach. The correct diagnosis is easily made upon opening the peritoneal sac; this also permits immediate treatment of the hernial sac and its contents. In fact, the use of a mesh prosthesis is the ideal treatment, owing to the large hernial defect that is usually present and the frequently associated severe damage to the overlying tissues of the anterior abdominal wall.

5. In obese patients, the preparatory surgical dissection and implantation of the giant preperitoneal mesh prosthesis are not unduly difficult. Furthermore, with this method it is impossible to overlook any hidden hernial defects. Also, in such patients the use of Trendelenburg's position will prove most helpful.

6. Simultaneous surgical treatment of associated intra- or extraperitoneal pelvic lesions—including varicoceles, hydroceles, and benign ovarian cysts—may be performed without undue risks.

Results

In a series of 2224 patients with groin hernias operated on during the 15-year period from 1970 to 1985, there were 349 (15.7%) recurrent or re-recurrent hernias. The bilaterality rates were 36.6% in primary hernias and 42.2% in recurrent hernias. Four techniques were employed—the Bassini operation (BO), the Cooper's ligament-McVay repair (CLR), the anterior inguinal patch repair (IP), and the use of the giant prosthesis through the midline preperitoneal approach (GPMPA). The numbers of cases and their respective percentages for the various techniques were the following: BO—2 (0.57%); CLR—30 (8.6%); IP—39 (11.2%); GPMPA—270 (77.4%). An additional 8 patients (2.3%) were treated with diverse suture techniques.

The postoperative course was excellent in the following: BO—2 (100.0%); CLR—28 (93.3%); IP—31 (79.48%); and GPMPA—261 (96.7%). Hematomas occurred in BO—0 (0.0%); CLR—2 (6.67%); IP—8 (20.5%); and GPMPA—9 (3.33%). Sepsis rates were BO—0 (0.0%); CLR—2 (6.66%); IP—3 (7.7%); and GPMPA—8 (3.0%). Accordingly, in our experience with the treatment of recurrent groin hernias, the most favorable results and the fewest complications have been observed with the use of the GPMPA.

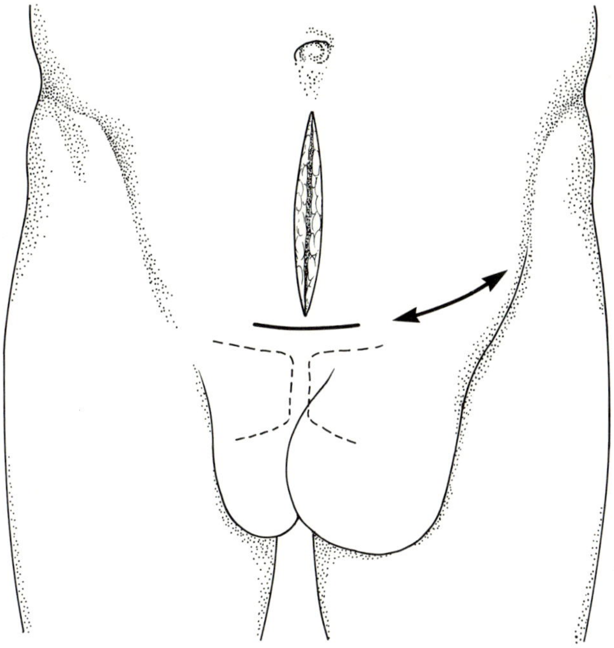

14 The separate incision, running either right or left as indicated (*arrowed line*), used to facilitate the reduction of the adherent contents within the retained sac of a large scrotal hernia.

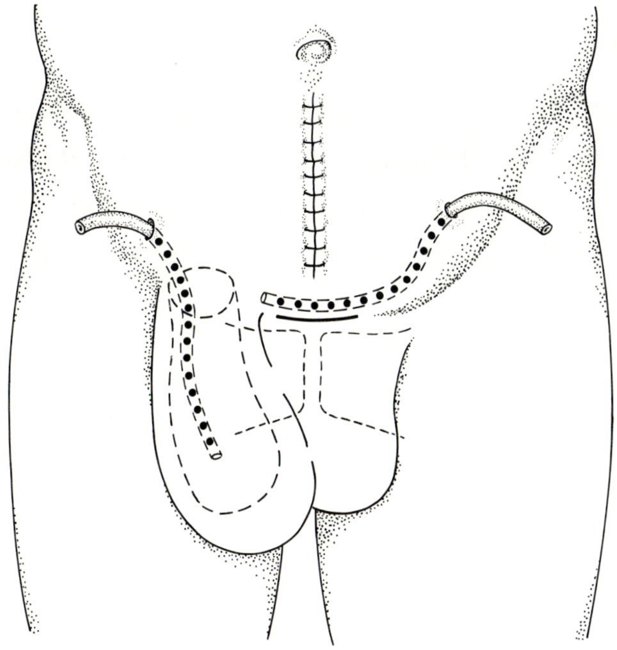

15 Schematic representation of the suction drain in the retained hernial sac (*right*), combined with the usual placement of the drain anterior to the prosthesis (*left*).

Follow-up Study

In the total of 2224 groin hernias that were repaired, 1669 (75.0%) patients were available for a follow-up study that ranged from a minimum of two years to a maximum of 10 years. This study included 344 (98.5%) of the 349 patients with recurrent and re-recurrent hernias that were treated.

In the 1669 hernia repairs that were evaluated, 113 had recurred for an overall recurrence rate of 6.8%. In the 344 recurrent hernias, there were 13 (3.8%) repeat recurrences. The incidence and rates of these re-recurrences, relative to the types of operations performed, were as follows: BO—1 of 2 (50.0%); CLR—5 of 30 (16.6%); IP—4 of 19 (21.0%); and GPMPA—3 of 270 (1.1%).

Remarks

1. The use of the GPMPA in the repair of recurrent and re-recurrent inguinal hernias is founded on correct anatomic principles. Inserted as described, the large piece of Dacron mesh acts as a permanent artificial endoabdominal fascial layer that prevents a hernial recurrence. With its use, the cure rate in the treatment of the most difficult types of groin hernias (the recurrent and the multiple re-recurrent) approaches the absolute (approximately 99%).

The operation is anatomically simple and is rapidly performed. The avascular cleavage of the retroparietal spaces provides good exposure of the hernial areas without the necessity of closing the hernial orifice or fixing the prosthesis with sutures. In summary, the basic essentials in performing the operation are a wide cleavage of the retroparietal areolar spaces and the use of an appropriately large piece of mesh to envelop the visceral sac and to reinforce the endoabdominal fascia bilaterally in the areas of the hernial orifices. Finally, the duration of the operation is optimal, requiring from 20 to 40 minutes for the repair of a bilateral hernia.

2. The primary goal in the use of GPMPA is the definitive curative treatment of recurrent and re-recurrent inguinal hernias, particularly in those patients in whom Poupart's and Cooper's ligaments have been destroyed. Furthermore, the preperitoneal route avoids the arduous and prolonged dissection of severely damaged tissues that is

REPAIR OF RECURRENT GROIN HERNIAS BY THE INSERTION OF GIANT MESH PROSTHESES THROUGH THE MIDLINE PREPERITONEAL APPROACH (GPMPA)

Continued

necessary when the anterior repair route is used. In fact, in some patients, the extent of tissue destruction precludes a curative result.

3. In the repair of recurrent and re-recurrent hernias with the use of large pieces of foreign material, infection is always a potential and serious complication due to the lowered resistance of the previously damaged tissues. Therefore, it is important to stress, again, that the surgeon must observe strict aseptic precautions—preoperatively, intraoperatively, and postoperatively—for the prevention of infection.

If a wound infection does occur, the wound is simply reopened, both superficially and deeply, for drainage. The prosthesis is not removed at this time. Its subsequent removal depends upon the appearance of the wound and the systemic response of the patient to the prescribed treatment. If the sepsis persists, which it rarely does, the mesh is removed. In one of the eight patients with sepsis, part of the prosthesis was removed. In the remaining seven patients, the wounds healed by second intention; none had a recurrence of the hernia.

The patient whose prosthesis was partly removed experienced a re-recurrence of the hernia of the same size as before the insertion of the mesh prosthesis. This was treated by a second prosthetic mesh repair using the Nyhus preperitoneal suprainguinal approach. The result, nine years later, is excellent.

Conclusion

Recurrent groin hernias may result from either repeated operative trauma or a collagen deficiency inherent in the fascia. In either circumstance, repair of the hernia by the use of a giant Dacron prosthesis, implanted through a lower midline preperitoneal approach, is an easily performed procedure that carries a nearly absolute curative reliability.

REFERENCES

Fruchaud H: *Anatomie Chirurgicale des Hernies de l'Aine.* Paris: C Doin & Cie, 1956.
Houdard C and Stoppa R: *Le Traitement Chirurgical des Hernies de l'Aine.* Paris: Masson, 1984.
Nyhus LM and Condon RE (eds): *Hernia,* 2nd ed. Philadelphia: JB Lippincott, 1978.
Stoppa R, Petit J, Abourachid H et al: Procédé original de plastie des hernies de l'aine: l'Interposition sans fixation d'une prothèse en tulle de dacron par voie médiane sous-péritonéale. Chirurgie *99*:119–123, 1973.
Stoppa R, Warlaumont C, Verhaeghe P, et al: Preperitoneal placement of Dacron mesh in the repair of groin hernias. Surg Rounds *6*(4):38–51, 1983.
Stoppa R, Rives J, Warlaumont C, et al: The use of Dacron in the repair of hernias of the groin. Surg Clin North Am *64*(2):269–285, 1984.

OPERATION 19

SEGMENTAL RESECTION OF THE SMALL INTESTINE: "OPEN" END-TO-END ANASTOMOSIS

Plate LXXIX
Plate LXXX
Plate LXXXI
Plate LXXXII

1 The irreversible compromise of the circulation to a segment of the small intestine is shown. The lines of transection of the bowel and the subjacent mesentery are indicated by the *broken lines*.

2, 3 By blunt dissection with a small clamp (**2**), an opening is made in an avascular portion of the mesentery immediately subjacent to the bowel wall at the site selected for its transection. Through this opening a catheter (14 French) is withdrawn (**3**).

4 Similarly, a second catheter (14 French) is used to encircle the bowel distally. Direction lines for transection of the mesentery are made through its serosal layer.

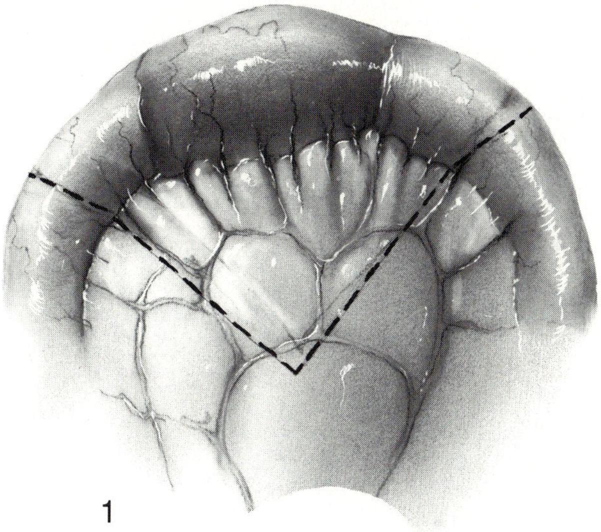

1

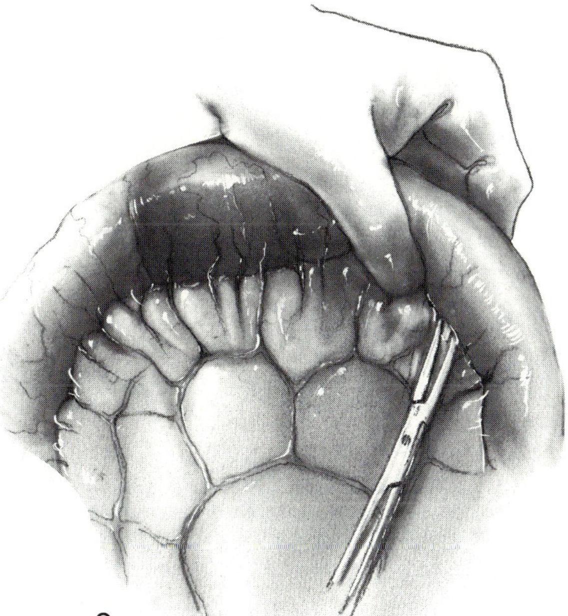

2

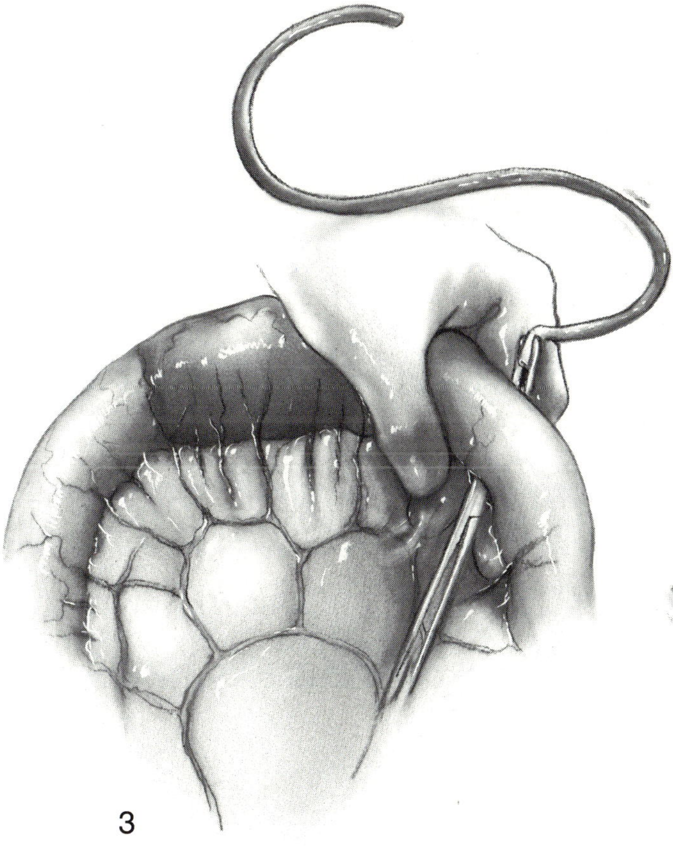

3

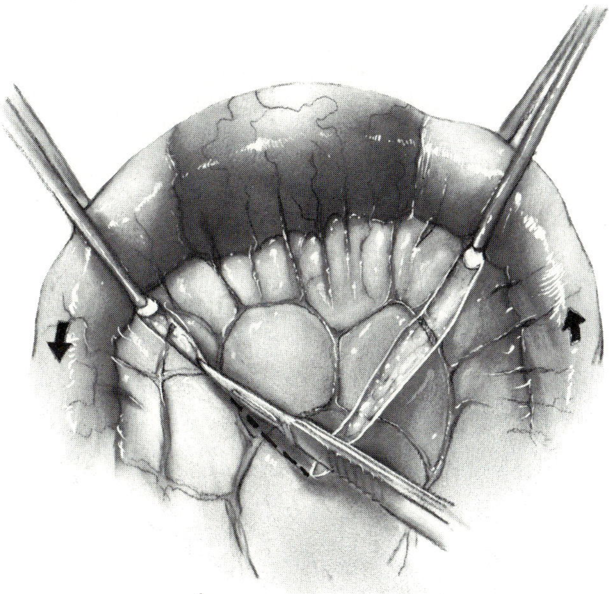

4

SEGMENTAL RESECTION OF THE SMALL INTESTINE: "OPEN" END-TO-END ANASTOMOSIS *Continued*

5, 6 The mesentery is serially clamped and severed by scissors dissection (**5**), and hemostasis is obtained with transfixion suture ligatures of 3-0 silk (**6**). In applying clamps to the mesentery, small bites of tissue should be taken and the clamps tightly locked to prevent slipping and resulting hemorrhage. In fatty areolar tissue, transfixion suture ligatures are used routinely for hemostasis.

7 The clamps on the cut margins of the mesentery of the bowel that is to remain are replaced by transfixion suture ligatures of silk (3-0); those on the segment of mesentery that is to be resected are replaced by simple ligatures of silk (3-0). The remaining attachment of the mesentery is doubly clamped and its severance is indicated by the *broken line*.

8 Following the completion of the transection of the mesentery and the ligation of its vessels, the operative field is declared contaminated. The field of contamination is defined with moist toweling and an appropriately colored (red) laparotomy sheet. The lumen of the bowel proximally is occluded with a rubber-covered intestinal clamp, and the bowel is doubly clamped at the sites of its transection. The transection of the bowel proximally is completed, and its severance distally with a scalpel is shown. The clamps are applied across the bowel at approximately a 60-degree angle obliquely to assure adequacy of the blood supply to the antimesenteric cut margin. The jaws of the noncrushing clamps (Potts') on the cut margins of the small intestine to be anastomosed are held in approximation but not locked. This is done to avoid unnecessary crushing trauma to the tissues.

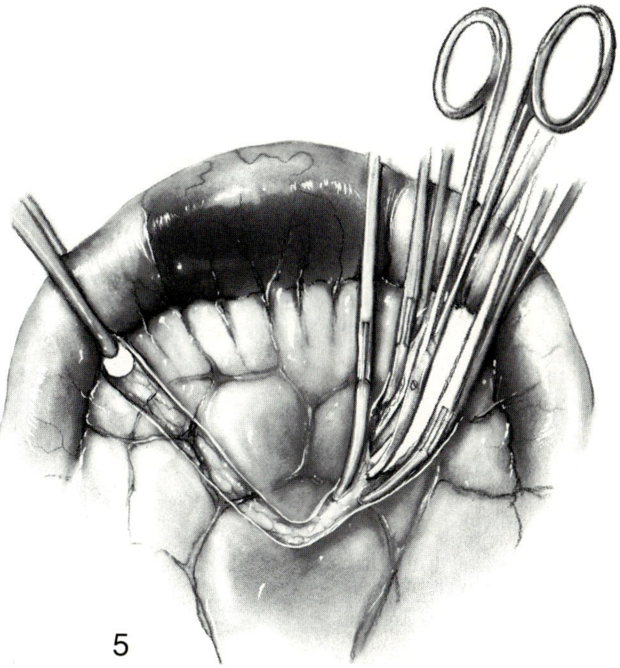

5

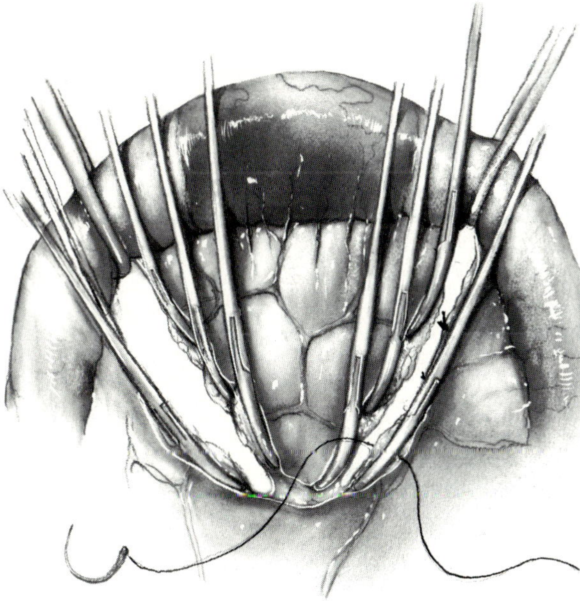

6

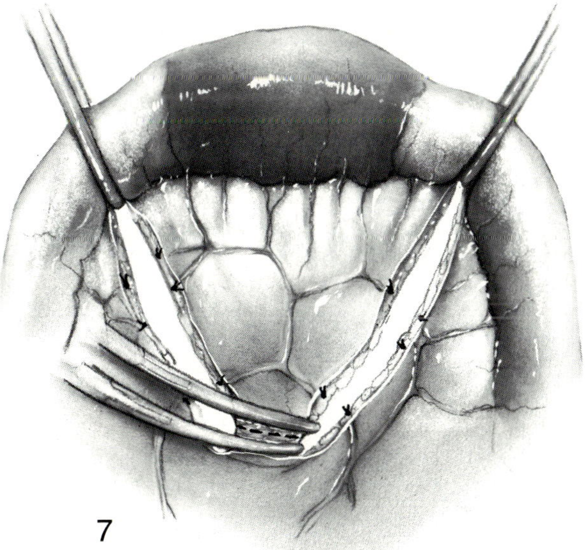

7

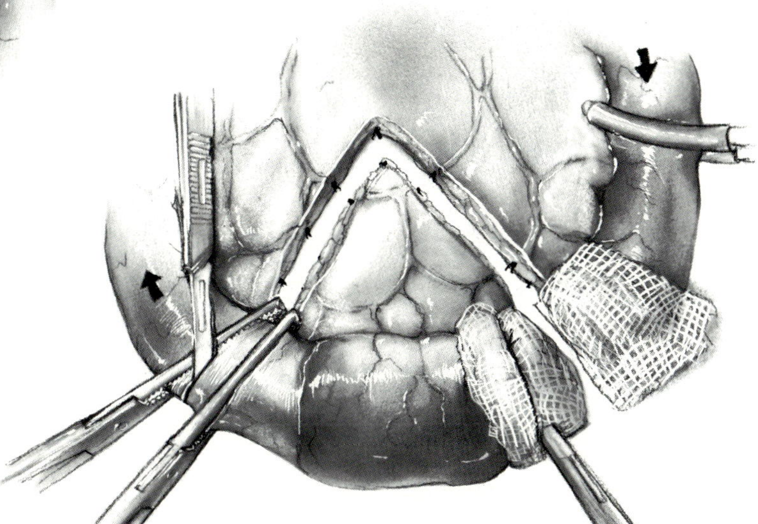

8

SEGMENTAL RESECTION OF THE SMALL INTESTINE: "OPEN" END-TO-END ANASTOMOSIS *Continued*

9 The end-to-end "open" anastomosis, the preferred technique, is begun. Prior to the anastomosis, adequacy of the circulation to the cut margins must be assured. This is indicated by the occurrence of fresh bleeding from, and the healthy appearance of, the unclamped cut margins. The antimesenteric margins of the transected small intestine are secured in Babcock clamps, and the mesenteric coaptation mattress suture (Lee) of fine (4-0) silk is inserted.

10 Similarly, a coaptation mattress suture of silk (4-0) with its loop on the mucosa is inserted for the approximation of the antimesenteric cut margins.

11 By traction on the untied coaptation sutures, the cut margins of the bowel are apposed, and a series of interrupted through-and-through everting mattress sutures of silk is inserted.

12 The coaptation and mattress sutures are tied, and the everted layers of the bowel wall are firmly approximated with simple interrupted sutures of fine (4-0) silk. Although the use of silk rather than fine (3-0) catgut for the inner or mucosal layer of the anastomosis is frequently condemned, no difficulty has been observed with its routine use.

13 The interrupted sutures of silk (4-0) are continued anteriorly and are inserted from the "inside out" to the "outside in" so that, when tied, the knots of these sutures are on the inside of the lumen and inversion of the bowel wall is obtained. Downward traction on the strands of the previously inserted suture facilitates this inversion.

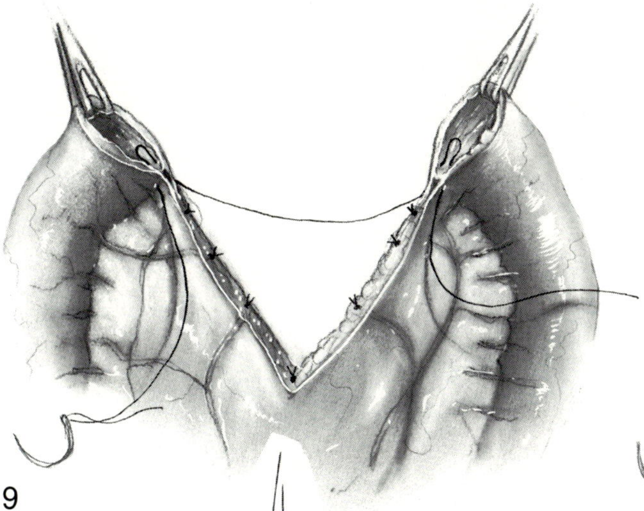

9

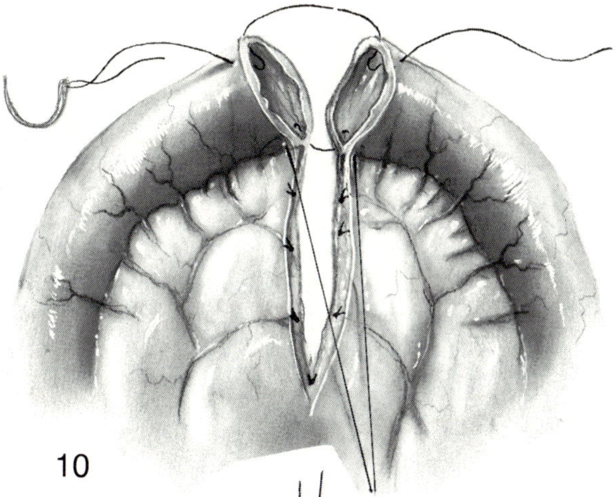

10

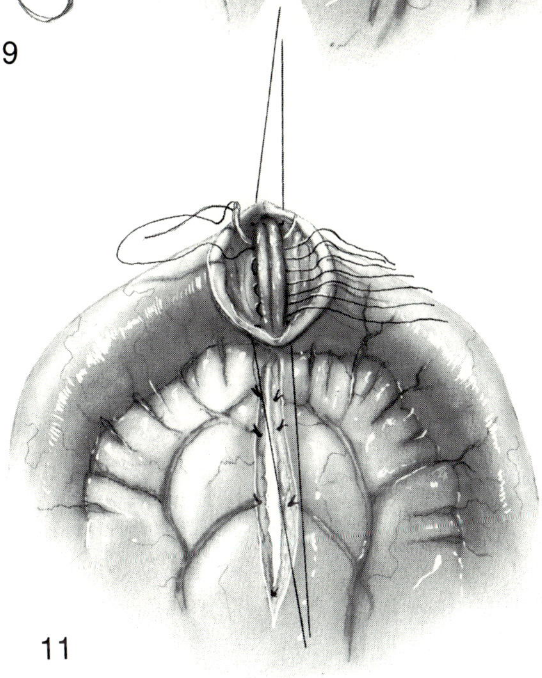

11

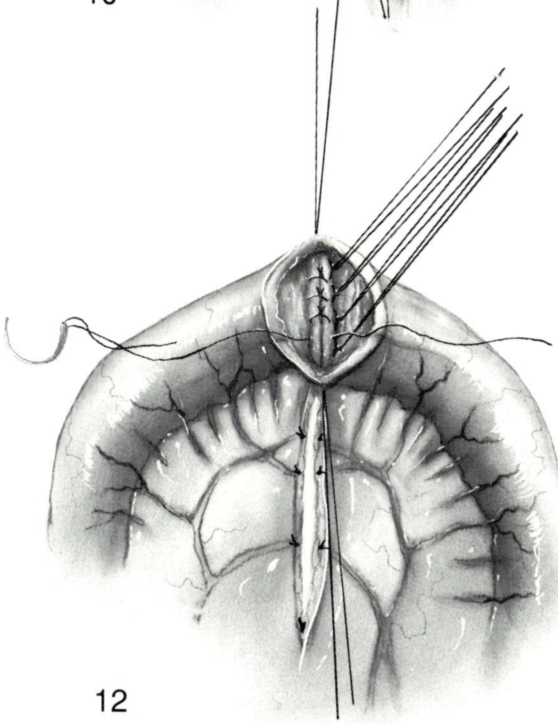

12

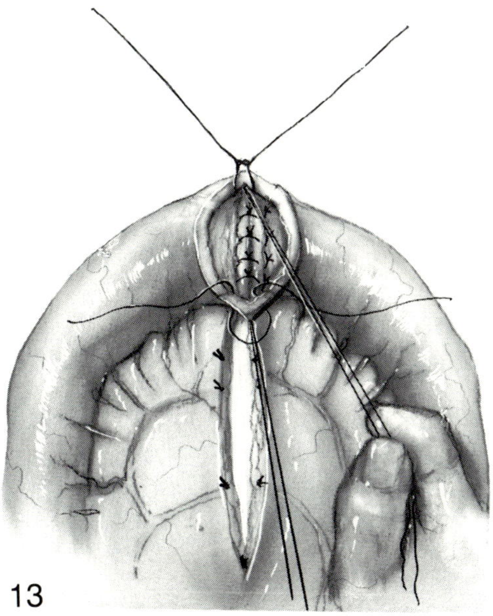

13

SEGMENTAL RESECTION OF THE SMALL INTESTINE: "OPEN" END-TO-END ANASTOMOSIS *Continued*

14 In their continuation anteriorly, the sutures are inserted alternately toward the midline to avoid an angle closure. The last two sutures are inserted and when tied, the first layer of the closure anteriorly is completed.

15 The last two sutures of the first layer anteriorly are tied and encircled by a reinforcing figure-of-eight mattress suture to assure an airtight and watertight closure.

16, 17 The second layer of sutures anteriorly, a series of interrupted seromuscular sutures (Lembert), is inserted (**16**) and continued as an additional reinforcing layer posteriorly (**17**).

18A In those instances in which an irreversible, linear circumferential compromise of the circulation of the bowel is caused by a constriction band, simple inversion by a series of interrupted seromuscular Lembert sutures may be employed. This technique is frequently referred to as Summers' stitch.

18, 19 Traction on the circumferential layer of seromuscular sutures is maintained (**18**) as each suture is tied to complete the anastomosis (**19**). The operative field is then declared clean. After a change of gloves by the surgical team and with a clean set of instruments, the opening in the mesentery is closed using interrupted sutures of fine (4-0) silk (**19**). Wound closure in layers, as previously depicted, completes the operation.

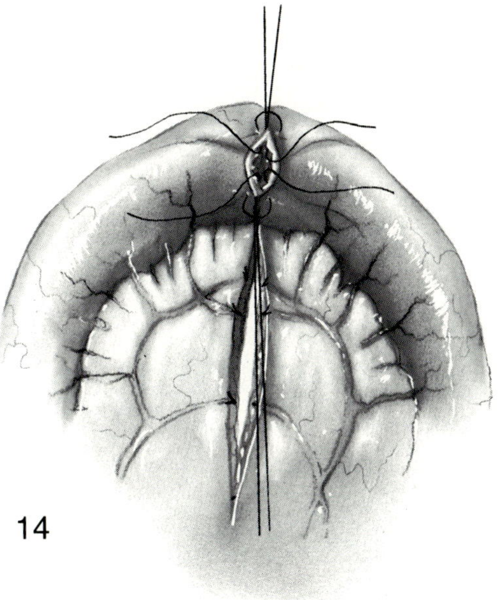

14

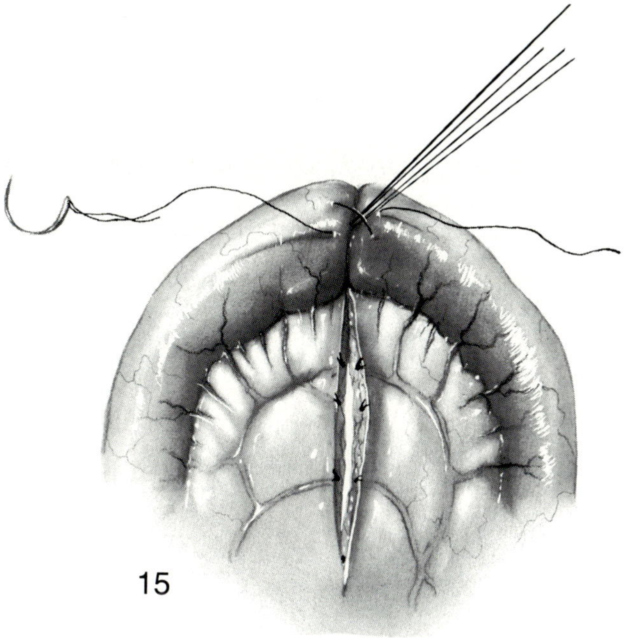

15

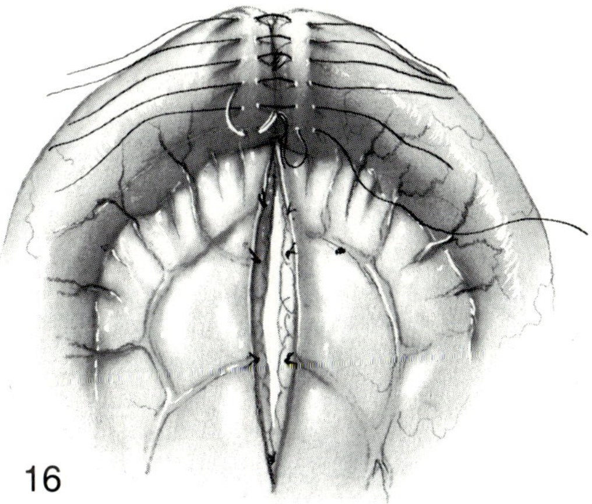

16

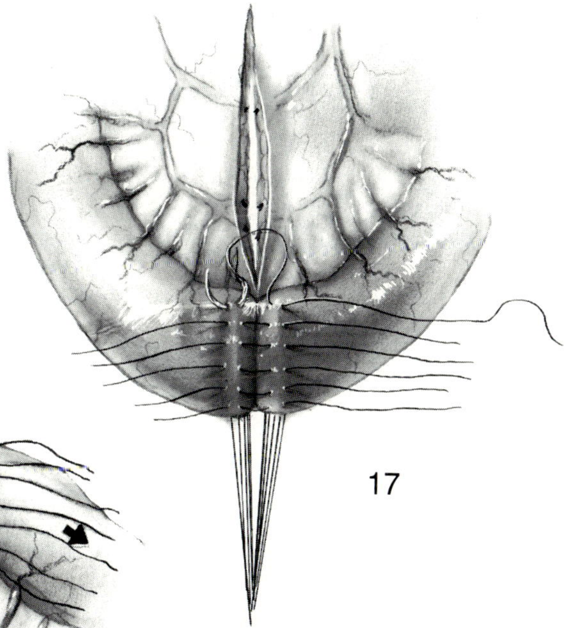

17

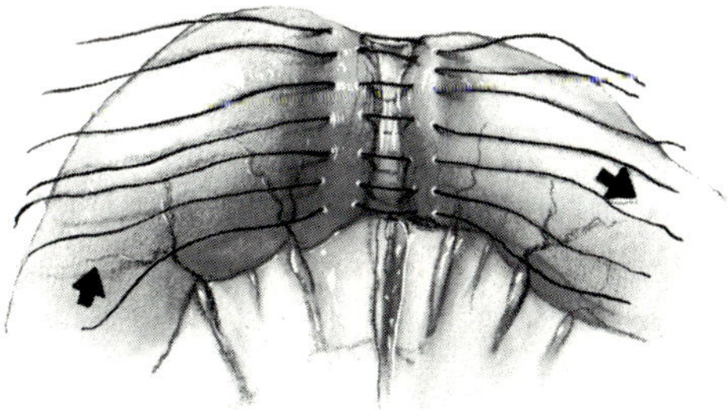

18A

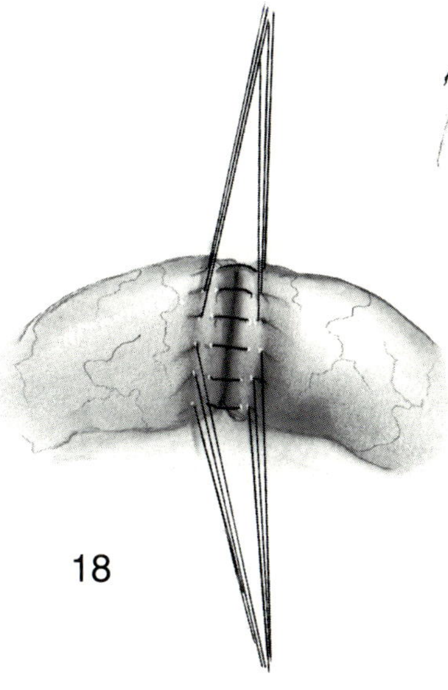

18

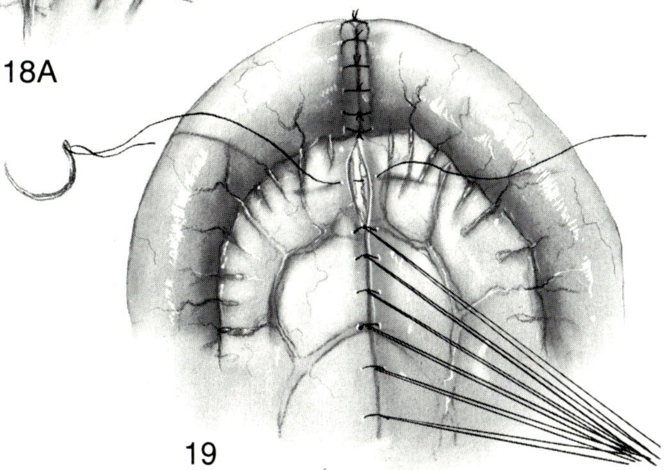

19

OPERATION 20

SEGMENTAL RESECTION OF THE SMALL INTESTINE: "CLOSED ASEPTIC" END-TO-END ANASTOMOSIS

Plate LXXXIII

1 The bowel on each side of the segment to be resected is doubly clamped. The sites of transection of the bowel and its subjacent mesentery are indicated by the *broken lines.*

2, 3 The segmental resection of the small intestine is completed (**2**), and with the minimal trauma occluding clamps firmly locked and carefully approximated, a series of interrupted seromuscular mattress sutures of silk (3-0) is inserted anteriorly (**3**).

4 The handles of the clamps are turned down to rotate the bowel 180 degrees on its longitudinal axis. A series of interrupted seromuscular mattress sutures of silk (3-0) is inserted posteriorly.

5 Traction is maintained on the strands of the untied, circumferentially placed, interrupted mattress sutures (3-0 silk) as the clamps are carefully and slowly withdrawn.

6 The mattress sutures are tied, and the opening on the antimesenteric surface of the bowel through which the clamps were withdrawn is closed with a seromuscular mattress suture of 3-0 silk.

7 The "aseptic" anastomosis is completed, and the opening in the mesentery is closed. By digital manipulation the agglutinated cut margins of the bowel are separated, and its lumen is restored. The importance of this maneuver in avoiding postoperative intestinal obstruction by a diaphragm cannot be overemphasized. Furthermore, careful inspection of the line of anastomosis, particularly along its mesenteric aspect, should be done to ensure that there is no leakage.

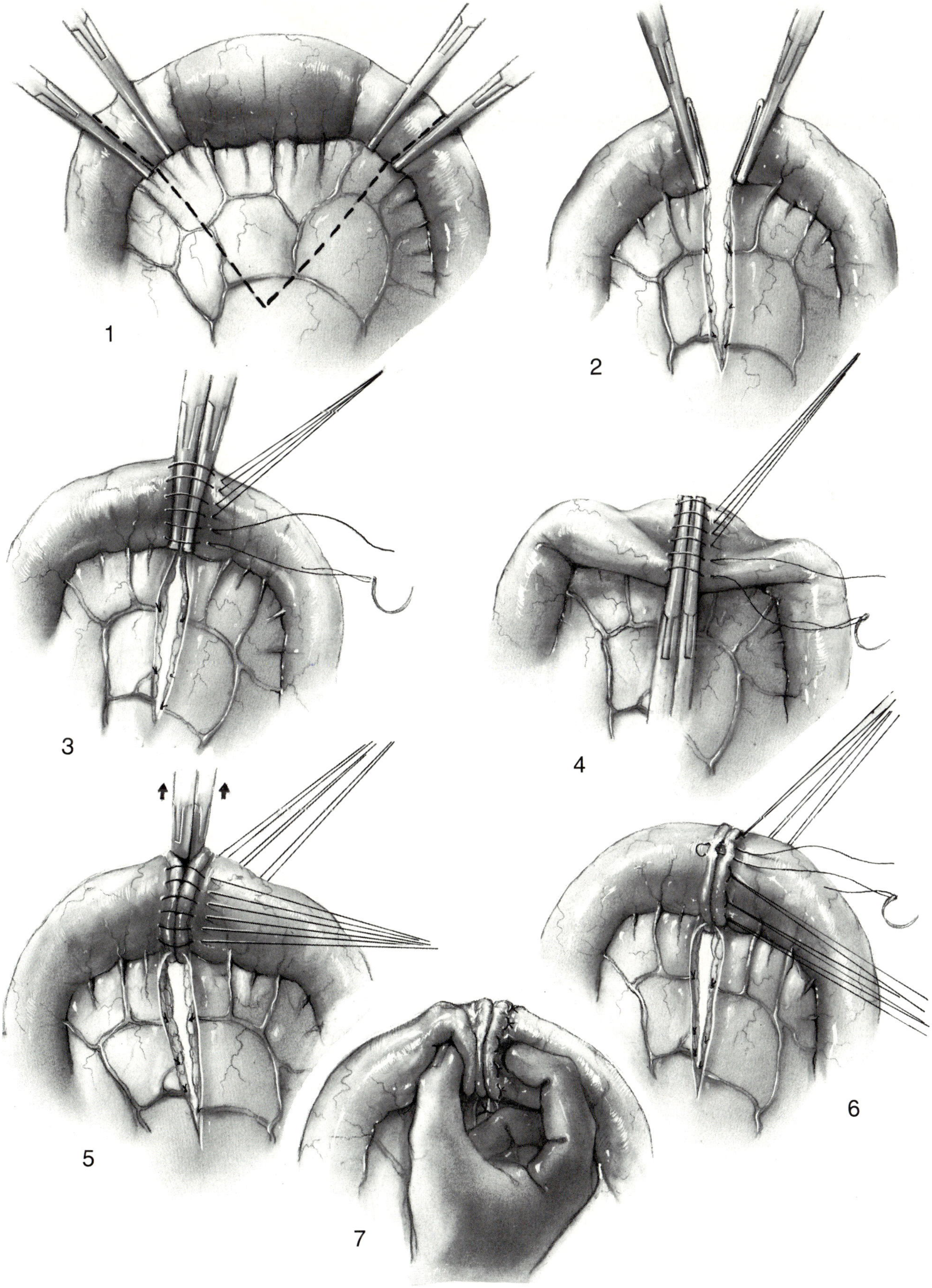
1
2
3
4
5
6
7

OPERATION 21

LARGE BOWEL RESECTION: "TUBE-WITHIN-A-TUBE" COLONIC (SIGMOID) ANASTOMOSIS

Plate LXXXIV
Plate LXXXV
Plate LXXXVI
Plate LXXXVII

In the performance of an intestinal anastomosis, many varied techniques have been described. The use of a one-layer inverting anastomosis has become increasingly popular because of the lessened degree of tissue trauma and the increase in size of the anastomotic lumen. Moreover, some surgeons elect to use the one-layer everting suture in preference to either the one- or two-layer inverting type.

The technique illustrated here is used routinely in all intestinal anastomoses with uniformly satisfactory results. It has all the proposed advantages of the one-layer anastomosis and none of the purported disadvantages of the two-layer union. Furthermore, the technique is also applicable to the closure of the duodenal stump, particularly when this presents a difficult problem.

The relationship of the mucosal and seromuscular layers in the intestinal wall is that of a "tube within a tube." Accordingly, for both anatomic and physiologic reasons each tube is sutured separately. Interrupted sutures may be used throughout or modified by the use of a continuous suture of 3-0 chromic catgut for the mucosa. In the suturing of the transected ends of the seromuscular layer, the submucosal tissue layer with its excellent holding power (emphasized by Halsted) is included. This layer is also included in the approximation of the mucosal layers.

In 1881 Wölfler used this technique for the suturing of the posterior seromuscular and mucosal layers in the performance of an end-to-end gastroduodenostomy following a partial gastrectomy for cancer of the pylorus (**1**).* He referred to the closure of the posterior mucosal layer as the "inner intestinal suture of Czerny" (**2**).

Anteriorly, however, a comparable "outer intestinal mucosal suture" was not used. Instead, the unsutured anterior mucosal layers of the stomach and duodenum were simply inverted into the lumen of the anastomotic stoma, using interrupted seromuscular sutures (**3**). A second reinforcing layer of serosal sutures was added to complete the Czerny-Lembert closure. The intestinal mattress suture of Jobert (**4**), which inverts the full thickness of the transected anterior layers of the anastomotic segments, is frequently but incorrectly depicted as the Czerny suture.

---

*Interestingly, this was the fourth partial gastrectomy done for cancer of the stomach. The first three were done by Wölfler's celebrated chief, Professor Theodor Billroth. The first of Billroth's three patients and Wölfler's patient survived.

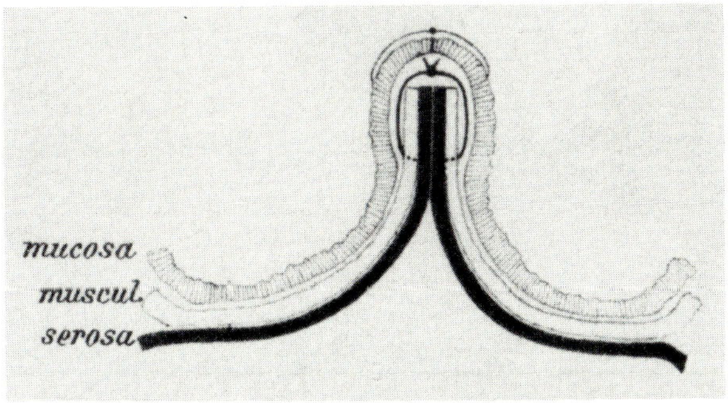

1 Diagrammatic coronal section of the posterior layers of an end-to-end gastroduodenostomy, depicting the separate closure of the seromuscular and mucosal layers.

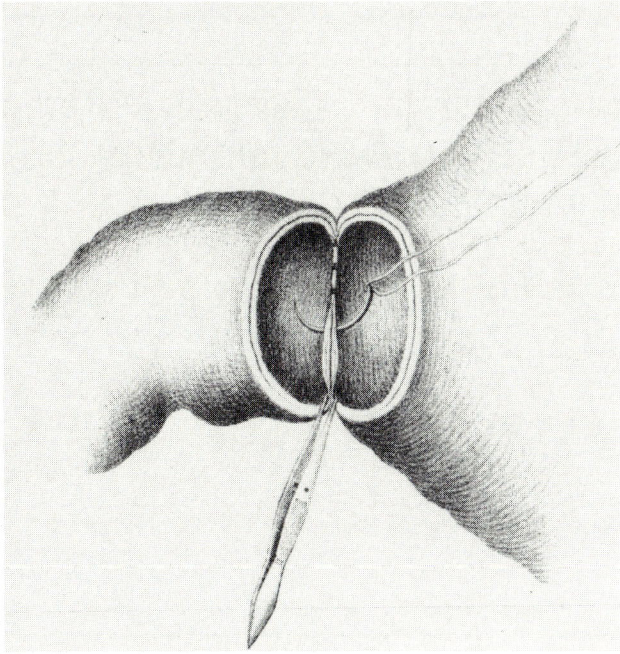

2 Suture of the posterior mucosal layers (inner intestinal suture of Czerny).

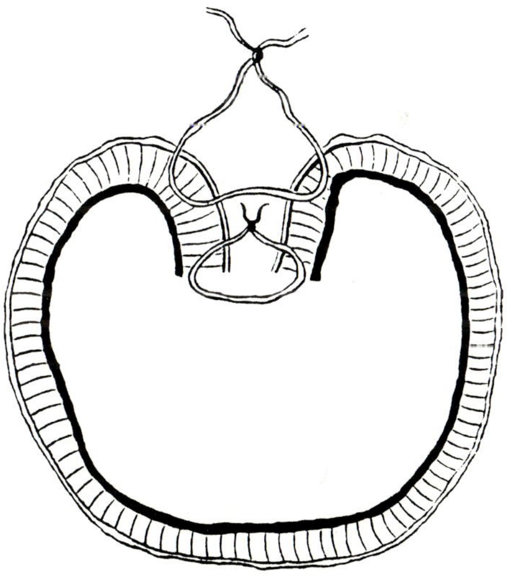

Czerny's Darmnaht.

3 The Czerny-Lembert suture for the two-layer anterior closure of the anastomosis. The unsutured transected ends of the mucosal layers are inverted into the lumen of the anastomosis instead of being united by an "outer intestinal mucosal suture." ("Darmnaht" = enterorrhaphy.)

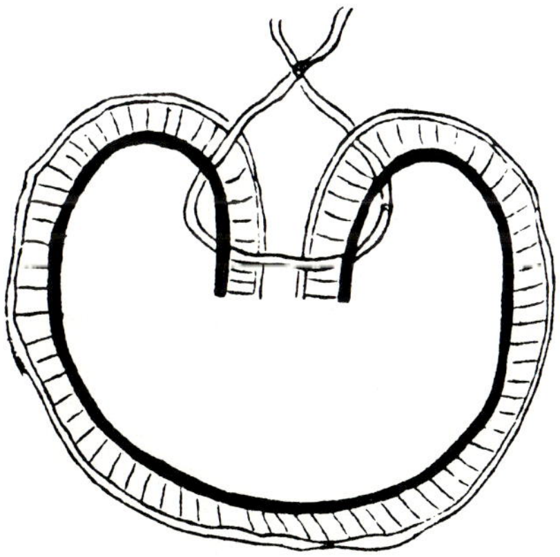

Jobert's Darmnaht.

4 The Jobert intestinal mattress suture for the one-layer, anterior, full-thickness closure of the anastomosis. The unsutured transected ends of both the mucosal and seromuscular layers are inverted into the lumen of the anastomosis.

LARGE BOWEL RESECTION: "TUBE-WITHIN-A-TUBE" COLONIC (SIGMOID) ANASTOMOSIS *Continued*

In the anatomic two-layer "tube-within-a-tube" anastomotic technique, the minimal tension on the suture line enhances a waterseal stoma. Furthermore, the exactness of the anatomic restoration precludes any compromise in the caliber of the anastomotic stoma, as is confirmed by study of postoperative barium roentgenograms.

5, 6, 7 The untied angle sutures for traction are in place, and the first posterior layer of the anastomosis is begun by the insertion of a series of interrupted sutures of 3-0 silk to approximate only the transected seromuscular layers of the colon (**5, 6**). When these sutures are tied, the posterior seromuscular layers are firmly approximated. The second posterior layer is started by the insertion of a continuous suture of 3-0 chromic catgut through the upper angle of the transected mucosal and submucosal layers (**7**).

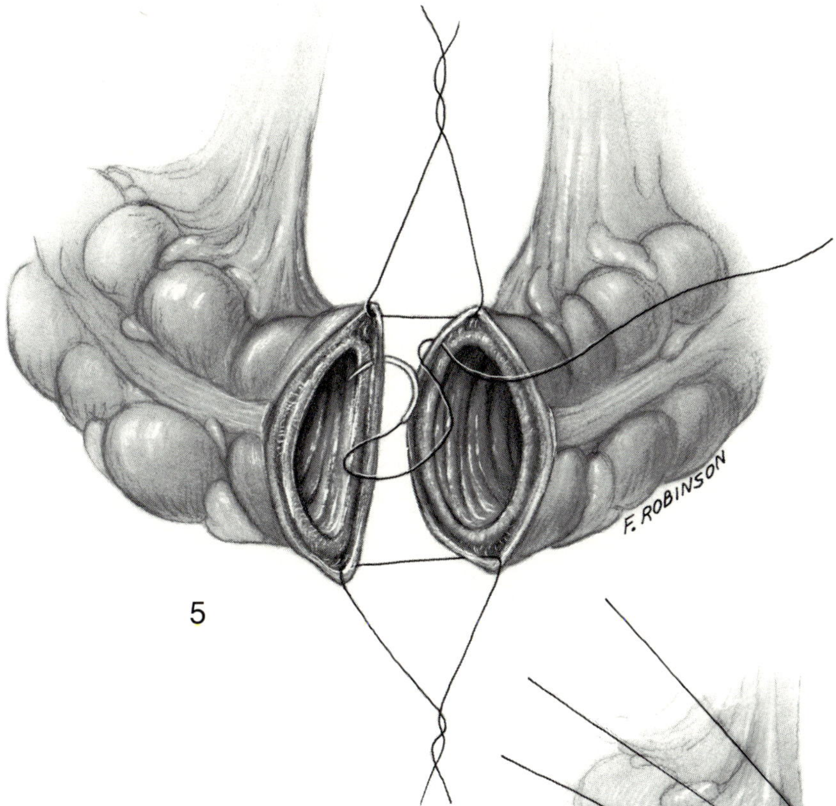

5

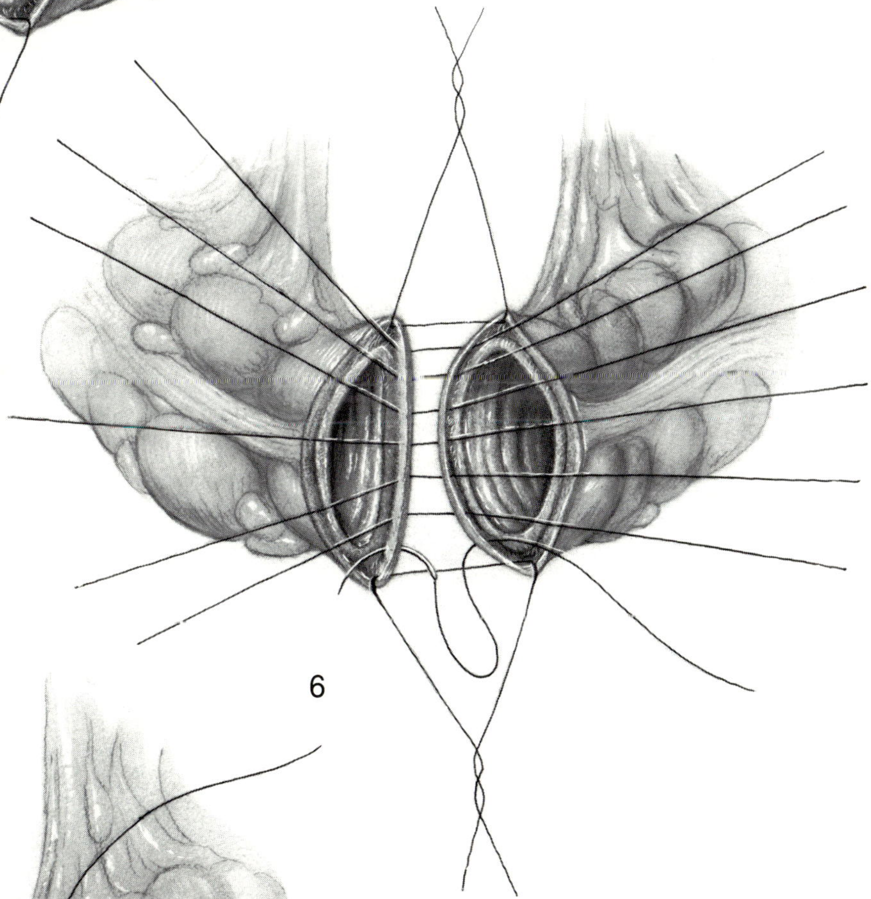

6

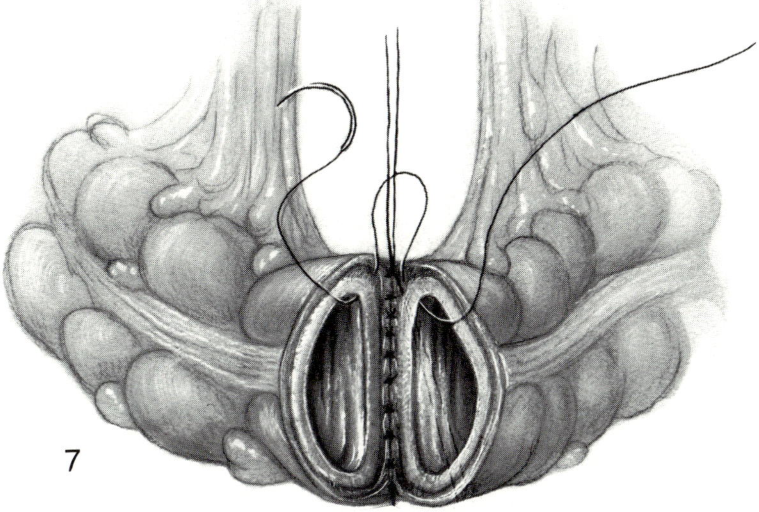

7

LARGE BOWEL RESECTION: "TUBE-WITHIN-A-TUBE" COLONIC (SIGMOID) ANASTOMOSIS *Continued*

8, 9, 10, 11, 12 The suture closure of the mucosal and submucosal layers is continued; each alternate suture is interlocked to prevent a pursestring effect on the suture line (**8**). The second posterior suture layer is completed, and the suture exits from the inside out at the lower angle of the proximal segment of the colon. It is then inserted into the lumen of the distal segment from the outside in and exits from the inside out to form a Connell or "loop on the mucosa" suture (**9**).

Similarly, a Connell suture is inserted into the lumen of the proximal end of the colon (**10**) and then into the lumen of the distal end (**11**). When this continuous suture strand (3-0 chromic catgut) is drawn taut, the lower angle of the anastomosis is readily inverted. The suture, interlocked at intervals, is then continued as the first anterior layer of the anastomosis. It approximates only the mucosal and submucosal layers to its termination in the center of the anastomosis (**12**).

In the upper angle of the anastomosis, downward traction is maintained on the anchor suture strand of the posterior (inner) mucosal suture (3-0); this facilitates the insertion of a second similar suture for the closure of the anterior (outer) mucosal and submucosal layers (**12**). When this suture is tied, the posterior anchor strand is cut and the suture is continued as an over-and-over stitch, joining its counterpart from below in the center of the first anterior layer of the anastomosis.

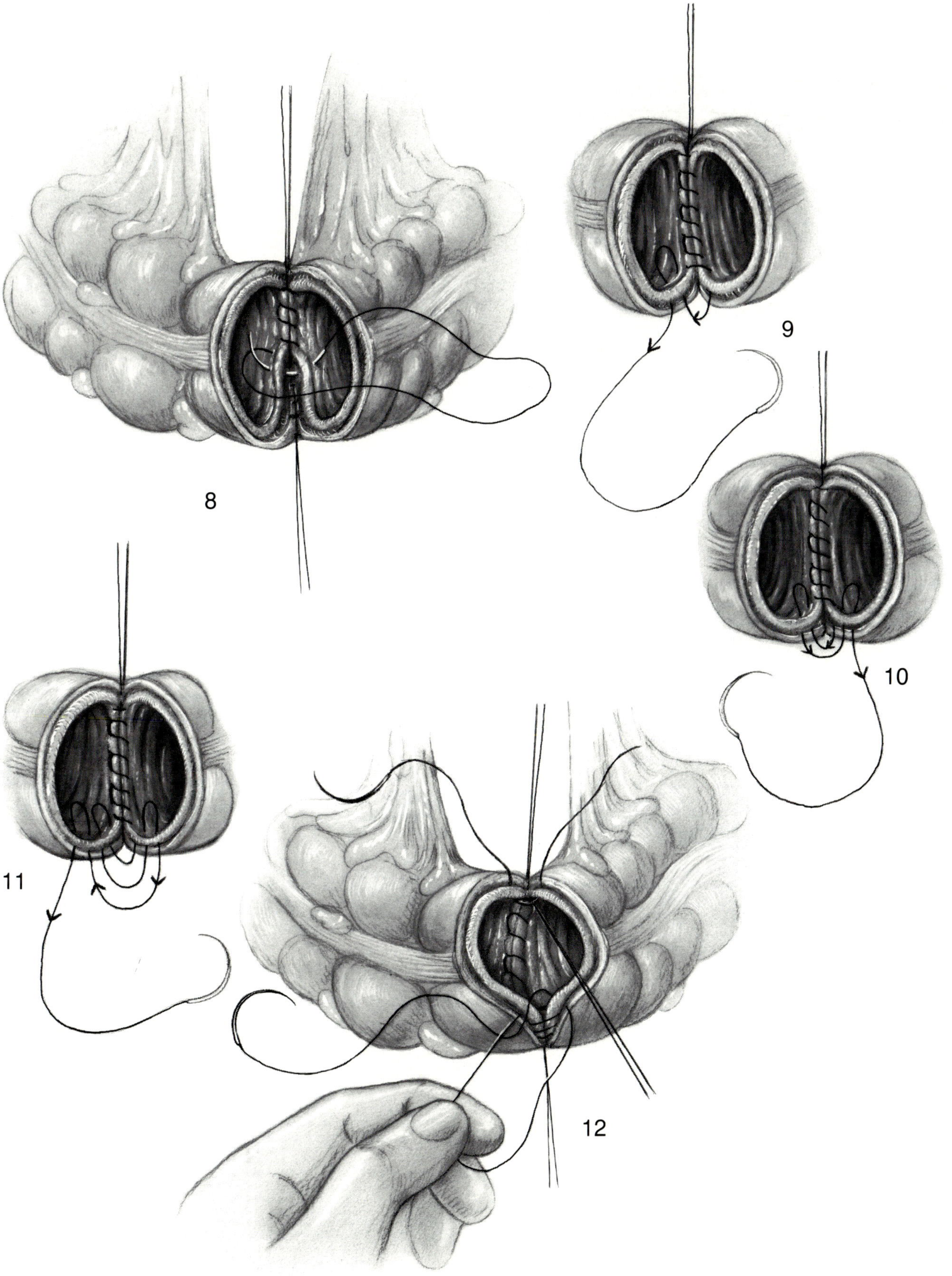
8
9
10
11
12

LARGE BOWEL RESECTION: "TUBE-WITHIN-A-TUBE" COLONIC (SIGMOID) ANASTOMOSIS *Continued*

13, 14, 15 The first anterior layer of the anastomosis, the approximation of the mucosal and submucosal layers, is completed. The upper and lower suture strands are tied in the center of the suture line to minimize the danger of leakage pursuant to an angle closure (**13**).

The second anterior suture layer is composed of a series of interrupted sutures of 3-0 silk, which approximates the transected seromuscular layers of the colon with minimal tension (**14**).

The completed two-layer end-to-end "tube-within-a-tube" anastomosis and the closure of the defect in the mesentery are depicted in **15**.

REFERENCES

Halsted, WS: Circular suture of the intestine. An experimental study. Am J Med Sci *94*:436–461, 1887.

Wölfler A: Ueber die von Herrn Professor Billroth ausgefuhrlen resectionen des carcinomatösen pylorus. Wein: Wilhelm Braumüller, 1881.

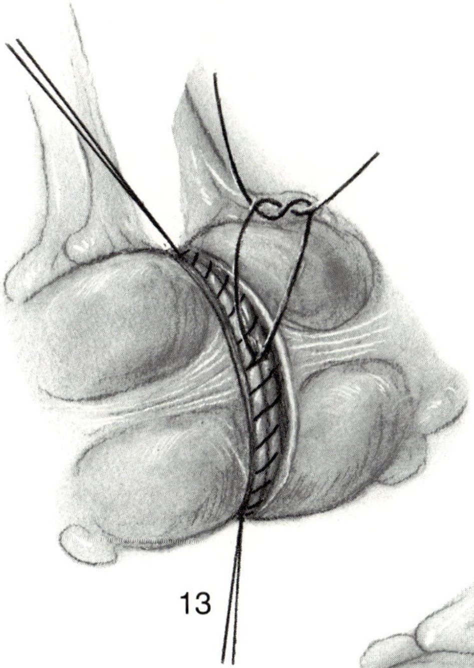

13

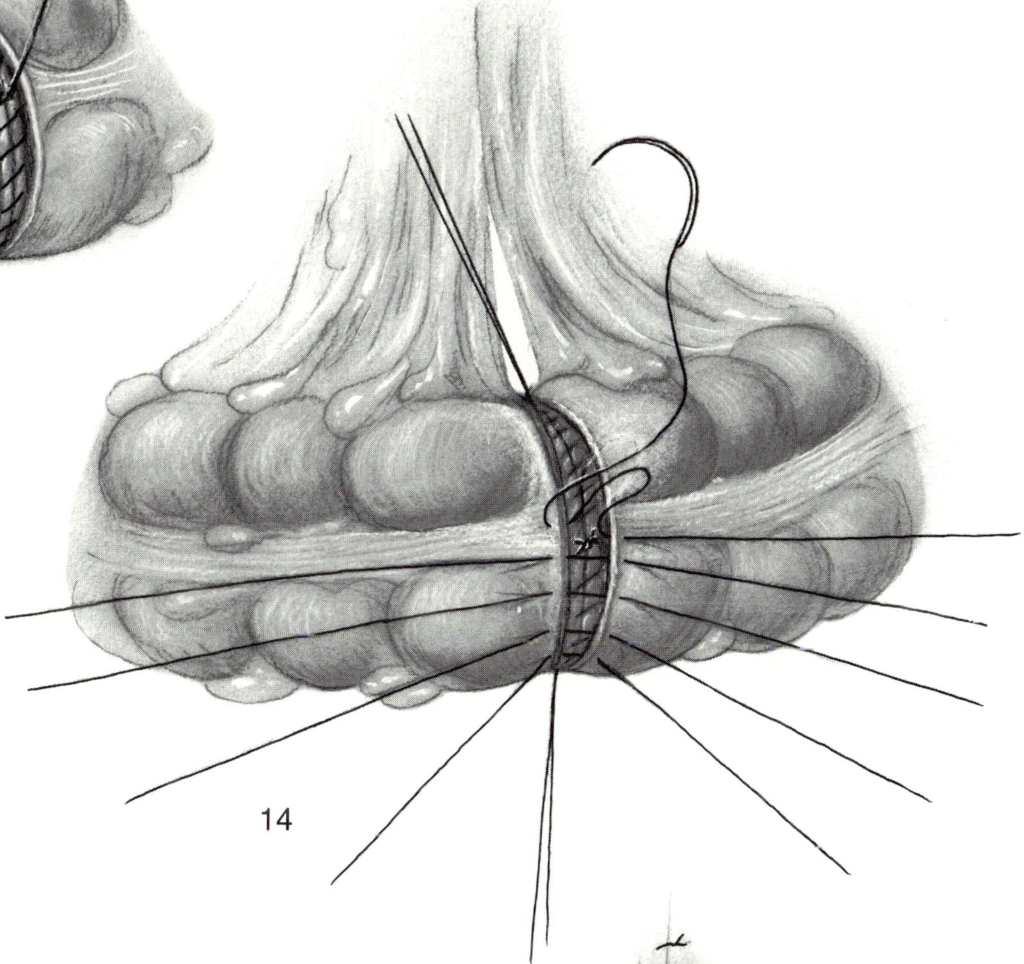

14

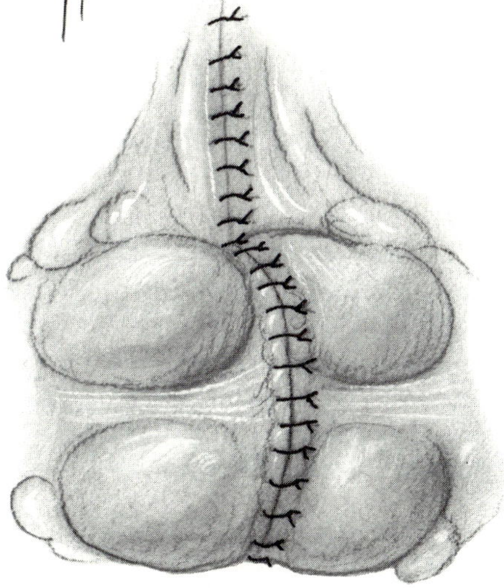

15

Appendix I

Illustrations from 18th and 19th Century Master Surgical Anatomists

ANTONIO DE GIMBERNAT (1734–1818)

Plate LXXXVIII
Plate LXXXIX

Antonio de Gimbernat, a brilliant and meticulous anatomist, was reputed to have dissected more cadavers than any man in Europe. From 1762 to 1774 he held the chair of anatomy at Barcelona; during that period he was also the surgeon of the Santa Cruz hospital in Barcelona. He visited Holland, Paris, Edinburgh, and London, where he attended a course of lectures by Hunter in 1777—on one occasion interrupting him to demonstrate a safe and simple method of operation for a crural hernia. His treatise *Nuevo Método de Operar en la Hernia Crural,* published in 1793, contains the first description of the ligament named after him. Beddoes translated the work into English in 1795, a German translation (by Schreger) was published in 1817, and G. Breschet translated it into French with additional notes in 1827. After returning from England, de Gimbernat became surgeon to King Charles IV of Spain (to whom his work was dedicated) and helped to found the Real Colegio de Cirugia de S. Carlos de Madrid in 1787. He is also known for his work on corneal ulcers.*

Gimbernat has been both cited and quoted frequently, in this text, and additional excerpts and quotations are used sparingly here. Because of its historical interest, however, a complete description of his "new method" of operating for a crural (femoral) hernia is presented.

Gimbernat emphasized the importance of understanding the "duplicature of the crural arch" in relation to the pathogenesis and treatment of the crural hernia. He described how the inferior band (pillar) of the crural arch (inguinal ligament) separates from the superior band to form the external inguinal ring and then inserts into the tubercle (spine) of the os pubis, which is the site of origin of the crest of the superior branch (ramus) of this bone. From this insertion, it continues inward along the crest (iliopectineal line) "from below upwards" to the end of the crest to form the "internal edge" of the duplicature of the crural arch.

In its termination this internal edge is in close approximation to the subjacent pectineus fascia and muscle at their sites of insertion and origin, respectively, to the inner (posterior) portion of the crest (iliopectineal line). The relationship between these two structures is illustrated in the Anatomic Supplement to Operation No. 13.

Concerning these structures, Gimbernat states, "In the internal lateral parts of the sheath [femoral] close to . . . where the insertion of the duplicature of the arch ends, and on the inside of the great secondary iliac [femoral] vein, there is a foramen (crural ring) . . . ." Since it is through this ring that the crural hernia passes, Gimbernat closes his description of the anatomy of the duplicature of the crural arch with the instruction to ". . . see the two plates at the end of this tract." However, a disparity exists between

*Biographical sketch courtesy of the Medical Librarian of the Rare Book Room, New York Academy of Medicine.

the text and the illustrations. Also, the terminology pertaining to the various anatomic structures frequently varies from present-day nomenclature. To prevent misinterpretation of Gimbernat's description of the anatomy of the structures concerned in the formation and surgical treatment of crural hernia, a further discussion follows.

In describing the technique for releasing the site of constriction of a crural hernia, Gimbernat states, "Cautiously press the bistoury to the end of the canal [of the sound]: and employing your two hands at once, carry both instruments close along the branch (ramus) to the body of the pubis, drawing them out at the same time." This agrees with the illustration in Plate LXXXIX, which shows the entire length of the internal border of the crural arch stripped from its insertion into the crest of the superior branch of the os pubis. However, the next sentence states, "By this easy operation you will divide the internal edge of the crural arch at its extremity. . . ." These final three words are open to interpretation. If they refer only to the division of the innermost or posterior extremity of "the internal edge," then Gimbernat is describing a partial division ". . . within four or five lines of the duplicature, the remainder continuing firmly attached . . . ." Although this does not agree with the illustration, it seems to be the correct interpretation of the operation as proposed by Gimbernat.

Before Gimbernat published his treatise, many surgical techniques had been recommended for the treatment of obstructed crural (femoral) hernias. They were, however, associated with excessively high morbidity and mortality rates. For these reasons, the supreme tribute to Gimbernat is the fact that the basic principle of the "simple and safe" operation that he proposed is accepted universally in the surgical treatment of the incarcerated or strangulated femoral hernia.

FROM *NEW METHOD OF OPERATING FOR THE FEMORAL HERNIA* (1795)

If the crural (femoral) hernia cannot be reduced, ". . . it is absolutely necessary to divide the part [the internal edge of the crural arch at its extremity—the innermost (posterior) part] that occasions the strangulations. For this purpose introduce, along the internal side of the intestine, a canulated or grooved sound, with a blunt end and a channel of sufficient depth. This is to be directed obliquely inwards, till it enter the crural ring, which will be known by the increased resistance; as also when its point rests upon the branch of the os pubis ("linea ileopectinea"; Cooper's ligament).

"Then suspend the introduction; and keeping the sound (with your left hand, if you are operating on the right side, and V.V.) firmly resting upon the branch of the os pubis, so that its back shall be turned towards the intestine and its canal to the symphysis pubis, introduce gently with your other hand into the groove of the sound a bistoury

ANTONIO DE GIMBERNAT (1734–1818)
Continued

with a narrow blade and blunt end, till it enter the ring: its entry will be known as before by a little increase of resistance.

"Cautiously press the bistoury to the end of the canal; and employing your two hands at once, carry both instruments along the branch to the body of the pubis, drawing them out at the same time. By this easy operation you will divide the internal edge of the crural arch at its extremity; and within four or five lines of its duplicature, the remainder continuing firmly attached by the inferior band or pillar, of which it is the continuation.

"This simple incision being thus made without the smallest danger, the internal border of the arch, which forms the strangulation, will be considerably relaxed and the parts will be reduced with the greatest ease.

"By this new method, the operation for the crural hernia, which the most celebrated surgeons have justly accounted extremely dangerous, is rendered the most simple and safe of all that are practiced in cases of strangulated hernia."

Gimbernat opposed transecting the inguinal ligament in the surgical treatment of crural (femoral) hernias, stating "The fallopian [inguinal] ligament is not at all concerned in this operation." He added, "The danger most to be dreaded is that of wounding the urinary bladder . . . but it cannot possibly be wounded if empty."

Both plates contained in Gimbernat's treatise are presented here. They are, however, inferior representations of applied surgical anatomy and have no practical value to the surgeon.

1 This is a preoperative sagittal view of the right side of the lower abdomen and pelvis. The duplicature of the crural arch and its insertion in the crest (crista) of the superior branch of os pubis is indicated (6). There is no visible anatomic continuity between the origin of the crural arch (15) and its duplicature (6).

The crural ring formed by the duplicature is depicted (7). It is in juxtaposition to the secondary iliac (femoral) vein and forms the medial boundary of the crural (femoral) sheath in which this vein is normally encased.

The "winged foot" and "bony" appearances of the duplicature and the width of the crevice between its internal edge and the crest are of particular interest.

2 This postoperative sagittal view can be compared with Plate LXXXVIII. The superior branch (ramus) of the os pubis (1) and the relationship of its crest (iliopectineal line) to the completely divided internal edge of the crural arch (2) are demonstrated.

Although the width of the crevice between the divided internal edge and the subjacent crest is only slightly increased in comparison to the preceding plate, two other significant changes have occurred. First, the "winged foot" appearance of the duplicature has been altered, but its "bony" image remains. Secondly, the concave curved base of the lateral portion of the duplicature, which formed the medial boundary of the crural ring, is not visible. This is the result of "dividing the internal edge of the crural arch at its extremity," as discussed earlier.

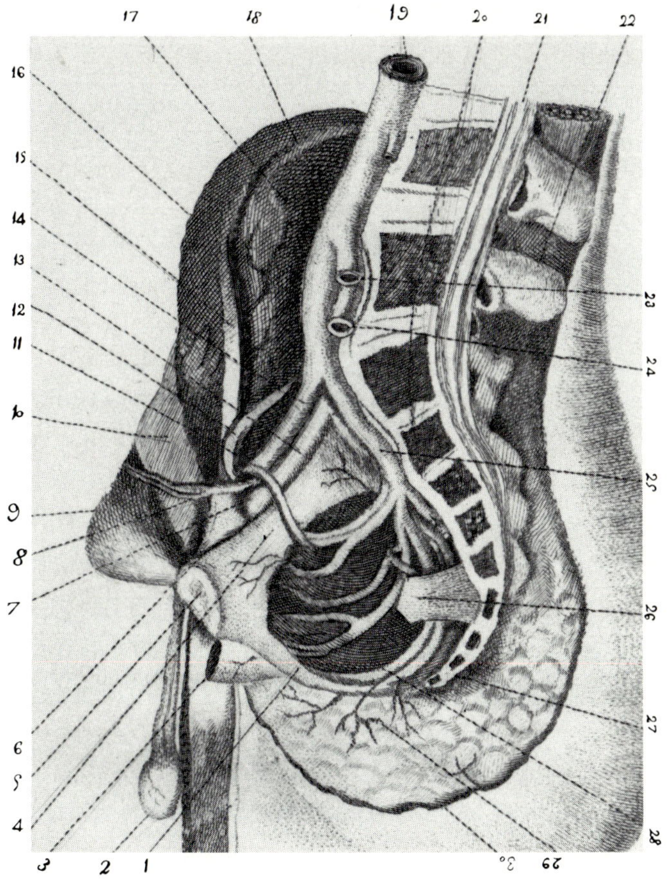

1

EXPLANATION of the PLATES.

Plate I, ſhews the pelvis vertically divided through its middle, with the two loweſt lumbar vertebræ, one of the nates, and a portion of the thigh with its integuments. The interior part of this right half of the pelvis is ſhewn for greater diſtinctneſs.

1. The inferior ramus, or branch, of the os pubis.
2. The teſticle.
3. Section of the corpus cavernoſum.
4. Superior ramus, or branch, of the os pubis.
5. The ſymphyſis pubis.
6. The duplicature of the crural arch, and its inſertion in the creſt of the os pubis.
7. The crural ring formed by this duplicature.
8. The epigaſtric veſſels.
9. Part of the rectus muſcle.
10. Aponeuroſis of the abdominal muſcles.
11. The vas deferens.
12. The ſpermatic veſſels, enveloped in cellular ſubſtance.
13. Great ſecondary iliac vein.
14. Great ſecondary iliac artery.
15. Crural arch at its origin.
16. Section of the abdominal muſcles.
17. The iliacus muſcle.
18. The creſt of the ilium.

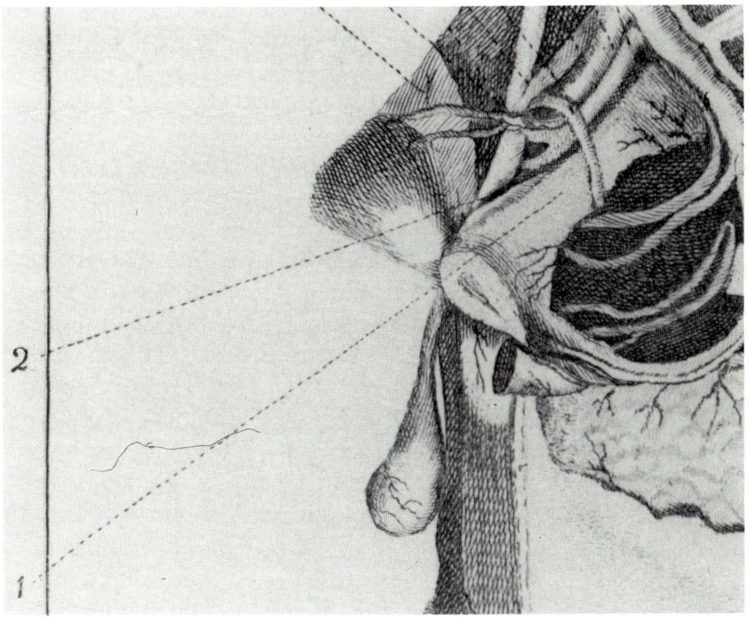

2

Plate II. The ſame ſide of the pelvis after the operation.

1. Superior branch of the os pubis.
2. Inciſion in the duplicature of the crural arch cloſe to the creſt of the os pubis, by which the crural ring is widened, and the internal margin of the arch is relaxed conſiderably.

PETRUS C. CAMPER (1722–1789)

Plate XC

Petrus C. Camper was born in Leiden, Holland on May 11, 1722 and died there on April 7, 1789, one month short of his 67th year. Knowledgeable in many of the disciplines related to the study of medicine, he held the positions of Professor of Medicine, Professor of Surgery, Professor of Pathology, and Professor of Anatomy and Demonstrator of Anatomy and Pathology. His lectures on forensic medicine and "medicina legalis" were exceedingly popular and well attended. In addition, he was a Professor of Philosophy and a Professor of Botany, as well as an artist, zoologist, archeologist, anthropologist, and paleontologist. In 1775 he became interested in politics, and in 1784 was elected to membership in the Congress of the Netherlands, ultimately becoming its President.[1]

In a belated tribute to Camper, Professor Cunningham, President of the British Society of Anthropologists, succinctly stated in 1907, "He was a man of the most brilliant talents, but it is a matter of regret, that he spread his energies over so many fields of intellectual activity."[2]

Although Camper will forever be known by the eponym "Camper's fascia," his most famous work is the Latin monograph entitled *Icones Herniarum*,[3] which consists of 16 pages and 14 plates pertaining to the surgical anatomy of inguinal hernia. Although completed in 1779, it was not published until 1801, 12 years after Camper's death in 1789.

Plate XIII of this work contains two figures, but only Figure I is reproduced here. The singular feature of this illustration is the sweeping turn-in of the crural arch as it courses medially over the uncovered (crural sheath removed) crural artery and vein. Because of the delay of 22 years between its completion and publication, the figure has historical significance.

In 1793, Gimbernat was the first to publish this specific anatomic characteristic of the crural ligament and referred to it in his "Description of the Crural Arch."[4] In 1807, Cooper referred to it as the third insertion of the tendon of the external oblique muscle ". . . into the ligament of the pubis over the linea ileopectinea. This last portion . . . forms a crescent shaped edge, which is turned towards the crural vein . . . ."[6]

Who then should be given historical priority for describing the characteristic anatomic turn-in of the medial portion of the crural ligament? When Camper completed his *Icones Herniarum* in 1779, Cooper was 11 years old. It is apparent, therefore, that recognition as the first to describe (not publish) the anatomic feature belongs to Camper or Gimbernat. Nothing is known about the former's years of preparation before the *Icones Herniarum* was completed in 1779. It is recorded, however, that Gimbernat visited London in 1777 to attend a course of lectures given by John Hunter. During one of these lectures, Hunter was discussing the technical difficulties and surgical risks in operating for crural hernia. Gimbernat took this occasion (to the subsequent delight

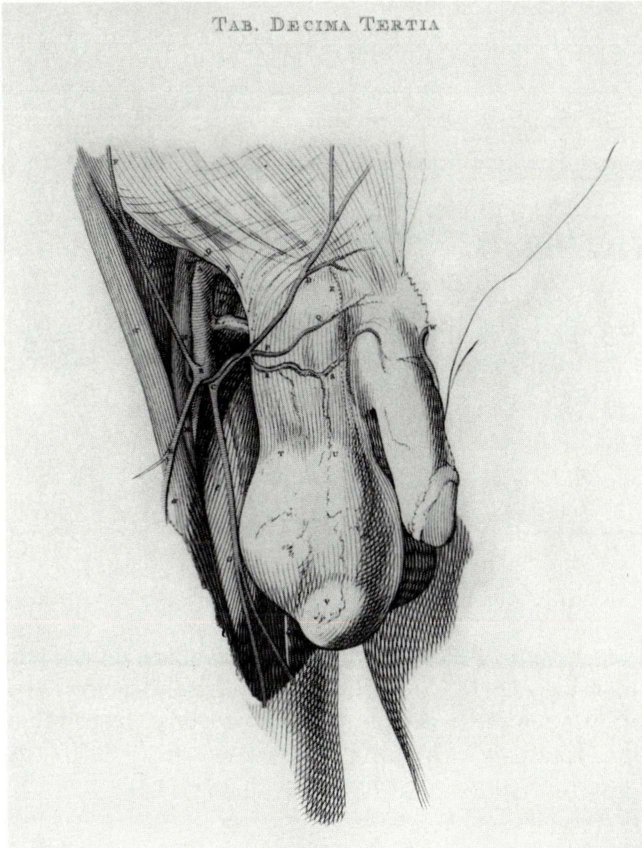

1

of Hunter) to demonstrate a safe and simple operation that he had performed for the first time in 1772. Furthermore, in 1793 Gimbernat wrote, "This part (crural arch), although it is remarkable, had been little examined, and less understood, till I demonstrated it for the first time in 1768. The ignorance of its true structure has occasioned such a variety of dangerous methods; and this is in reality, the reason why surgery has not made the smallest progress in the treatment of this accident [incarcerated or strangulated femoral hernia]."[5]

Accordingly, it is believed that Gimbernat should be given full credit as the first not only to write but also to publish a description of the crural arch.

1 This illustration clearly depicts the twisting turn-in of the medial portion of the crural ligament as it proceeds medially to its insertion into the pubic tubercle. Unfortunately, the fascia lata has been removed; therefore, its intimate adherence and concomitant turn-in with this portion of the crural ligament to form the lacunar (fascial) part of Gimbernat's ligament are not seen.

The other parts of the illustration, with the exception of the crural and superficial pudendal vessels, are not of surgical significance. Furthermore, the labels and their specific legends are difficult to correlate. In general, the illustration is not well done.

REFERENCES

1. Biographical sketch from *Biographisches Lexikon der Hervorragenden Ärzte. Aller Zeiten und Völker.* Vienna and Leipzig: Urban & Schwarzenberg, 1884, pp. 652–653.
2. Cunningham Prof: *Nieuw Nederlandsch Biogenfisch Woordenboek.* Leiden: AW Sijthoff's Uitgevers–Maatschappi, 1911, p. 555.
3. Camperi Petrie: *Icones Herniarum.* Frankfurt: Varrentrapp and Wenner, 1801.
4. De Gimbernat D: *Nuevo Método de Operar en la Hernia Crural.* Madrid: Ibarra, 1793.
5. De Gimbernat D: *New Method of Operating for the Femoral Hernia.* (English translation by Thomas Beddoes.) London: Johnson, 1795.
6. Cooper AP: *The Anatomy and Surgical Treatment of Crural and Umbilical Hernia, Part II.* London: Longman & Co, 1807, p. 2.

ASTLEY PASTON COOPER
(1768–1841)

Plate XCI
Plate XCII
Plate XCIII
Plate XCIV
Plate XCV
Plate XCVI

The old axiom, "Progress is made by standing on the shoulders of our predecessors," applies most appropriately to Sir Astley Paston Cooper, who was both a surgeon and a renowned anatomist. It seems fitting, therefore, to commemorate his contributions to the surgical anatomy of inguinal (1804) and crural (1807) hernias by including excerpts from both of these texts—in particular, his description of the transversalis fascia (which he named the fascia transversalis).

FROM *THE ANATOMY AND SURGICAL TREATMENT OF INGUINAL AND CONGENITAL HERNIA* (1804)

"The direction of the abdominal rings is obliquely upwards and outwards, in a line from the pubis to the spinous process of the ilium. Though called a ring, it is not a true circle, for the diameter in length, which is the direction from the pubis to the transverse column, is about one inch; but the breadth, from one column of tendon to the other, is only half an inch. The center of this aperture is one inch and a quarter from the symphysis. A fascia [currently referred to as the external spermatic fascia] which originates from the tendon of the external oblique muscle . . . and uniting with the spermatic cord, accompanies it in its descent into the scrotum, to which, as well to the spermatic sord [*sic*], it closely adheres.

"Surgeons have . . . generally believed that the aperture was continued into the abdomen immediately behind the ring. This however is not the case, for all direct passage of the spermatic cord into this cavity is shut out by tendons and a fascia, which are probably intended as a guard against protrusions of the contents of the belly.

"Poupart's ligament, or crural arch, is connected to the spine of the ilium, whence it passes down in a vaulted form over the femoral vessels, and terminates on the inner side of those vessels in a semicircular sweep, from which extends a triangular portion connected with the spinous process of the pubis, and extending from it to the upper part of the symphysis pubis . . . If there had been no other defence to the lower part than that afforded by this arch, few persons would escape herniae . . .

"Three different fasciae are connected with Poupart's ligament, two of which pass upwards and one downwards . . . .

"The fascia which passes . . . downwards, is the fascia lata of the thigh, which, being continued from the crural arch and from the pubis, gives a strong covering to the muscles of the thigh. . . Secondly, a thinner fascia* is sent upward from the crural arch immediately behind the abdominal muscles, to which it gives a lining similar to that tendinous expansion which covers them on the fore part. This is the fascia which leaves an opening from the abdomen for the spermatic cord in the male, and for the round ligament of the uterus in the female. It is continued from Poupart's ligament, and passes upwards to the inner side of the transversalis muscle and its tendon, to which it is united by a cellular membrane; and it is extended from thence on the inner side of the same muscle to the upper part of the abdomen, but becomes thinner as it ascends. Above the middle of Poupart's ligament it passes on each side of the spermatic cord, leaving a hole for its passage. The lower part of this hole has a thin tendinous margin; its upper part is shut by the internal oblique and transversalis muscle. From the edge of this fascia a thinner is sent off, which unites itself to the spermatic cord. A part of the same fascia descends from the middle of Poupart's ligament, and becomes united to the femoral artery and vein, and a part is fixed to the pubis.

"The strength of the fascia differs in different subjects . . . but in all cases of inguinal herniae it becomes of considerable strength and thickness, especially on its inner edge; and if it had not existed the bowels would, in the erect posture, be always capable of passing under the edge of the transversalis muscle, so that without it no person could be free from inguinal hernia.

"Through the opening [internal or deep ring], which I have just described, and through the abdominal ring [external or subcutaneous ring; also called the saphena opening] of the external oblique muscle, the spermatic cord passes down to the testis.

"The vas deferens on each side arises from the posterior part of the testicle, to which it is the excretory duct; and, with the cord, passes into the abdomen; here it quits the spermatic artery and vein, sinks into the cavity of the pelvis and runs behind the bladder to open into the urethra.

"These three† vessels together with their appropriate absorbents and nerves, receive a double covering of peritoneum from the part at which they quit the abdomen, which closely unites them together. This covering is called the Tunica Vaginalis of the Spermatic Cord. Just above the testis the two layers of the tunic recede from each other, so as to form a bag for the purpose of covering this organ, and this is named the Tunica Vaginalis Testis."

---

*This is Cooper's original description of the transversalis fascia. He described it again in 1807.
†These are not three vessels but two—the spermatic artery and vein—and the vas deferens.

ASTLEY PASTON COOPER (1768–1841)
Continued

THIS Plate is intended to shew the insertions of the external oblique muscles, the formation of the abdominal rings, and of two of the fasciæ which are connected with Poupart's ligament, as well as the course of the spermatic cord under the edges of the internal oblique and transverse muscles, before it reaches the abdominal ring.

a. Symphisis pubis.

b b. Anterior and superior spinous process of the ilium.

c c. External oblique muscles.

d. Linea alba extending down to the symphisis pubis, and formed by the union of the tendinous fibres of the two oblique and transverse muscles.

e e. Lineæ semilunares, formed by the union of the tendinous fibres of the external and internal oblique and transverse muscles.

f f. The abdominal rings, formed by the separation of two columns of tendinous fibres; the upper inserted at *a* into each pubis; the lower inserted into the pubis at *h*. after passing behind the spermatic cord.

g. The origin of some tendinous fibres which proceed from the anterior spinous process of the ilium, and crossing the columns of tendon, assist in uniting them above the abdominal ring.

i i. Poupart's ligament, or the crural arch, which is extended from the anterior spinous process of the ilium at *b*, to the pubis at *h*, receiving the lower column of tendon, which forms a part of the abdominal ring, and which passes behind the cord to be inserted from the spinous process to the crest of the pubis.

k. The fascia lata of the thigh, which is continued from Poupart's ligament, and seen turning in under the femoral vessels near the middle of the fore part of the thigh.

l. Is the saphæna major vein of the leg going through the fascia to enter the femoral vein.

m. Another part of the same fascia which arises from Poupart's ligament, and joins with the fascia lata, which it assists in forming.

n. The tendon of the external oblique muscle cut open to shew the parts which are situated behind it.

o. The internal oblique muscle, its lower edge which arises from Poupart's ligament, is raised and turned to shew the parts behind it. It is inserted into the pubis behind the upper column of tendon which forms the abdominal ring.

p. The transversalis. Its lower edge also arises from Poupart's ligament, but is here raised and turned up. It in its natural state runs over the cord to be inserted into the pubis behind the abdominal ring, which it serves as a valve to close behind.

q. A fascia, connected with Poupart's ligament, which runs upwards to the transversalis, and unites itself to the posterior part of the transverse muscle and its tendon, and thus prevents the bowels from slipping between the lower edge of the muscle and Poupart's ligament, or between the fibres of the muscle itself.

That portion of the fascia which is placed between the spinous process of the ilium at *b*, and the hole *r* is strong; but that between the hole *r* and the pubis, is often little more than condensed cellular membrane, as that part is strengthened by the tendon of the transversalis, and by the epigastric artery.

A portion of the fascia *q* is fixed in the pubis, and another part of it passes behind Poupart's ligament to unite with the femoral vessels.

r. The place at which the spermatic cord goes into the abdomen. The fascia situated on its outer side and lower part, is of considerable density, but becoming thin upon its inner side, so as to shew the epigastric artery and vein behind it; from the edge of the fascia a thinner is sent off which unites itself to the spermatic cord, which fascia in this dissection has been removed.

s. The epigastric artery and vein, situated behind the fascia, at first on the inner side, and afterwards behind the spermatic cord.

t t. The spermatic cord, near two inches of which is above and to the outer side of the abdominal ring, and still not in the abdomen; it is also seen below the ring, running to the testicle.

1

1 This plate shows a completed cadaver dissection of the lower half of the anterior abdominal wall and subjacent parts of the thighs. The description, "the course of the spermatic cord under the edges of the internal oblique and transverse muscles, before it reaches the abdominal ring" is anatomically reversed. It would be preferable to state, "the course of the spermatic cord from the internal ring under the edges of the internal oblique and transverse muscles, before it reaches the scrotum."

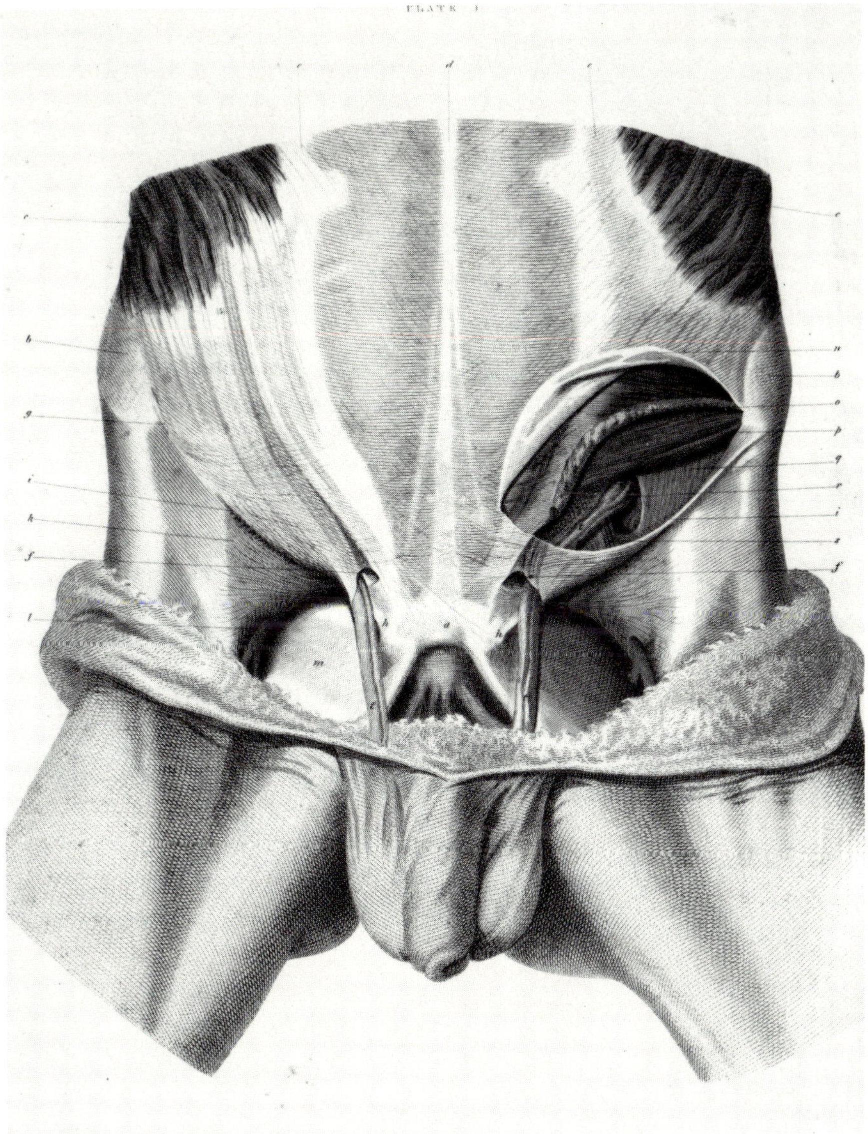

1

ASTLEY PASTON COOPER
(1768–1841)
Continued

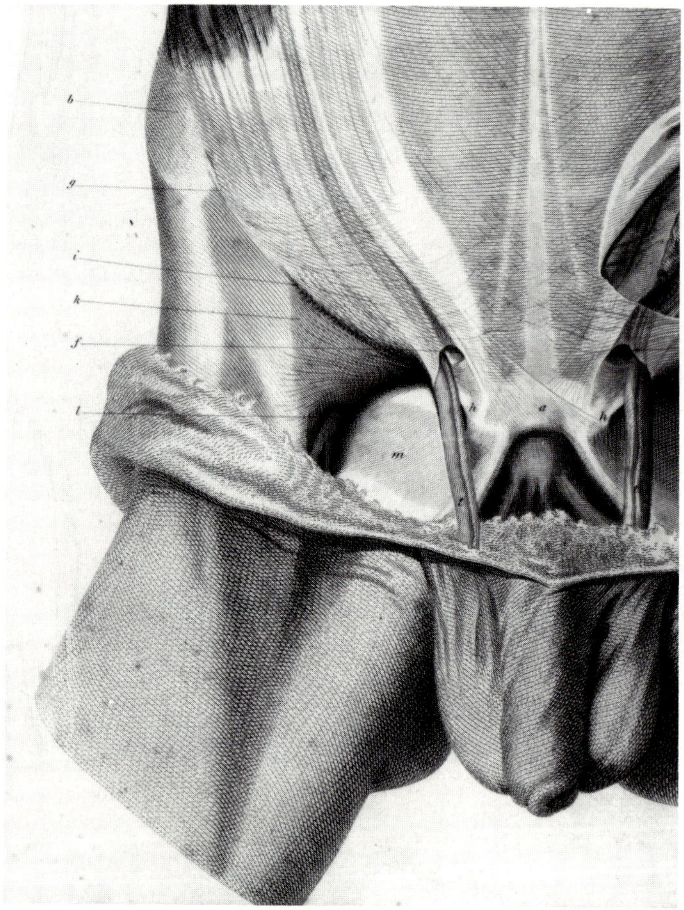

2

2 This close-up view of the right side depicts the turn-in of the medial portion of the crural arch (inguinal ligament) and the subjacent attached portion of the fascia lata to form the superficial (tendinous) and deep (lacunar) parts, respectively, of Gimbernat's ligament.*

3 An enlarged close-up view of the lower portions of the groin areas in **1.**

---

*Interestingly, in this regard William Lawrence (a contemporary of Cooper) stated, "Where the attachment of the fascia to the crural arch terminates, it forms a distinct semilunar or crescent-shaped fold." To this he added a footnote: "This part is represented in the first plate of Mr. Cooper's work on inguinal hernia, although it is not marked by any letter of reference."[2]

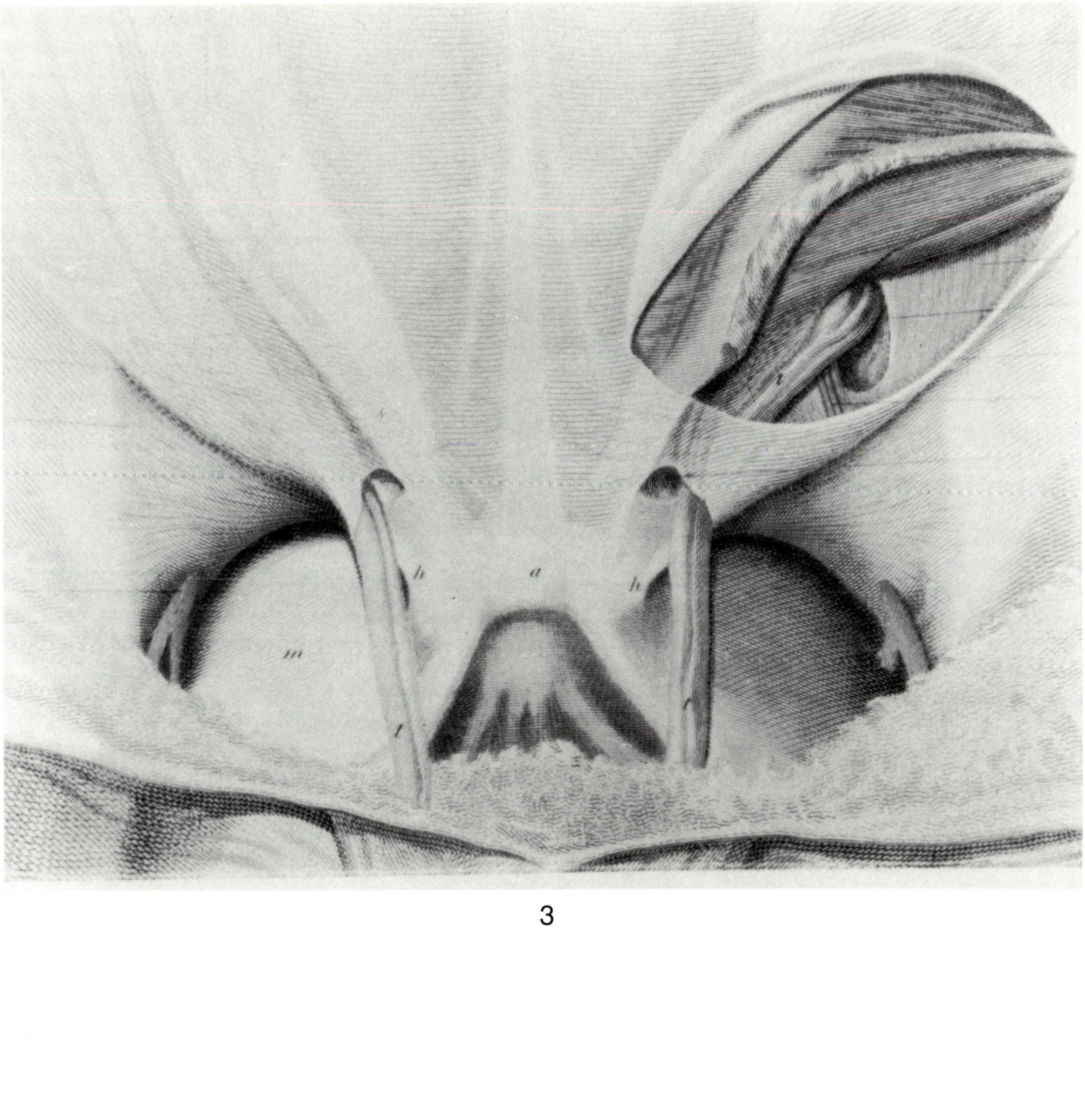

3

ASTLEY PASTON COOPER (1768–1841)

Continued

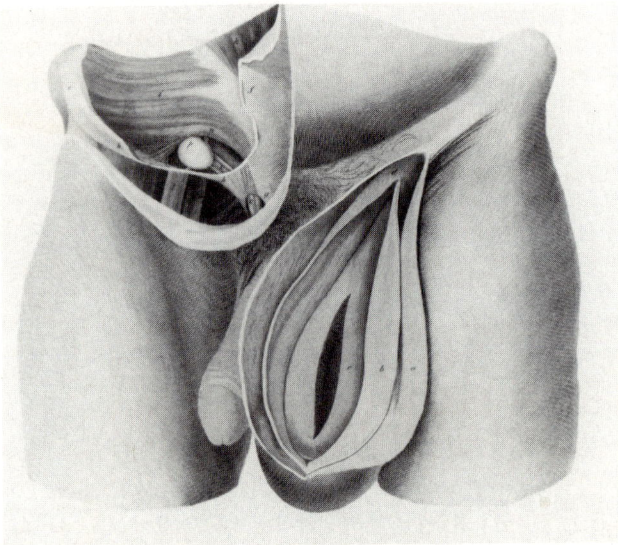

4

SHEWS two inguinal herniæ. That on the left side, having existed many years, has descended into the scrotum and become of great magnitude. That on the left side, is in an incipient state, and shews the distance from the abdominal ring, at which it first protrudes from the abdomen.

a. Common integuments cut through and turned back.
b. The fascia, which is extended from the external oblique muscle over the spermatic cord, in the healthy state; and over the hernial sac, when it descends into the scrotum. To the inner side of this fascia the cremaster muscle adheres.
c. The hernial sac cut open.
d. Abdominal ring, concealed in some degree by the fascia which passes over it.
e. Anterior and superior spinous process of the ilium.
f. Tendon of the external oblique muscle.
g. Abdominal ring on the right side.
h h. Poupart's ligament.
i. Internal oblique muscle passing above the hernial sac.
k. The rectus muscle.
l. Femoral artery.
m. Femoral vein.
n. Epigastric artery passing behind the hernial sac.
o o. Spermatic cord above and below the abdominal ring.
p. Sac of an incipient inguinal hernia, situated as usual, below the edges of the internal oblique and transverse muscles, and above the middle of Poupart's ligament.

4, 5, 6, 7, 8 This illustration of the right inguinal region was selected for its excellent depiction of the arched transverse distribution of the fasciculi of the internal oblique muscle *(i)* and their distance from Poupart's ligament *(h)*. (In the introductory paragraph to the legends, the third sentence beginning "That on the left side" should read "That on the right side.") This agrees with the intraoperative surgical anatomy of the right internal oblique muscle as shown by Frank Robinson (see Plate VI, Fig. 33). Both of these illustrations mirror the fasciculi of the internal oblique muscle as depicted in the intraoperative color photograph **(5)** taken during the initial stages of an anterior repair of a right direct inguinal hernia. This demonstrates the importance of illustrations *and* photographs as anatomic guides for the practicing surgeon. All too frequently artistic licenses are taken, and the resulting illustrations fail to conform with surgical anatomy.

In the drawing by Max Brödel **(6)**, a consummate medical artist and the true "father" of medical art illustration in America, the internal oblique muscle is depicted as closely packed fibers that course parallel and in juxtaposition to the inguinal ligament to terminate in a conjoint tendon with seemingly excellent holding power.[1] At operation, however, the loosely separated fasciculi of the internal oblique muscle invariably are arched transversely and at a distance from the inguinal ligament **(7)**. Fatty areolar tissue is often interposed between the lowermost fasciculi, further lessening their holding power **(8)**. The author has never observed a conjoint tendon in the anterior repair of inguinal hernias. It is concluded, therefore, that the use of the internal oblique muscle as a supportive structure in the anterior repair of inguinal hernias is both unanatomic and unphysiologic and cannot be advocated.

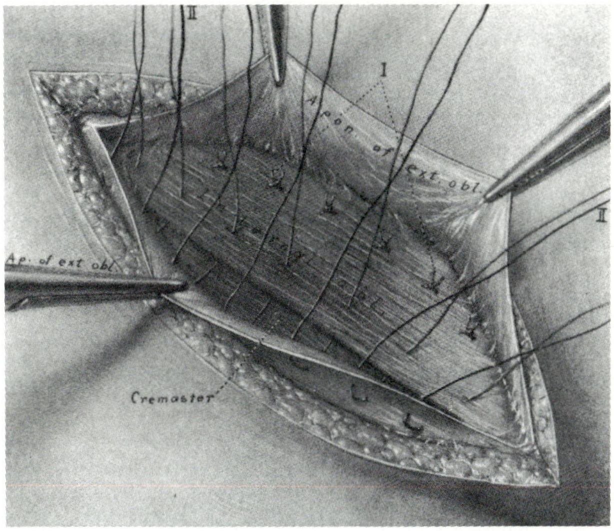

6

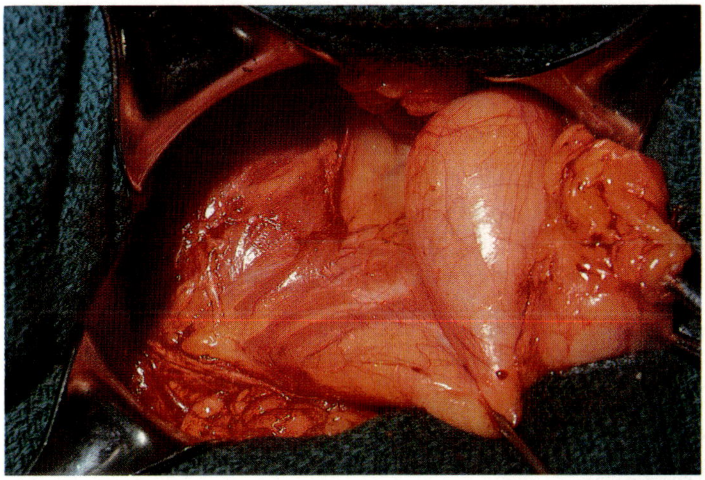

5

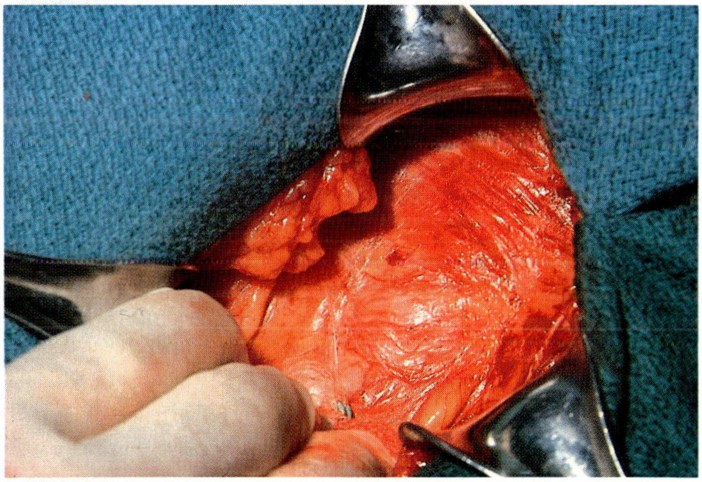

7

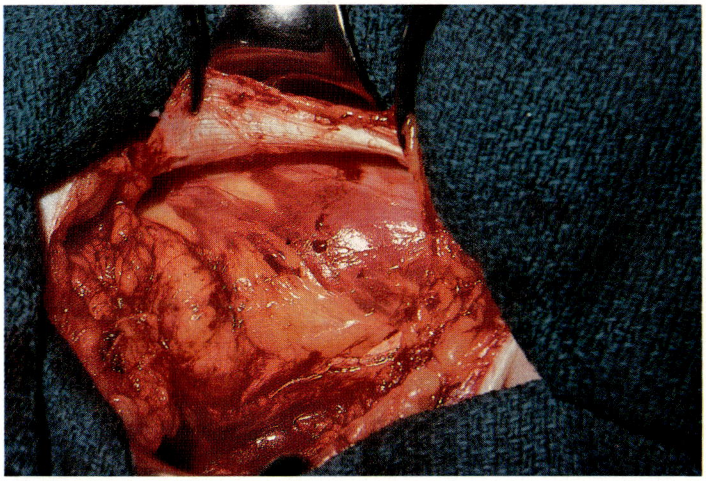

8

ASTLEY PASTON COOPER (1768–1841)
Continued

FROM *THE ANATOMY AND SURGICAL TREATMENT OF CRURAL AND UMBILICAL HERNIA* (1807)

"The pubis is covered by a ligamentous substance, which forms a particularly strong production above the linea ileopectinea, extending from the tuberosity of the pubis outwards, and projecting beyond the bone above that line [Cooper's ligament]. Into this process the external oblique muscle is inserted . . . .

"The lower tendinous edge of the external oblique muscle has generally been called *Poupart's ligament,* but is now more commonly named the Crural Arch. This arch is stretched from the anterior superior spinous process of the ilium to the tuberosity of the pubis, into which a part of it is fixed, whence it proceeds forward to the symphysis pubis, where the remainder is inserted.

"It appears . . . that the lower part of the tendon of the external oblique muscle has three distinct insertions; first, into the symphysis, and this forms the superior column of the external abdominal ring; secondly, into the tuberosity of the pubis, which forms the lower column of the ring; and thirdly, into the ligament of the pubis over the linea ileopectinea. This last portion by its conjunction with the ligament of the pubis forms a crescent-shaped edge, which is turned towards the crural vein . . . about the distance of five-eighths of an inch from it.

"When the fascia lata is first laid bare, it . . . is found to form a sharp crescent-shaped edge; . . . This fascia passes over the crural vessels, and its principal use is to cover the femoral artery and vein and thus strengthen the sheath in which they are contained . . . .

"The anterior part of this sheath [femoral] is formed by a thin fascia that appears . . . to arise from the crural arch, but may be detached from it by passing the finger behind the arch, where it will be found to be a continuation of the fascia which lines the transversalis muscle; but as it passes under the posterior edge of the arch it closely adheres to it . . . The whole of this fascia . . . might be described as arising from the crural arch and dividing into two portions; one, ascending to the transversalis muscle, the other, descending to form the crural sheath. The anterior part of the sheath in which the crural vessels are contained, is joined to the fascia transversalis, and when it is removed the crural artery and vein are laid bare.

"When the sheath is cut open the crural artery and vein are exposed. These vessels pass down within the sheath for about two inches, after which they carry with them a closely investing fascia, derived from the fascia lata, which accompanies them in their course down the thigh. The sheath is therefore formed like a funnel; it is large above, but contracted around the artery and vein below.

"Anteriorly to the crural arch is situated . . . another fascia . . . and it ascends to the posterior part of the transversalis muscle; it is . . . firmly fixed to the ligament of the pubis, and is extended over the pubis into the cavity of the pelvis; it rises to the tendon of the transversalis muscle on the inner side of the spermatic cord, and is firmly attached to the linea semilunaris.

"This anterior fascia, which is described in the first part of this work, should be

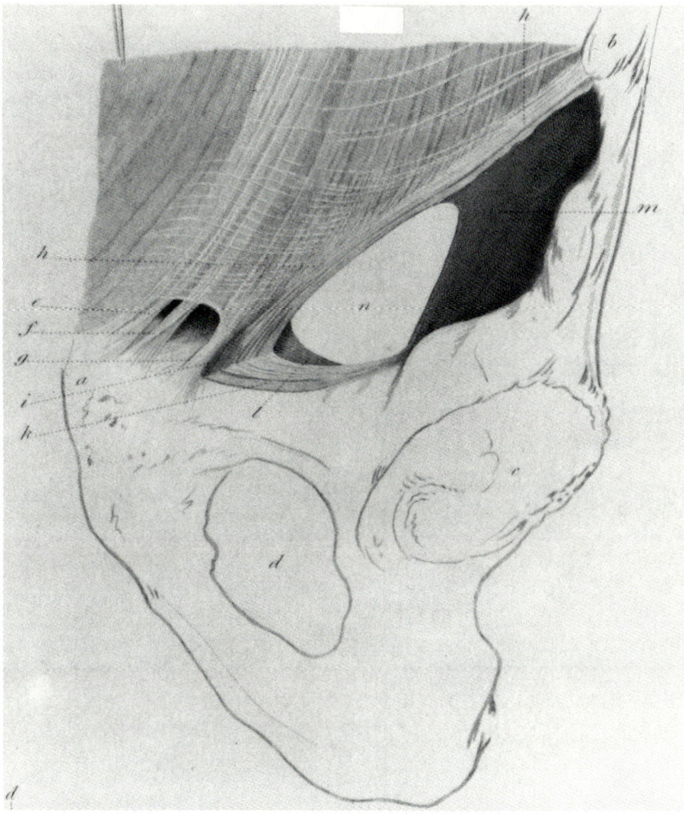

Shews the insertions of the external oblique muscle into the pubis and its ligament, and the fascia iliaca, or GIMBERNAT'S fascia.

a. Pubis.
b. Spine of the ilium.
c. Acetabulum.
d. Thyroid foramen.
e. Column of tendon. *f.* Another column. *g.* A third column, making together two apertures at the abdominal ring in the female, which is not uncommon.
h. Anterior edge of the crural arch, or POUPART'S ligament.
i. Third insertion of the external oblique muscle.
k. Ligament of the pubis, into which the external oblique *i* is inserted.
l. Portion of fascia transversalis, and tendon of the rectus, passing behind the insertion of the external oblique.
m. Fascia iliaca passing from the crural arch over the iliacus internus muscle.
n. Orifice of the crural sheath, for the passage of the crural artery vein and absorbent vessels.

9

called the *fascia transversalis;* it lines the posterior part of that muscle, and there prevents the viscera from descending between the fibers of the abdominal muscles, but leaves an opening for the passage of the spermatic cord and round ligament, which I have ventured to name the *internal abdominal ring.* This fascia sends a process before the external iliac artery and vein, and another between them, which unites one passing from the fascia iliaca, and these vessels are then united to the crural arch.

"Each of these fasciae sends down a portion of its substance under the crural arch, to form the crural sheath for the artery and vein. The fascia iliaca sends the posterior part, the fascia transversalis the anterior, and by the union of these on each side the lateral portions of the sheath are produced.

"The space called the crural ring, is . . . between the crural vein, which forms its outer part, and the crescent-shaped edge of the insertion of the external oblique muscle into the ligament of the pubis, anteriorly by the inner edge of the crural arch, and posteriorly by the pubis and the ligament which covers it. It is lined by the fasciae which form the sheath . . . .

" . . . When the finger is thrust down through the crural space, the lunated or semilunar edge of the fascia lata may be distinctly felt."*

9 This illustration is purposely included because it is the only one in which Gimbernat is mentioned. It is ironic, however, that Cooper should link Gimbernat's name to the fascia iliaca and not to the ligament that he described in his monograph *Nuevo Método de Operar en la Hernia Crural* (1793). This "new method" was the severance of the ligament that is universally known as Gimbernat's ligament. Cooper obviously had knowledge of Gimbernat's work and its English translation, as is shown by his reference to Gimbernat and by his subsequent performance of the operation originally described by Gimbernat.

*This finding of Cooper's confirms the fixed relation of the fascial or lacunar portion of Gimbernat's ligament to the medial wall of the femoral sheath, as described in this atlas.

ASTLEY PASTON COOPER (1768–1841)

Continued

Shews the crural sheath.

a. Pubis.
b. Ilium.
c. Abdominal muscles drawn up.
d. Transversalis muscle.
e. Its tendon.
f. Seat of the posterior edge of the crural arch.
gg. Fascia transversalis.
h Inner portion of the same fascia.
i. Fascia iliaca.
k. Crural sheath
l. Crural artery,
m. Crural vein.
n. Saphæna major vein.
o. Anterior crural nerve.
p. Fascia lata turned back.
q. Tendon of the external oblique muscle, drawn down.

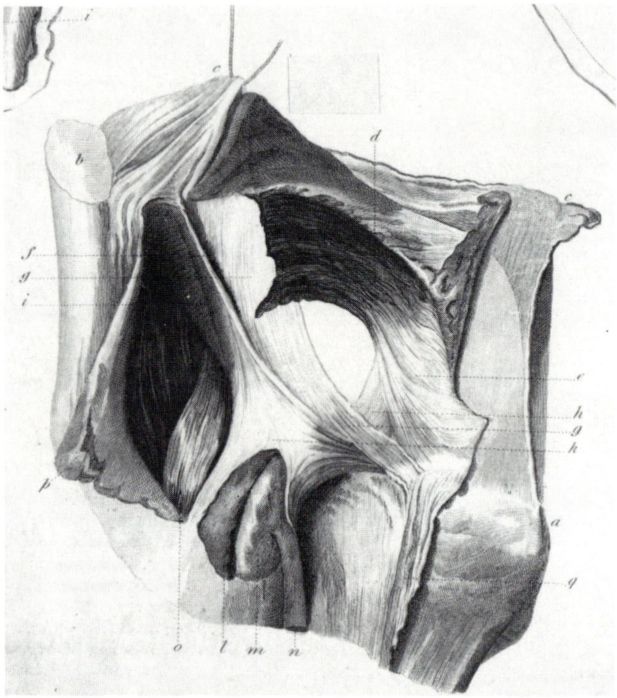

10

Yet in his writings on the subject of femoral hernia, Cooper, for reasons unknown, never referred to "Gimbernat's ligament."

There are, also, errors of anatomy in the artist's illustration. The ligament of the pubis *(k)* (Cooper's ligament) is incorrectly depicted as superficial and anterior, rather than deep and posterior, to the crural arch. Furthermore, it is shown in a horizontal rather than a diagonal plane in relation to the crural arch. In addition, the "external oblique" is not being inserted into the ligament of the pubis as described *(k)*. Because of these errors, this illustration has no practical application for the surgeon.

10 Although it is not described in the legends, this illustration shows nicely the twisting turn-in of the medial portion of the crural arch and its attached fascia lata to form the deep or lateral (lacunar) part of Gimbernat's ligament. Its relationship to the crural sheath *(k)* and the fascia of the posterior inguinal wall (*e* and *g*) is clearly visible.

11 In this illustration, the "third insertion of the external oblique" *(g)* corresponds to the lateral or lacunar part of Gimbernat's ligament. Although in *m* it is stated, "The division in the crural hernia is made at the upper and inner parts," in Plate XCVI (**13** and **14**) the division is made through the center of its crescentic margin, as originally described by Gimbernat.

12 This is a good anatomic illustration, particularly in comparison to the distorted anatomy in Plate XCIII, Fig. **9**. Particularly to be noted is the diagonal plane relationship between the "posterior edge of the crural arch" *(n)* and "the linea ileopectinea" *(c)*.

The twisting turn-in of "the third insertion of the external oblique into the ligament of the pubis [Cooper's ligament]" *(g)* is clearly depicted. This was previously described

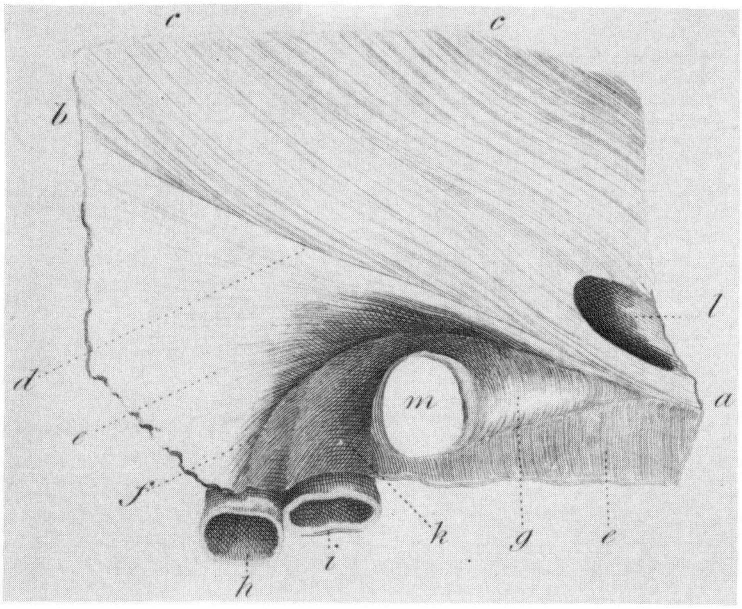

Crural hernial sac removed to shew the hole by which it descends in the female.

a. Seat of the pubis.
b. Crural arch extending towards the ilium.
cc. Abdominal muscles.
d. Crural arch.
ee. Fascia lata.
f. Semilunar edge of the fascia lata.
g. Third insertion of the external oblique.
h. Crural artery.
i. Crural vein.
k. Crural sheath.
l. Abdominal ring.

11

12

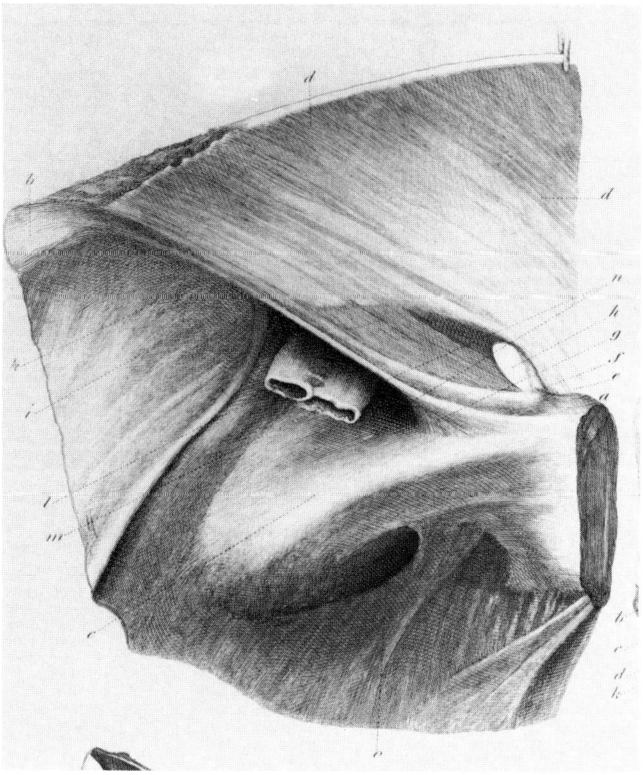

Posterior view of the external oblique muscle, of the external iliac artery and vein, and of the fascia iliaca.

a. Symphisis pubis.
b. Spinous process of the ilium.
c. Pubis at the linea ileo pectinea.
d. External oblique muscle and its tendon.
e. Superior column of the tendon of the abdominal ring.
f. Insertion of the inferior column of the ring into the tubercle of the pubis.
g. The third insertion of the external oblique into the ligament of the pubis, from whence it is extended towards the symphisis.
h. Abdominal ring.
i. The fascia iliaca extending over the iliacus internus and psoas muscles.
k. The junction of the fascia iliaca with the posterior edge of the crural arch, and it is seen extending near to the external iliac artery.
l. External iliac artery.
m. External iliac vein.
[These vessels pass through an oval space, which is the beginning of the crural sheath, which is bounded internally by the third insertion of the external oblique muscle, externally by the fascia iliaca joining to the posterior edge of the crural arch, behind by the process of the same fascia, and before by the posterior edge of the crural arch.]
n. Posterior edge of the crural arch extending from the pubis to the ilium. That part of it which is included between the two lines from *n*, forms the posterior stricture in large crural herniæ.
o. Thyroideal foramen.

ASTLEY PASTON COOPER (1768–1841)

Continued

Anterior view of a crural hernia operated on by cutting directly inwards.

- *a.* Symphisis pubis.
- *b.* Spine of the ilium.
- *cc.* Abdominal muscles.
- *d.* Crural arch.
- *e.* Abdominal ring.
- *f.* Lower column of the ring inserted into the tubercle of the pubis.
- *g.* Fascia lata.
- *h.* Saphæna major vein.
- *i.* Fascia propria, or protruded crural sheath.
- *k.* Hernial sac included in the former.
- *l.* Insertion of the external oblique muscle into the ligament of the pubis, divided in the operation.

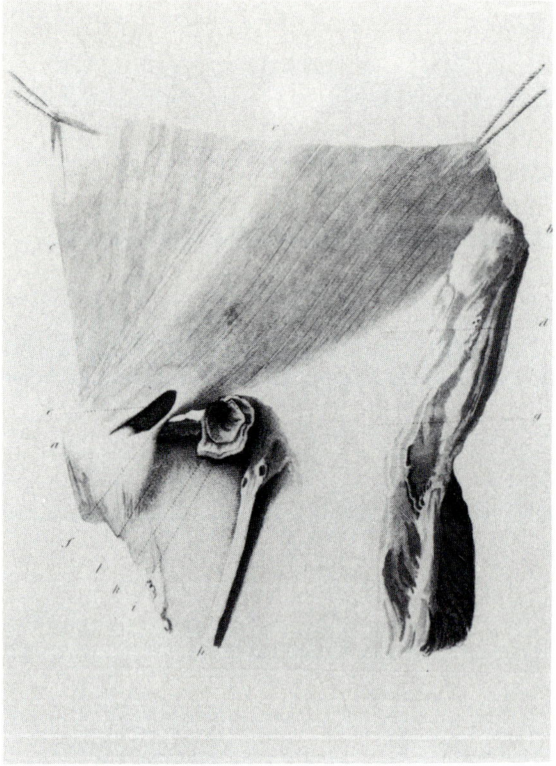

13

13, 14 These two illustrations—an anterior (**13**) and a posterior view (**14**)—were made from a postoperative and postmortem cadaver dissection. Each clearly shows Gimbernat's method of operating for crural hernia by cutting the inner edge of the duplicature of the crural arch.

REFERENCES

1. Burket, WC (ed): *Surgical Papers by William Stewart Halsted* (Vol. 1). Baltimore: Johns Hopkins, 1952.
2. Lawrence, W: *A Treatise on Ruptures*. Philadelphia: Edward Parker, 1811, p. 279.

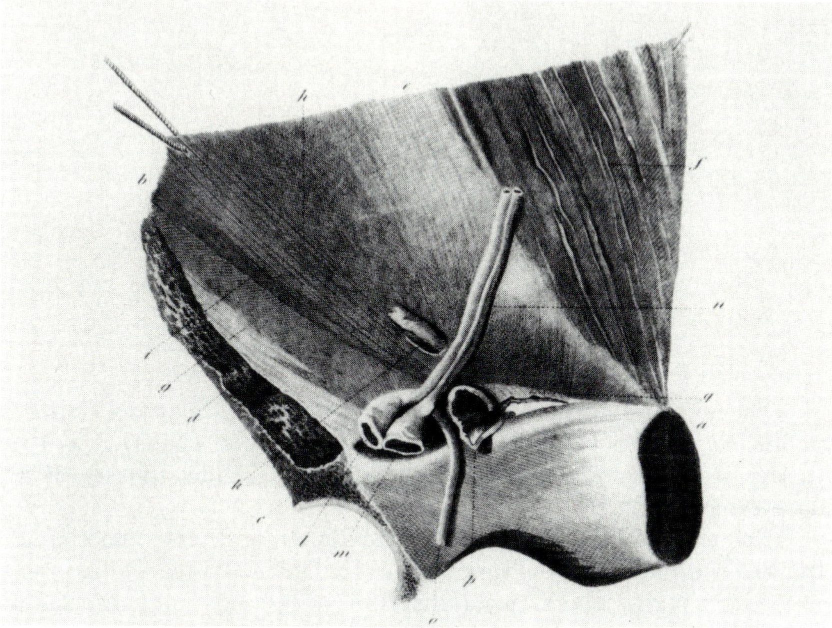

14

Posterior view of the same.

a. Symphisis pubis.

b. Spine of the ilium.

c. Ilium.

d. Iliacus internus.

e. Abdominal muscles.

f. Rectus abdominis.

g. Fascia iliaca.

h. Fascia transversalis.

i. Junction of the two fascia at the posterior edge of the crural arch.

k. Internal abdominal ring, and the round ligament passing through it.

l. Iliac artery.

m. Iliác vein.

n. Epigastric artery and vein.

o. Obturator artery passing from the epigastric, but taking its course on the outer side of the hernial sac.

p. Hernial sac.

q. The insertion of the external oblique muscle, which had been divided in the operation inwards.

ANTONIO SCARPA (1747?–1832)

Plate XCVII

The following illustrations are reproduced from Scarpa's *Traité Pratique des Hernies*, published in Paris in 1812. An English translation appeared in 1814.

1 In this illustration, made from a cadaver dissection, the sac of a femoral hernia has been removed, leaving a dark oval space.

The letter *p* indicates the site of union of the internal portion of the fascia lata with the external border of the ligament of Fallopius (Poupart's ligament). This point lies in immediate juxtaposition to the insertion of this ligament into the pubic tubercle *(c)*. Of particular interest in this diagram is the depiction of the anatomic relationship of the epigastric artery *(s)* and veins *(t)*. This artery is frequently and incorrectly depicted with only one accompanying vein instead of two.

The letter *q* in the diagram depicts the narrow band of fascia lata, formed by the superior extremity of the falciform ligament, that is adherent to the external border of the ligament of Fallopius. It is commonly known as Hey's ligament after the English surgeon who described it. This ligament is anterosuperior to Gimbernat's ligament *(m)* and forms the anterior boundary of the femoral hernial orifice.

This orifice, described by Lytle, is the site of the opening in the "blind" lower end of the femoral sheath where the sac of a femoral hernia protrudes. The orifice surrounds the neck of the sac; its medial boundary, the crescentic lateral margin of Gimbernat's ligament, is the cause of constriction in an incarcerated or strangulated femoral hernia. The remaining two boundaries of the orifice are the pectineus fascia and its underlying muscle posteriorly, and laterally the falciform edge of the fascia lata of the thigh.

The ligament of Fallopius *(l)* is elevated on a hook, and the twisting turn-in (Gimbernat's duplicature of the crural arch) of its insertion into the "linea iliopectinea" is visible *(m)*. Its lateral extremity or base is joined by the internal portion of the fascia lata of the thigh *(o)* to form the medial boundary of the femoral sheath. In addition, this union forms an anatomic barrier between the abdomen and thigh, as originally described by Gimbernat.[1]

The internal portion of the fascia lata of the thigh continues laterally and behind the femoral vessels *(q)* to join with the iliac fascia in forming the posterior wall of the femoral sheath. This anatomic disposition of the fascia lata of the thigh *(o, q)* is more clearly demonstrated in **2**.

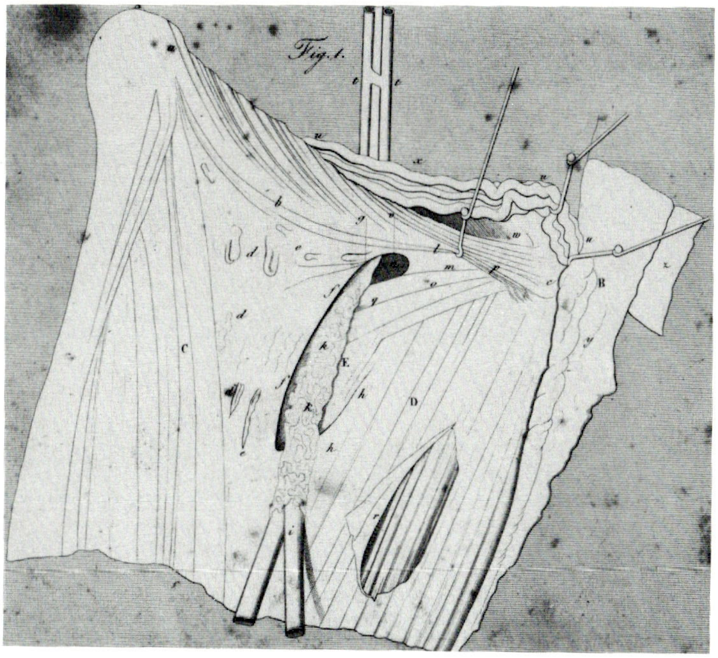

PLANCHE XII.

FIGURE I.

A.	Epine antérieure et supérieure de l'os iliaque.
B.	Os du pubis.
C.	Portion *latérale externe* de l'aponévrose *fascia-lata*.
D.	Portion *latérale interne* de cette même aponévrose.
a. b. c.	Ligament de Fallope.
d. d. d.	Ouvertures de l'aponévrose *fascia-lata* qui donnent passage à de petits vaisseaux sanguins sous-cutanés, ainsi qu'à quelques vaisseaux lymphatiques superficiels et profonds.
e. e.	Paroi antérieure de la gaîne aponévrotique des vaisseaux fémoraux, formée par l'aponévrose *fascia-lata*.
f. f.	Repli *falciforme* de l'aponévrose *fascia-lata*.
g.	Extrémité supérieure du repli falciforme, qui se recourbe au-dessous du ligament de Fallope et va s'unir à l'angle supérieur et antérieur du ligament de Gimbernat.
h. h.	Extrémité inférieure du repli falciforme, qui se recourbe en haut et limite inférieurement la fosse *ovale*.
i.	Tronc de la veine saphène.
k. k.	Tissu cellulaire *fibreux et réticulaire*, qui recouvre le côté interne de la grosse veine fémorale dans le point où elle n'est pas recouverte par le repli *falciforme* de l'aponévrose *fascia-lata*.
l.	Ligament de Fallope, qui est soulevé par un crochet, afin de laisser voir le ligament de Gimbernat.
m.	Ligament triangulaire de Gimbernat.
n.	Anneau *crural*.
o.	Portion *latérale interne* de l'aponévrose *fascia-lata*, qui s'insère le long de l'axe longitudinal du ligament de Gimbernat.
p.	Union de la portion plus mince de l'aponévrose *fascia-lata* avec le bord externe du ligament de Fallope, près son insertion au pubis.
q.	Portion *latérale interne* de l'aponévrose *fascia-lata*, qui, après s'être unie à l'axe longitudinal du ligament de Gimbernat, passe derrière les vaisseaux fémoraux, et contribue, en partie, à la formation de la gaîne aponévrotique qui les enveloppe.
r.	Section de la portion *interne* de l'aponévrose *fascia-lata*, qui fait voir que son épaisseur est moindre que celle de la portion *externe* de la même aponévrose.
s.	Artère épigastrique.
t. t.	Veines épigastriques.
v.	Angle supérieur et antérieur du ligament de Gimbernat.
u. u. u.	Cordon spermatique.
w.	Anneau inguinal ouvert suivant sa longueur. Le pilier inférieur de l'anneau inguinal, avant de s'attacher au pubis, reçoit dans un sillon le cordon spermatique.
x.	Artère spermatique.
y.	Tissu cellulaire du scrotum.
z.	Racine du pénis.

Supplément.

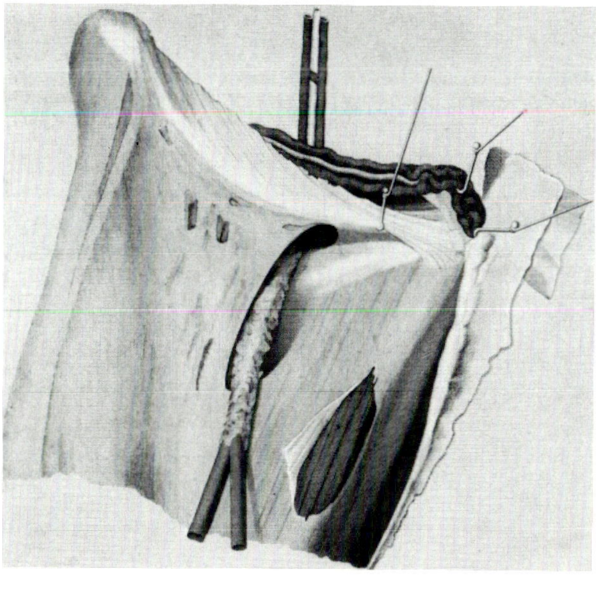

1

ANTONIO SCARPA (1747?–1832) *Continued*

a. a. a.	Ligament de Fallope.
b. b. b.	Portion interne, ou pubienne, de l'aponévrose *fascia-lata*, qui a été coupée près de son insertion à l'axe longitudinal du ligament de Gimbernat.
c.	Portion supérieure du ligament de Gimbernat, qu'on voit au-dessus de l'insertion de l'aponévrose *fascia-lata* à l'axe longitudinal du ligament de Gimbernat.
d.	Portion inférieure du ligament de Gimbernat, qu'on voit au-dessous de l'insertion de l'aponévrose *fascia-lata* à l'axe longitudinal du ligament de Gimbernat. Cette région est remplie par l'origine du muscle pectiné, qui s'attache à la crête de la branche horizontale du pubis, à laquelle le bord inférieur et interne du ligament de Gimbernat s'insère également.
e.	Anneau *crural.*
f.	Artère fémorale qui a été coupée.
g.	Veine fémorale qui a été coupée.
h.	Aponévrose iliaque.
i.	Aponévrose iliaque qui descend derrière les vaisseaux fémoraux, au-dessous de l'arcade fémorale, pour former la paroi postérieure de la gaîne aponévrotique de ces vaisseaux; de manière que les aponévroses iliaque et *fascia-lata* se confondent entre elles.
l. l. l.	Portion de l'aponévrose *fascia-lata* réunie au ligament de Fallope, et qui s'étend depuis l'épine antérieure et supérieure de l'os des iles jusqu'à l'éminence ilio-pectiné.
m.	Insertion commune des aponévroses iliaque et *fascia-lata* à l'éminence ilio-pectiné.
n.	Trou *obturateur.*
o.	Angle supérieur et antérieur du ligament de Gimbernat.
p.	Cloison aponévrotique, qui sépare l'artère de la veine fémorale.

2 This illustration is a view of the external surface of the right side of the pelvis. It depicts nicely the interrelation of its bony framework with the structures that compose the femoral arcade.

Laterally, the iliac fascia *(i)* descends behind the femoral vessels and beneath the femoral arcade. Medially, the fascia lata *(b)* courses below and then behind the femoral vessels, where it blends with the iliac fascia to form the composite posterior boundary of the femoral arcade. In addition, the conjoint insertion of the iliac fascia and the fascia lata into the iliopectineal eminence is depicted *(m)*. Finally, the relationship between Gimbernat's ligament and the fascia lata, shown in **1**, is again in evidence *(b, c)*.

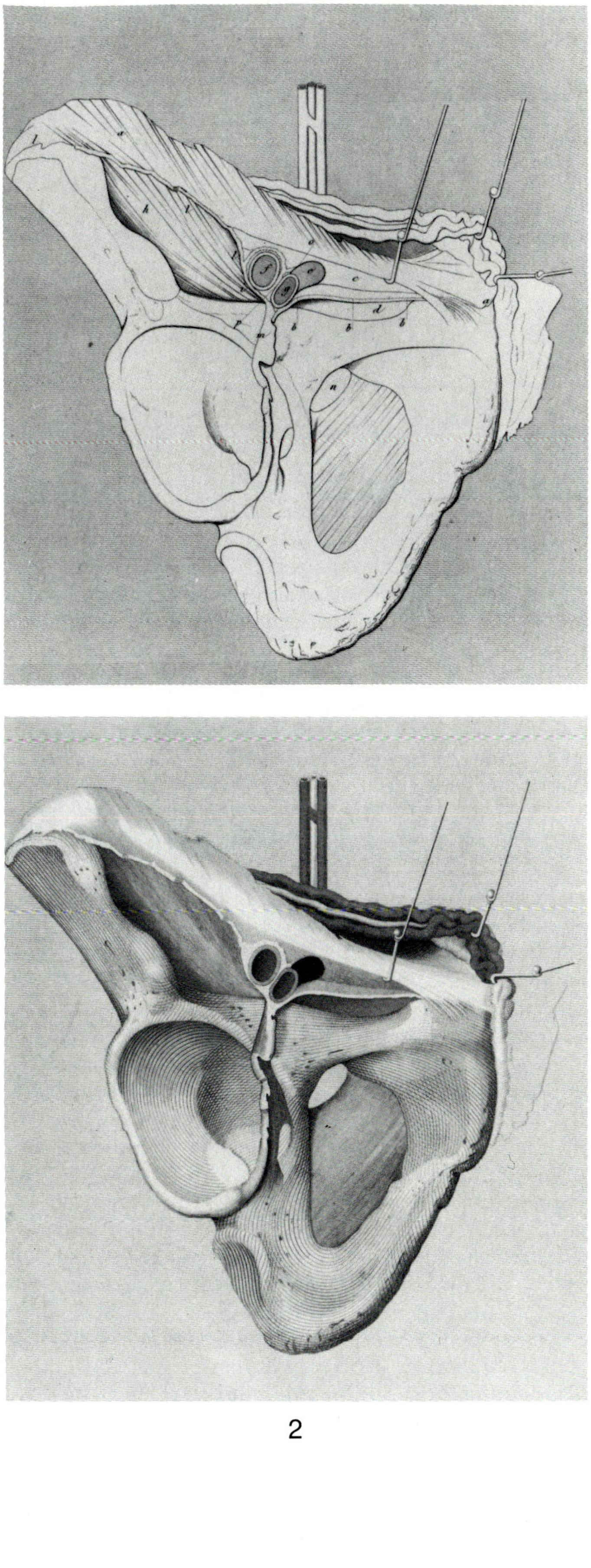

2

FRANZ K. HESSELBACH
(1759–1816)

Plate XCVIII
Plate IC

Franz Kaspar Hesselbach, a German surgeon, published his monograph *Ortu et Progressu Herniarum* in 1816.

1 This illustration from a cadaver dissection (male) demonstrates the internal (preperitoneal) anatomy of the right inguinofemoral region. A primary feature of this view is indicated by *b*, described in the accompanying legends (not shown here) as the "firm internal fibres of the inguinal ligament." Three years later (1819), Cloquet called a similar structure the "posterior surface of the crural arch." Thereafter, a multiplicity of other "reasonable facsimiles" were described (see the section on Jules Cloquet).

Another important structure is *h*, the "lacuna" in immediate juxtaposition to the femoral vein. It is depicted more fully in **2** *(m)*, which substantiates the fact that the lacunar ligament, as first described by Gimbernat in 1793, forms the boundary of the medial wall of the femoral sheath. Hesselbach did not use the eponym "Gimbernat's ligament," which was already widely accepted by 1816.

2 This illustration, which offers a better view of the lacunar ligament *(m)*, also shows the triangular area on the back of the right side of the lower portion of the anterior abdominal wall. This area is now commonly referred to as "Hesselbach's triangle." Its boundaries are medially and superiorly the lateral border of the lower portion of the rectus abdominis muscle *(B)*; laterally and superiorly the inferior epigastric vein *(i)* and artery *(h)*; and inferiorly the medial or inner part of the inguinal ligament, which forms its base but is not visible in this posterior (preperitoneal) view.

3 This is a preperitoneal view of the back of the right inguinofemoral region. It demonstrates in particular the orifice of the triangular fossa *(a)* that characteristically results from the protrusion of a direct inguinal hernia. The boundaries of Hesselbach's triangle are accentuated in varying degrees, depending upon the size of the hernia.

The relationship of the internal ring to the U-shaped sling of the transversalis fascia and its respective crura (the internal crus medially and the external crus laterally) is clearly visible. Also shown is the relationship of the internal crus *(b)* to the inferior (deep) epigastric vessels (see **4**).

4 This photograph shows the back of the lower portion of the anterior abdominal wall, in a 7½-month-old fetus. The relationship of the internal crus of the transversalis fascial sling to the inferior (deep) epigastric vessels (parallel black line) is visible on the right side. The point at which the uncovered inferior epigastric vessels (caudad) are covered by the posterior rectus sheath (cephalad) is marked by the visible semilunar line of Douglas (linea semicircularis). Cephalad, the inferior epigastric artery anastomoses with the superior epigastric artery, a branch of the internal thoracic (internal mammary) artery. The concomitant veins are tributaries of the external iliac vein.

Of special interest is the suspension of the gubernaculum testis by the transversalis fascial sling and its relationship to the internal (deep) ring. Note also the backward

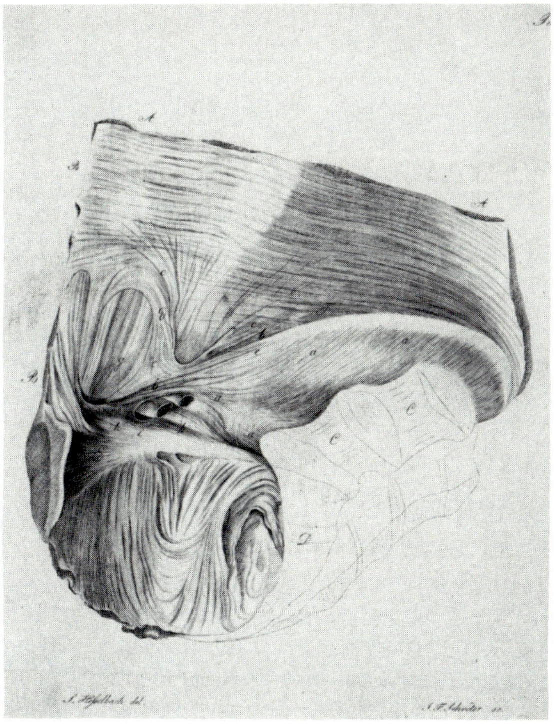

1

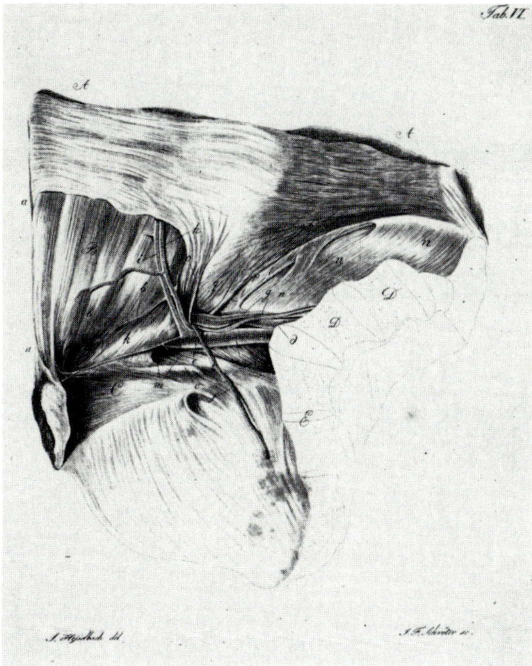

2

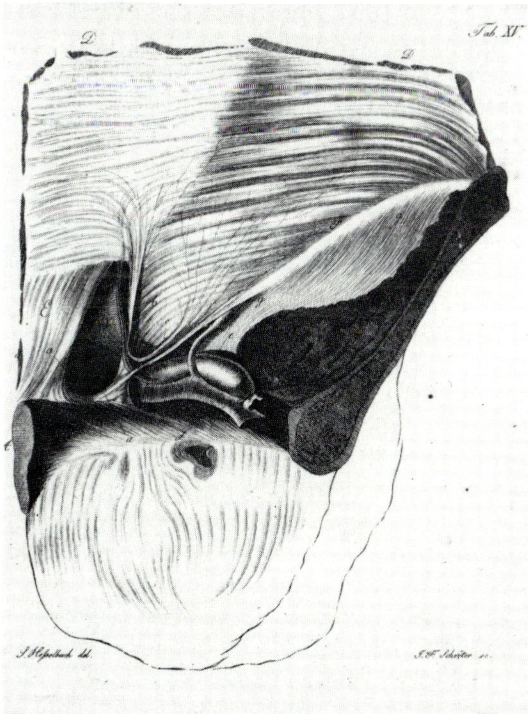

3

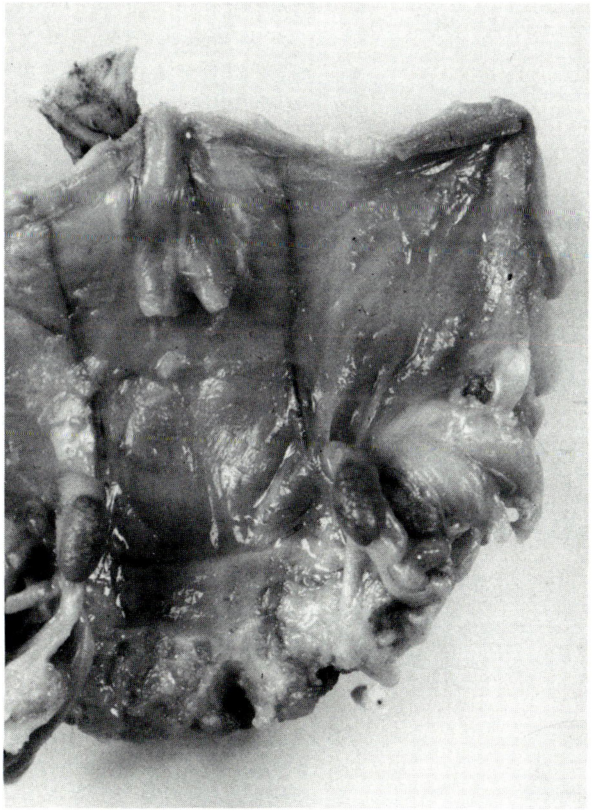

4

bulge of the posterior wall of the inguinal canal, caused by compression from the overlying swollen gubernaculum.

The large size of the truncated internal iliac arteries (hypogastric) on each side of the back of the lower portion of the anterior abdominal wall can also be seen. They converge to form the umbilical artery, which passes through the umbilicus. (Courtesy of WJ Lytle.)

JULES CLOQUET (1780–1883)

Plate C
Plate CI

In 1819, Cloquet published his work entitled *Recherches sur les Causes et l'Anatomie des Hernies Abdominales.* Figure 3 from this work is reproduced here.

1 The primary feature of this illustration, which merits the full discussion that follows, is the "posterior surface of the crural arch" identified by the letter *L*.

In 1836, 17 years after Cloquet's original publication, Alexander Thomson, an expatriate anatomist and surgeon from London who was practicing in Paris, described a "reasonable facsimile" of this structure as the "bandalette iliopubienne" (see Section I, Surgical Anatomy). Later, Testut **(2)**,[8] Polya **(3)**,[7] and Fruchaud **(4)**[1] each used the same designation for similar facsimiles. In the United States, it is commonly named the "iliopubic tract," as described by Nyhus **(5)**.[4] In 1954, however, Mikkelsen[3] used the same anatomic description as Cloquet in describing the preperitoneal approach for the repair of a femoral hernia, except that he labeled it "Poupart's ligament." This name is synonymous with both the "inguinal ligament" and the "crural arch."

Regardless of the name applied to this structure, it can be seen only in the posterior (preperitoneal) approach for the repair of a groin hernia. This fact is believed to be the reason for the difficulty in surgically identifying the iliopubic tract when the anterior (inguinal) approach is used.

With the exception of Fruchaud,[2] the various artists' conceptions of the anatomic disposition of the iliopubic tract anteriorly are not discernible during operation. This has proved most confusing to the surgeon and explains why McVay and Mikkelsen have referred to the iliopubic tract as an "illusion" and a "will-o'-the wisp," respectively. Its identification as "the retraction of the inguinal ligament,"[5] as illustrated in **7**, does not conform to the surgical anatomy of the posterior inguinal wall as described in this atlas (see Plate V, Fig. 24). This confusion in the identity of the iliopubic tract in the anterior (inguinal) approach stems from the failure to use its correct anatomic and "surgical" name—the inferior segment of the fascia of the posterior inguinal wall. This segment comprises two layers; the aponeurotic expansion of the transversus abdominis muscle anteriorly and the transversalis fascia posteriorly. It inserts into the iliopectineal line (Cooper's ligament), although at this site its hidden posterior component (the transversalis fascia) constitutes an intimate adherence rather than a true insertion, since it continues into the pelvic cavity as the endoabdominal fascia (Cooper).

The disparities in anatomic representations of the iliopubic tract from the preperitoneal (posterior) approach are reflected in this sampling of illustrations.

2 This illustration from Testut demonstrates the anatomic inter-relationships of Cooper's ligament (5), Gimbernat's ligament (7), and the *bandalette iliopubienne* (8) (iliopubic tract). The distance between the iliopubic tract and Cooper's ligament is noteworthy. (From Testut, LT: *Traité d'Anatomie Humaine. Quatrième Edition.* Paris: Octave Doin, 1899, p. 819.)

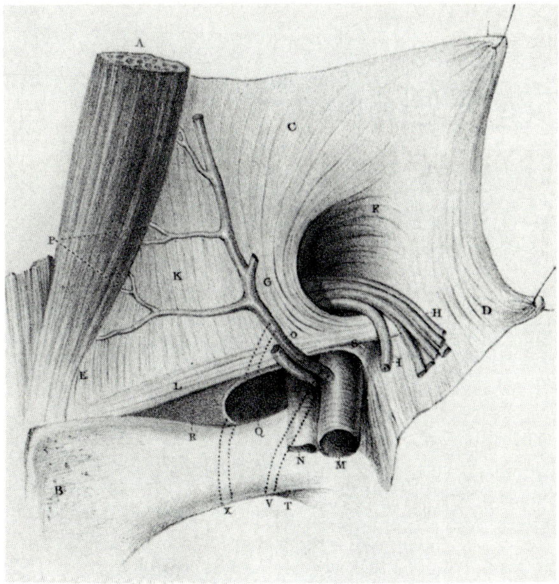

1

Posterior View of the Superior Openings of the Inguinal and Crural Canals, on the right side.

A. Part of the rectus abdominis.
B. Posterior surface of the pubes.
C. Fascia transversalis.
D. Fascia iliaca continuous with the fascia transversalis.
E. Fascia transversalis continuous below with the tendon of the rectus, and with the crural arch.
F. Superior opening of the inguinal canal, formed by the fascia transversalis.
G. Fasciculus of fibres, forming the inner margin of the superior opening of the inguinal canal.
H. Spermatic vessels.
I. Vas deferens joining the other vessels of the cord at an acute angle.
K. Triangular space, bounded externally by the epigastric artery; internally, by the rectus muscle; and inferiorly, by the crural arch. In this situation internal inguinal hernia takes place.
L. Posterior surface of the crural arch.
M External iliac artery.
N. External iliac vein.
O. Epigastric artery. The epigastric vein has been divided.
P. Branches of the epigastric artery to rectus muscle.
Q. Superior opening of the crural canal.
R. Gimbernat's ligament.
S. Concave fibrous fold, forming the external angle of the superior opening of the crural canal, and situated opposite to Gimbernat's ligament.
T. Upper part of the obturator foramen.
V. Dotted outline, indicating the course which the obturator artery most frequently takes, when it arises from the epigastric. Here the obturator artery would be situated to the outer side of the sac of a femoral hernia.
X. Dotted outline, indicating the course of the obturator artery, when the common trunk which furnishes this artery and the epigastric is of considerable length. In such a case, the obturator artery descends behind Gimbernat's ligament, and passes first above, and then on the inner side of the neck of the sac in femoral hernia.

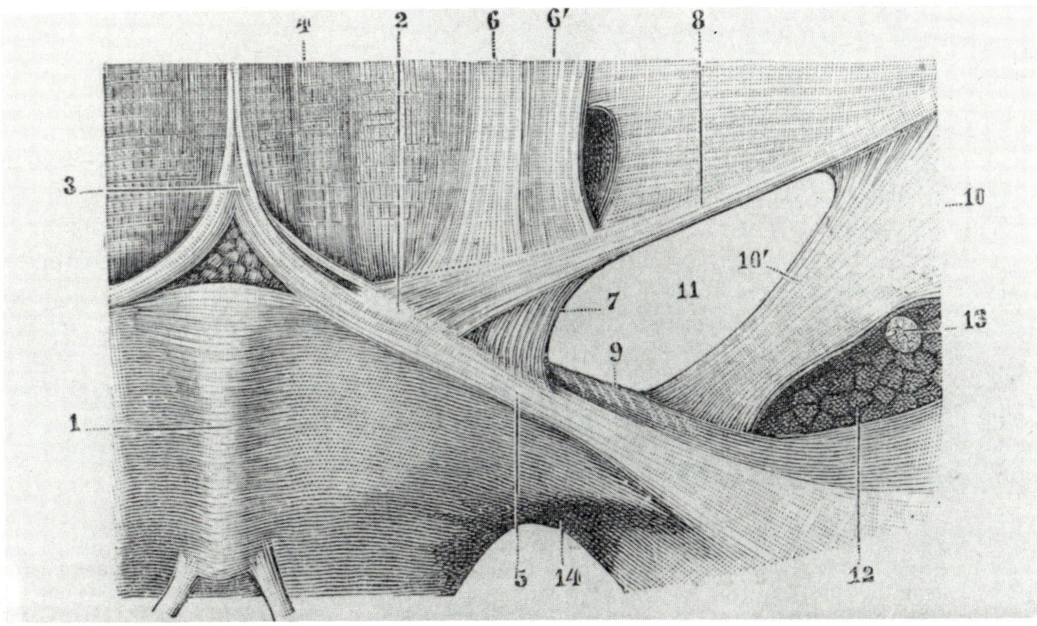

2

JULES CLOQUET
(1780–1883)
Continued

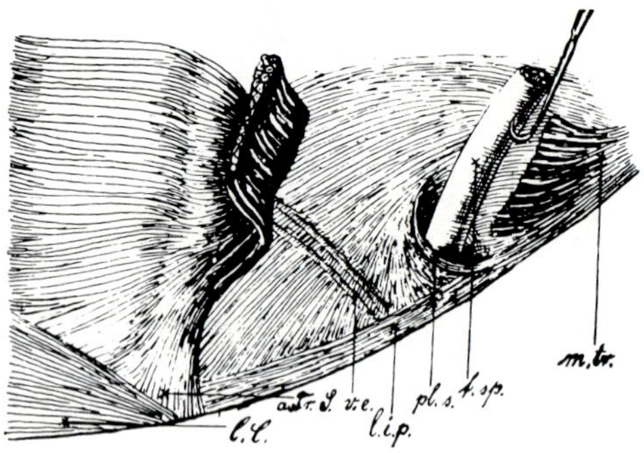

3

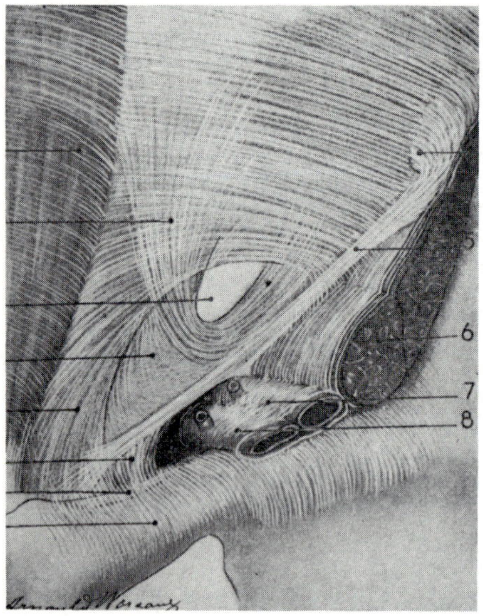

4

3 Polya's preperitoneal representation of the iliopubic tract, the "ligament iliopubicum" (l.i.p.), is shown. (From Polya, E: Die Ursachen der Recidive nach Radicaloperation des Leistenbruches. Arch klin Chir *99*:816, 1912.)

4 The posterior or preperitoneal appearance of the *bandalette iliopubienne* (5) is shown by Fruchaud. (From Fruchaud, H: *Anatomie Chirurgicale des Hernies de l'Aine*. Paris: C Doin & Cie, 1956, p. 131.)

5 This illustration shows the anatomic structures as seen from the preperitoneal approach. (From Nyhus, LM, Condon, RE, and Harkins, HN: Clinical experiences with preperitoneal hernial repair for all types of hernia of the groin. Am J Surg *100*:234–244, 1960.)

6 The iliopubic tract (6) and its lateral extension as the anterior femoral sheath (5) are depicted. However, the acute turn-in of the iliopubic tract and its insertion into Cooper's ligament (7) is not shown. Instead, it is simply replaced with an oblong black defect that is not identified. The neighboring transversalis fascia (12) and the aponeurosis of the transversus abdominis muscle (13) are clearly visible. (From Fruchaud, H: *Le Traitement Chirurgical des Hernies de l'Aine Chez l'Adulte*. Paris: C Doin & Cie, 1956.)

7 This intraoperative exposure of the iliopubic tract from the anterior (inguinal) approach has not been observed by the author. (From Nyhus, LM, and Harkins, HN: *Hernia*. Philadelphia: JB Lippincott, 1964, p. 107.)

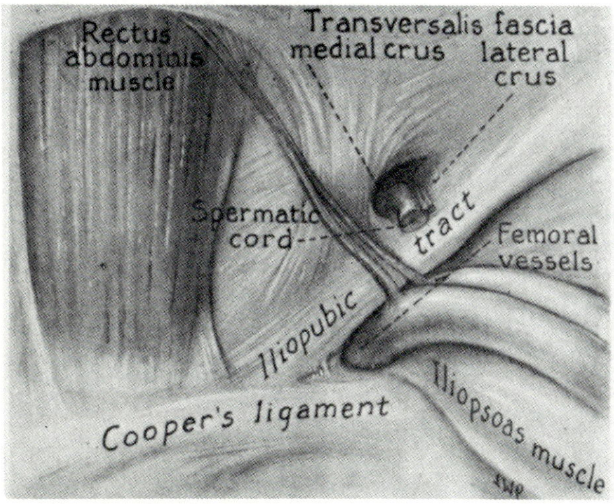
Rectus
abdominis
muscle
Transversalis fascia
medial crus
lateral
crus
Spermatic
cord
tract
Femoral
vessels
Iliopubic
Cooper's ligament
Iliopsoas muscle

5

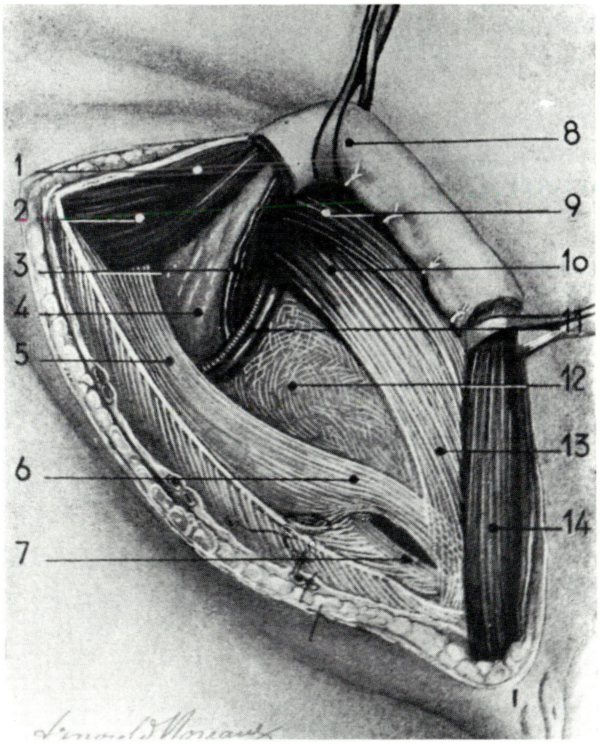
1
2
3
4
5
6
7
8
9
10
11
12
13
14

6

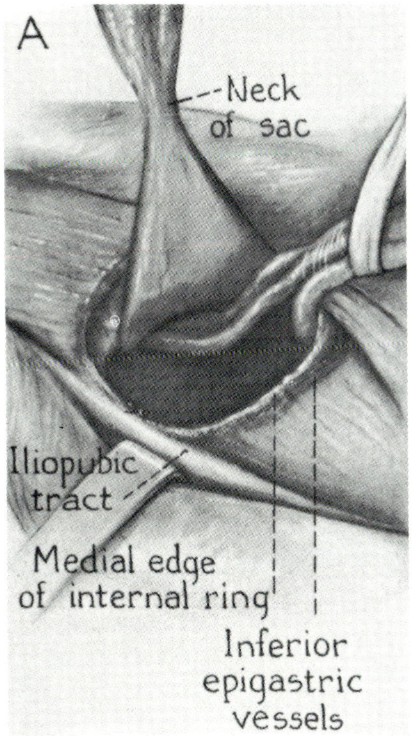
A
Neck
of sac
Iliopubic
tract
Medial edge
of internal ring
Inferior
epigastric
vessels

7

JULES CLOQUET (1780–1883)
Continued

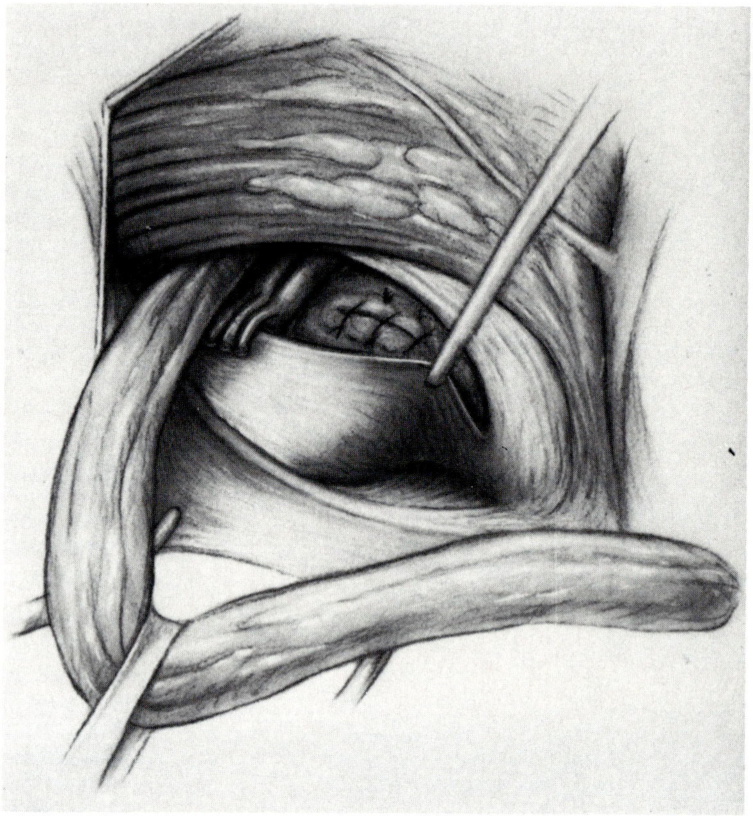

8

8, 9, 10 The inferior segment of the fascia of the posterior inguinal wall, the "new iliopubic tract," held in tissue forceps, is being retracted upward to show the turn-in as it proceeds to insert into Cooper's ligament. Its relationship to the subjacent pyriform fossa is also visible.

REFERENCES

1. Fruchaud, H: *Anatomie Chirurgicale des Hernies de l'Aine*. Paris: C Doin & Cie, 1956.
2. Fruchaud, H: *Le Traitement Chirurgical des Hernies de l'Aine Chez l'Adulte*. Paris: C Doin & Cie, 1956.
3. Mikkelsen, WP, and Berne, CJ: Femoral hernioplasty: Supra-pubic extraperitoneal (Cheatle-Henry) approach. Surgery *35*:743, 1954.
4. Nyhus, LM, Condon, RE, and Harkins, HN: Clinical experiences with preperitoneal hernial repair for all types of hernia of the groin. Am J Surg *100*:234–244, 1960.
5. Nyhus, LM, and Harkins, HN: *Hernia*. Philadelphia: JB Lippincott, 1964, p. 108.
6. Nyhus, LM, and Harkins, HN: *Hernia*. Philadelphia: JB Lippincott, 1964, p. 107.
7. Polya, E: Die Ursachen der Recidive nach Radicaloperation des Leistenbruches. Arch klin Chir *99*:816, 1912.
8. Testut, LT: *Traité d'Anatomie Humaine. Quatrième Edition*. Paris: Octave Doin, 1899, p. 819.

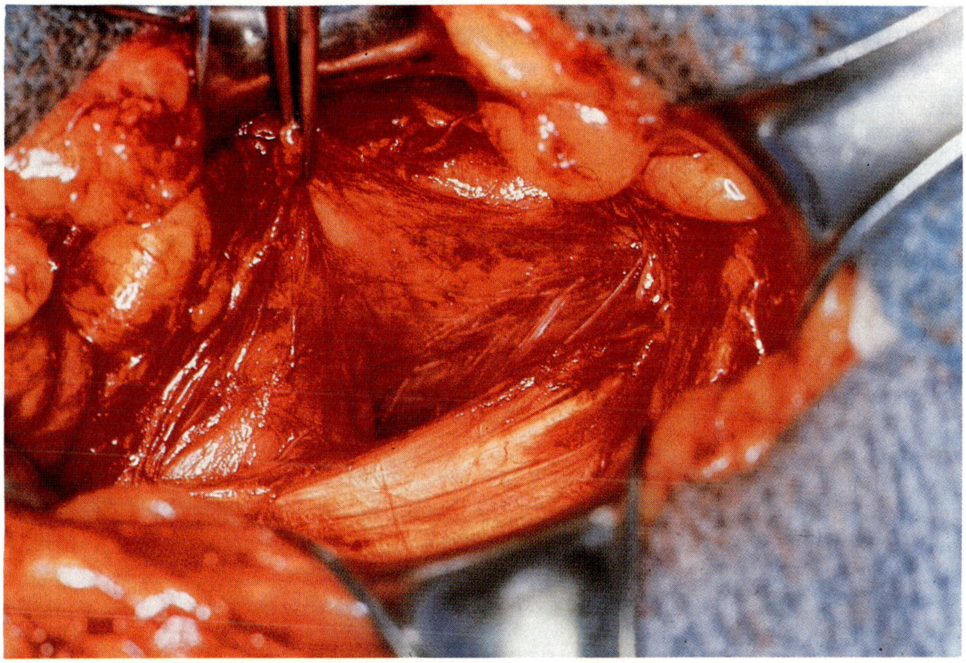

9

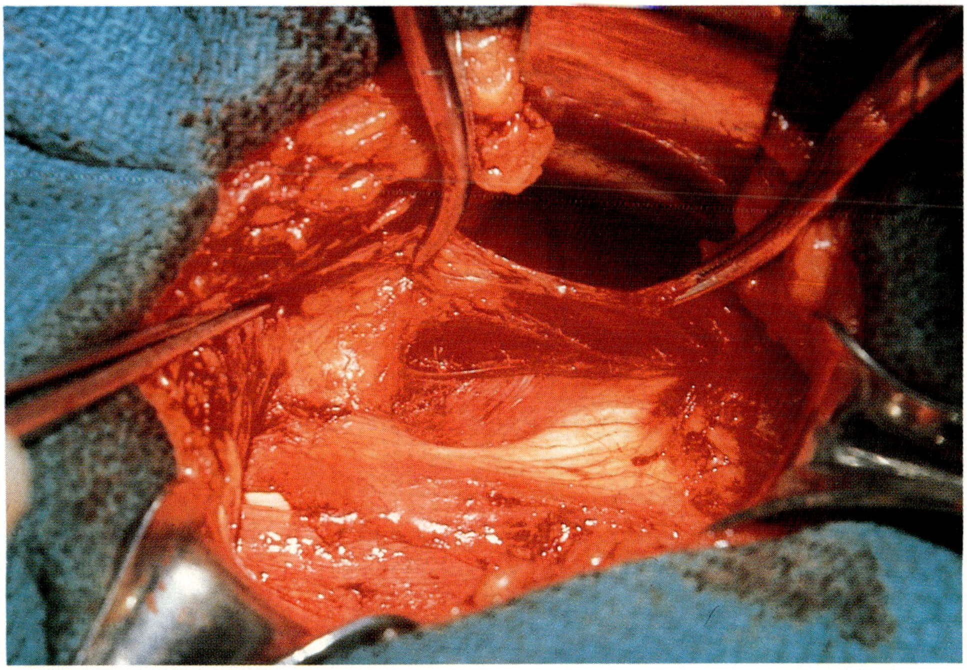

10

JOHN GAY
(1791–1870)

Plate CII

The following illustrations are reproduced from Gay's treatise *On Femoral Rupture*, published in London in 1848.

1 In this drawing, the abrupt twisting turn-in of the medial portion of the crural arch and its attached segment of fascia lata (femoral aponeurosis) is shown. Previously, it had been depicted by Cooper (see Plate XCI) but was not referred to in his text.

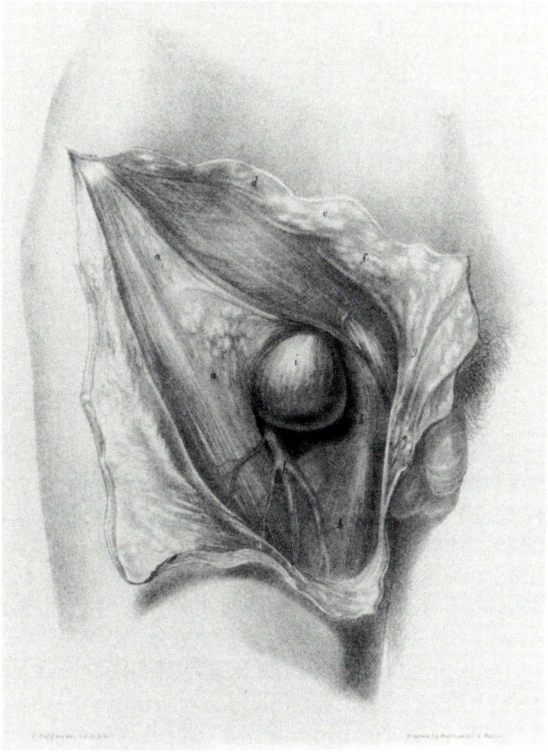

1

The hernial sac and parts, the subject of this drawing, were discovered in the course of a dissection. The tumour did not present those external indications that led to a suspicion of its existence, until the superficial and cribriform fasciæ had been cut through. The engraving was made from a cast and drawing of the parts taken by Mr. E. Wilson, and is well adapted to show the parts prior to their alterations by the processes of disease. The sac is denuded of its fascia propria. Any further description, but for the sake of junior students, would be superfluous.

a a.—Upper layer of the iliac portion of fascia lata.

b b.—Pubic portion of the same fascia, or *pectineal* fascia, forming the floor of the *femoral* fossa. Pl. ii. *l*.

c.—Falciform process, and portion of the border of the saphenous opening.

d.—External or semilunar portion of the same border.

e.—Burn's ligament, or pubic portion of the arch formed by the lower border of the same opening.

f.—Inferior pillar of the external abdominal ring; or that portion of the crural arch which terminates upon the tuberosity of the pubis and adjoining portion of the ileo-pectineal ridge.

g.—Spermatic cord.

h.—Saphenous vein.

i.—Hernial tumour.

A black line shows the situation and direction of the incision which is made through the integuments into the *femoral fossa*, for the new operation. See Plate iii. fig. 2, *e*.

JOHN GAY
(1791–1870)
Continued

2 The label *f* is identified as "Portion of Gimbernat's ligament, formed by the outer pillar of the external abdominal ring." This is incorrect, since the portion of Gimbernat's ligament that is shown is formed by Gimbernat's "duplicature of the crural arch." In fact, its origin in continuity from the medial transected segment of the crural arch and its insertion into the linea iliopectinea (Cooper's ligament) are visible *(f)*. The origin of the lateral (deep) or lacunar portion of Gimbernat's ligament from the fascia lata *(g)* may also be seen.

The knife blade is shown in dotted outline "behind those seats of stricture." This is an error, since in simple incarcerated or strangulated femoral hernias there is only one seat of stricture—the crescentic margin of the lacunar ligament. In fact, its transection is the essence of the "new method" of operating for femoral hernia, as described by Gimbernat.

The transverse disposition of the fasciculi of the internal oblique muscle and their relationship to the underlying and caudad portions of the transversalis (transversus abdominis) muscle and fascia are clearly shown.

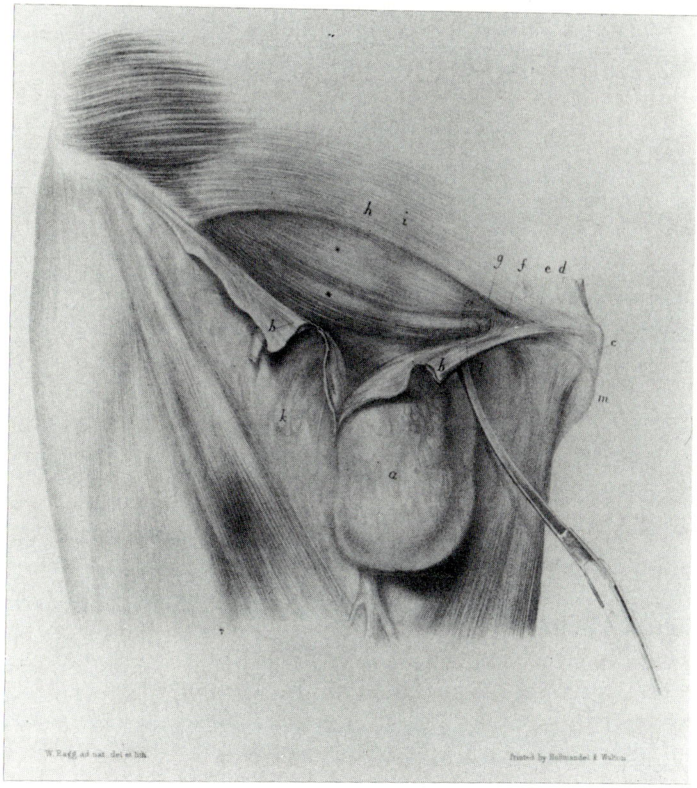

2

Represents a hernial tumour and the adjacent parts of the thigh, as they are displayed by the removal of the superficial fascia and the contents of the *femoral fossa.* The crural arch and upper layer of the iliac portion of the fascia lata have been divided and turned back, to show the deep layer of that fascia, and its relations to Hey's ligament. The knife is passed from the femoral fossa behind those seats of stricture, which are here seen.

a.—The hernial tumour with its cribriform covering.

b b.—The crural arch divided and turned back.

c.—Pubic insertion of the tendon of the external oblique muscle.

d.—Tendon of rectus.

e.—Pubic attachment of the conjoined tendons of the internal oblique and transversalis muscles.

f.—Portion of Gimbernat's ligament, formed by the outer pillar of the external abdominal ring.

b

g.—Portion of Gimbernat's ligament, formed by the falciform process of the fascia lata.

h.—Situation of the band of fibres belonging to the internal inguinal ligament of Hesselbach, below the *under layer* of the iliac fascia lata.

i.—The femoral, or Hey's ligament; or the *deep crural arch.*

k.—Upper lamina of the iliac portion of the fascia lata, divided vertically and thrown back, in order to display the *deep lamina,* with Hey's ligament, and its continuity to the arched margin of the internal oblique muscle.

l.—The femoral fossa.

m.—Process from the deep abdominal fascia which completes the upper arched border of the saphenous opening on the pubic side.

3 Although the anatomic structures in this illustration are unduly magnified and out of normal proportion, they are essentially self-explanatory. Particular attention is directed to *n*, which indicates "the crural [femoral] canal." The crural ligament has been transected, and the proximity of its medial segment and the attached lacunar portion of Gimbernat's ligament is visible. In the intact state, both cadaveric and living, the lateral crescentic margin of the lacunar ligament is in juxtaposition to the medial wall of the femoral sheath and forms its medial boundary (see the Anatomic Supplement to Repair of a Femoral Hernia).

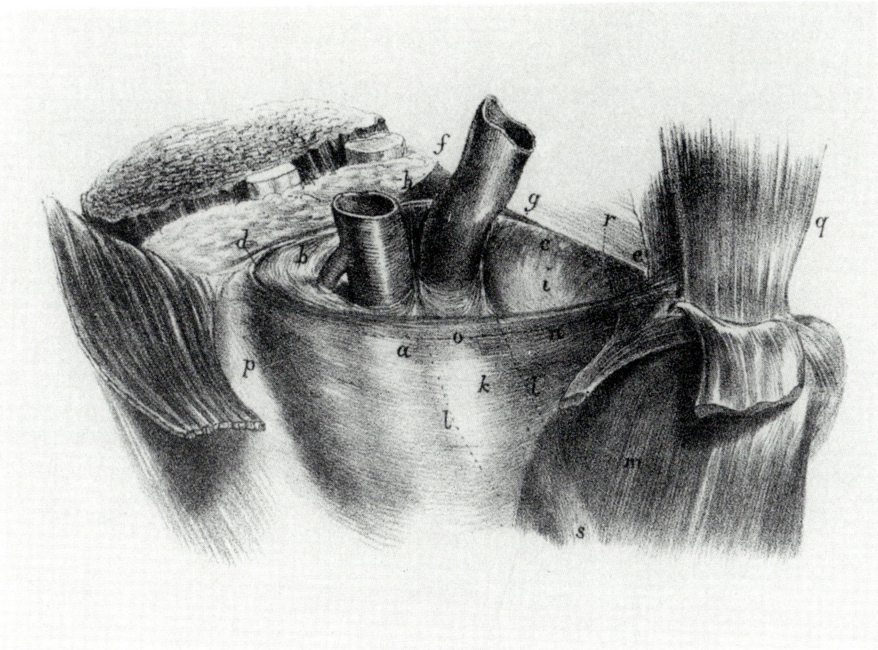

3

a.—The *front* wall of the femoral sheath, as displayed on the careful removal of the iliac fascia lata.

b, c.—Its iliac and pubic *walls.*

d, e, f.—The *angles* formed by the union of these walls.

g, h.—The *septa* by which the sheath is divided.

i.—The *upper orifice* of the crural canal, or *crural ring.*

k.—The venous compartment of the sheath.

l l.—Lines shewing the *direction* of the septa of the sheath,—the outer one being between the artery and vein.

m.—The front margin of the *lower* orifice of the sheath.

n.—The *crural canal.*

o.—Dotted line, showing the relative position of Hey's ligament to the front wall of the sheath.

p.—The band of fibres appertaining to the front wall of the sheath, described as the "fibræ crassiores" of the internal inguinal ligament of Hesselbach ; also seen in Plate ii., *h.*

q.—Tendon of the rectus.

r.—The pubic margin of the *crural ring* : the septum crural had been pushed before a hernial sac, by which the canal had been occupied.

s.—The terminal portion of the saphenous vein.

APPENDIX II

THE REVOLUTIONARY ERA IN THE SURGICAL TREATMENT OF HERNIA

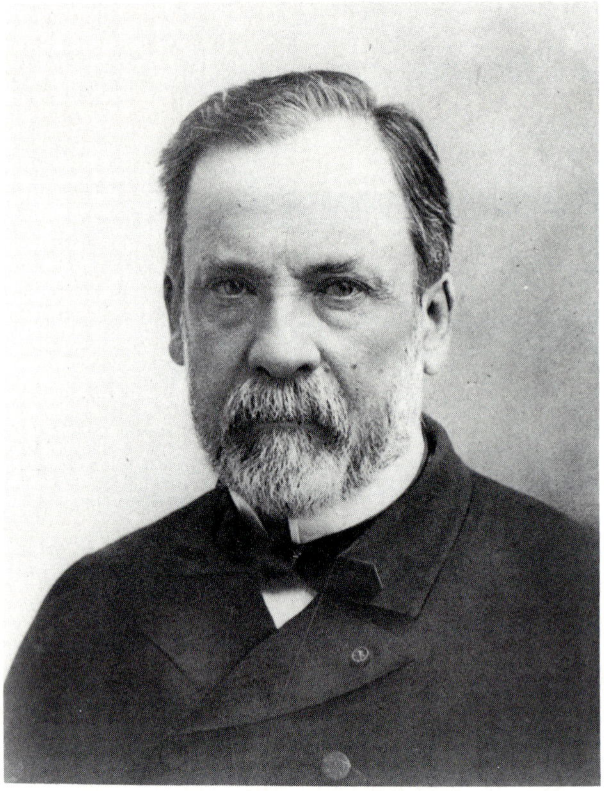

Figure 1. Louis Pasteur.

The revolutionary era in the surgical treatment of hernia was made possible by three revolutionary discoveries.

The first was the use of ether as a general anesthetic. It was publicly administered for the first time by William T. G. Morton of Boston on October 16, 1846, in an operation performed in the Massachusetts General Hospital by Joseph Collins Warren for the removal of a benign tumor of the left side of the neck in a young man.

Warren's skepticism about the "unknown anesthetic" was enhanced by the delay in the start of the operation until he was told by Morton, "Your patient is ready." Upon completing the operation, Warren's memorable words were "Gentlemen, this is no humbug."

On November 4, 1847, Sir James Y. Simpson, Professor of Obstetrics in Edinburgh, introduced the use of chloroform for the delivery of his obstetric patients. Its use was rapidly extended to general surgical patients.

The second discovery was by Louis Pasteur of Paris (Fig. 1), a world-renowned chemist, who by 1860 had demonstrated conclusively that lactic acid fermentation and the fermentation of both wine and beer were caused by the presence of living micro-organisms that were carried on dust particles in the air (the germ theory). Furthermore, he demonstrated that micro-organisms were the cause of putrefaction and decay and were ubiquitous. From his studies of the various types of fermentation, begun in 1856, Pasteur also concluded that the generally accepted theory of spontaneous generation as the cause of fermentation ". . . is a chimera."

The third discovery was that of Joseph Lister, who in 1867 established the principles of antisepsis and asepsis in the care of wounds (Figs. 2 and 3).

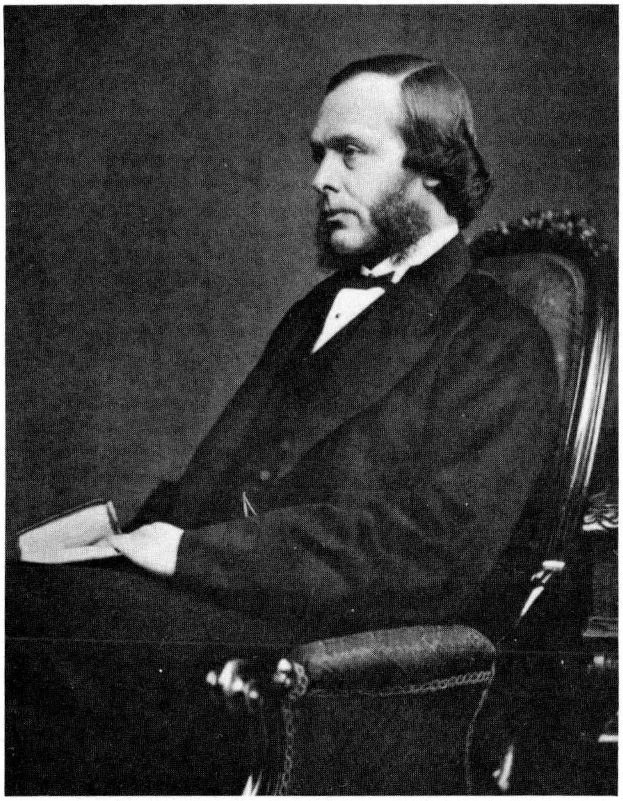

Figure 2. Joseph Lister in 1867 at the age of 40.

THE LANCET, SEPT. 21, 1867. 353

ON THE ANTISEPTIC PRINCIPLE IN THE PRACTICE OF SURGERY.*

BY JOSEPH LISTER, ESQ., F.R.S.,
PROFESSOR OF SURGERY IN THE UNIVERSITY OF GLASGOW.

IN the course of an extended investigation into the nature of inflammation, and the healthy and morbid conditions of the blood in relation to it, I arrived, several years ago, at the conclusion that the essential cause of suppuration in wounds is decomposition, brought about by the influence of the atmosphere upon blood or serum retained within them, and, in the case of contused wounds, upon portions of tissue destroyed by the violence of the injury.

To prevent the occurrence of suppuration, with all its attendant risks, was an object manifestly desirable; but till lately apparently unattainable, since it seemed hopeless to attempt to exclude the oxygen, which was universally regarded as the agent by which putrefaction was effected. But when it had been shown by the researches of Pasteur that the septic property of the atmosphere depended, not on the oxygen or any gaseous constituent, but on minute organisms suspended in it, which owed their energy to their vitality, it occurred to me that decomposition in the injured part might be avoided without excluding the air, by applying as a dressing some material capable of destroying the life of the floating particles.

Upon this principle I have based a practice of which I will now attempt to give a short account.

* A paper read before the British Medical Association in Dublin on the 9th of August, 1867.

Figure 3. Title page of Lister's first publication, which appeared in *The Lancet* on September 21, 1867.

Most interesting in these contemporary discoveries is the close personal relationship that was established between Pasteur and Lister (Fig. 4). Lister, of course, was intensely interested in the clinical study of wound infections but had no specific knowledge of either their cause or prevention; therefore, all of the treatments prescribed were empiric.

Fortuitously, in 1865 Lister read Pasteur's pamphlets on the presence of living micro-organisms that were associated with the various fermentation processes. The fact that these micro-organisms were shown to be the cause of putrefaction and decay proved to be of particular clinical interest to Lister. Fortified with this newly acquired knowledge, he hypothesized that the presence of micro-organisms transmitted "on the dust particles in the air" could be the cause of suppuration in open wounds, both surgical and nonsurgical. If this were true, the primary goal was to determine the method by which these micro-organisms could be destroyed. Lister brought his research to Pasteur's attention in a letter written in 1874.

Edinburgh, 10 February 1874

My Dear Sir,

Allow me to send you a brochure that enumerates some of the researches on a subject that you have elucidated so well: The Theory of germs and fermentation. I would like to think that you would be interested to know that I have written about an organism which you were the first to study in your *Memoires on the fermentation called lactic*.

I do not know if you are familiar with the Annals of British Surgery. In case you have read them, you may have found, from time to time, news about an antiseptic system, that for the past nine years, I have been trying to bring to perfection.

Allow me to take this occasion to thank you for demonstrating to me, by your brilliant researches, the truth of the germ theory of putrefaction and in so doing giving me the only principle that could lead to the final idea of the antiseptic system.

If you ever pass by Edinburgh, you will be gratified to see in our hospital how much mankind has profited from your work. I must also add how gratifying it would be for me to show you what surgery here owes you.

Please excuse my frankness that was inspired by our mutual love of Science, and please accept my deepest respect.

Yours very sincerely,
JOSEPH LISTER*

*Translation from French courtesy of Souheil Kandalaft, M.D.

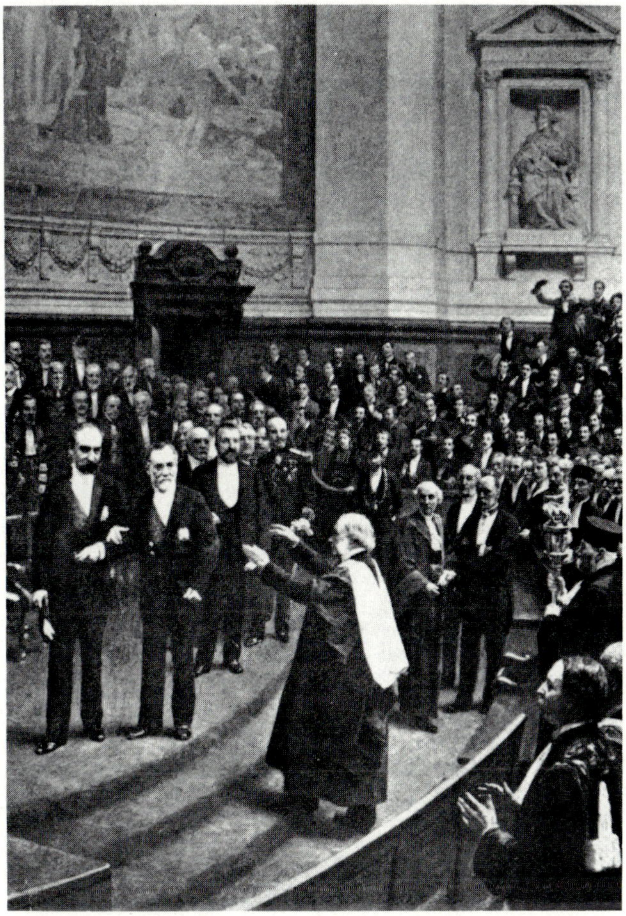

Figure 4. Jubilee on Pasteur's 70th birthday, held on December 27, 1892, in the Sorbonne. Lister, with arms outstretched, is walking up the steps to embrace Pasteur.

Having learned of the effectiveness of carbolic acid as a disinfectant for sewage at Carlisle, Lister selected it for use as an antiseptic in both the prevention and treatment of infections in surgical wounds. In addition to the "antiseptic dressings," a carbolic spray for use in the operating room was designed. Generally, however, by 1890 both the carbolic acid dressings and spray were discontinued and replaced by strict asepsis for the prevention of infection in the surgical wound.

The clouding of the definitions of antisepsis and asepsis was dispelled by the statement of Sir Rickman Godlee, a surgeon (who was both Lister's nephew and his biographer): ". . . the word antiseptic may seem to imply, the old struggle against putrefaction . . . in a wound." Instead, "It was an effort to prevent the occurrence of putrefaction . . . by eliminating decomposition altogether, that is, a true aseptic surgery; and if he [Lister] had from the first, adopted the word aseptic which appears to more closely connote his principle than the word antiseptic, some misunderstandings of later years could never have arisen."

Ironically, Lister's great discovery was not generally accepted in Great Britain for nearly 25 years, although it was almost immediately embraced in Europe and America. La Rochefoucauld's Maxim: "The greater our knowledge of the past, the greater become our powers of invention, and the more apt that invention will prove original" is no better exemplified than in the relationship between the discoveries of Pasteur and Lister.

HENRY O. MARCY (1837–1924)

Plate CIII
Plate CIV

Henry O. Marcy of Boston is justly famed for his two scientific contributions to the practice of surgery. As a disciple of Joseph Lister of London, he brought back to America the fundamental principles of antisepsis and asepsis that Lister originated and practiced. The second contribution was his classic work *The Anatomy and Surgical Treatment of Hernia*, published in 1892. In the preface to this work he stated, "The subject of hernia is invested with new interest owing to the revolutionary methods of modern surgery, which make operative measures comparatively safe when undertaken with proper aseptic precautions which were formerly fraught with the greatest danger."

In 1871, Marcy reported on the first two patients (both women) upon whom he operated successfully for the radical cure of strangulated inguinal hernias, utilizing Lister's principles of antisepsis and asepsis in conjunction with the use of buried carbolized catgut sutures.[1] In each patient, following the release of the constriction and reduction of the hernial contents, the unopened sac was replaced and the inguinal canal was closed by two or three catgut sutures, "taken deeply through the pillars of the ring."

In 1878, he performed for the first time the radical cure of a reducible inguinal hernia, using the same technique.[2] Two months before (December, 1877), however, Marcy had operated upon this patient for a strangulated inguinal hernia on the opposite side (right); following its reduction, the neck of the sac was closed with catgut sutures and the redundant portion of the sac was excised. (Apparently, this was the first time that he had treated the hernial sac in this manner.) The suture closure of the internal ring and the overlying structures of the abdominal wall completed the operation.

In 1887, he reported a series of over 30 consecutive operations for the elective radical cure of hernia and stressed the importance of dissection of the sac to its base (neck), excision of the redundant hernial sac, and the secure closure of the pillars of the internal ring around the spermatic cord to restore the obliquity of the inguinal canal.[3] Tendon sutures, obtained from the tail of the kangaroo, were used for the closures of the neck of the sac and the pillars of the internal ring, "since its parallel fibers do not readily fray."

Marcy is frequently credited as the first surgeon in America to perform a suture reconstruction of the divided posterior wall of the inguinal canal. This claim is given credence by the excellence and clarity of the surgical technique portrayed in the illustrations reproduced here. However, although he considered the restoration of the obliquity of the canal the most important step in the operation for cure of an inguinal hernia, there is some difficulty in correctly interpreting the relevant illustrations and text.

In **1**, the first stitch of a double continuous tendon suture, which will reunite the visibly divided posterior wall of the inguinal canal, is being inserted. In **2**, the suture approximation of the divided fascial margins has been continued upward to its site of termination at the exit of the spermatic cord. This exit is indicated by the adjacent oval space. It can only be concluded that the obliquity of the inguinal canal is restored by the suture closure of its completely divided posterior wall. However, apart from the short legends accompanying them, these figures are neither cited nor described in the text.

In contrast, illustrations **3** and **4** are identified both by the accompanying legends and the text, which are in complete accord. In the text Marcy writes, "It is . . . of the first importance to reunite these tissues (which constitute the posterior wall of the canal) about the cord at its exit from the abdominal cavity. This is accomplished without difficulty by lifting the cord from the inguinal canal [**3**] and elevating it at its exit to the upper border of the internal ring. Having done this, the tissues comprising the posterior wall of the canal are carefully brought into juxtaposition by a continuous double-tendon suture [**4**] . . . The base or posterior portion of the canal having been re-enforced and elongated by the closing from below upward of the internal ring, the cord is replaced . . . ."

In the closure and reformation of the external wall of the inguinal canal, the conjoined tendon is sutured to Poupart's ligament. This is in contrast to the suture approximation of the "three part layer"—the internal oblique muscle, the transverse (transversus abdominis) muscle, and the "vertical fascia (transversalis) of Cooper"—to the deep part of Poupart's ligament, as described by Bassini in the formation of a "new" posterior wall of the inguinal canal. He continues, "In this way the canal is . . . elongated, and the transversalis fascia is intrafolded and . . . thickened."

In **3** and **4**, the reunion of "these tissues about the cord" is accomplished by the simple inversion of the thinned and weakened fascia that constitutes the posterior wall of the canal. Neither in the text nor in the "Diagrams showing . . . the author's method of closure of the parts, and restoration of the canal" is the posterior wall described as divided. The reader is thus presented with a dilemma—did Marcy divide and close the fascia that forms the posterior wall of the inguinal canal, as is clearly shown in **1** and **2**, or did he simply gather together the attenuated fascia of the posterior wall by imbrication with an inverting double-tendon continuous suture as depicted in **4** through **8**? Despite the evidence of **1** and **2**, it is believed that Marcy actually advocated the latter technique.

HENRY O. MARCY (1837–1924)

Continued

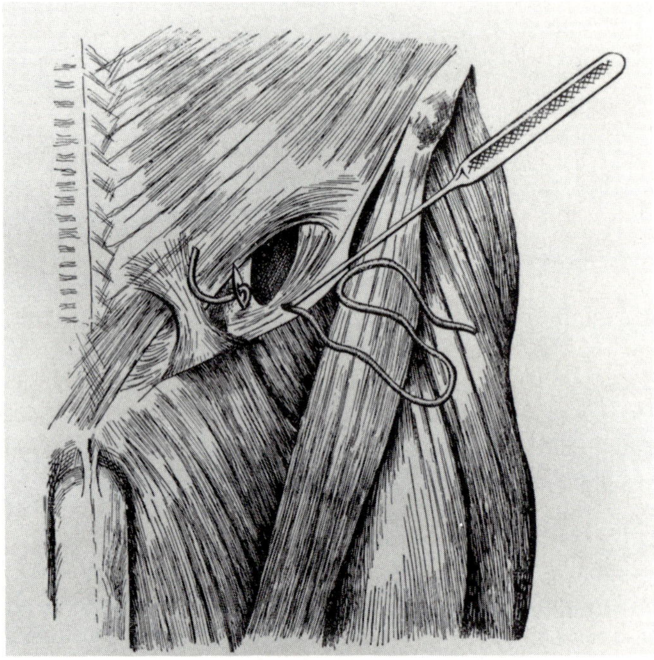

1

The following legends are from Marcy's classic work.[4]

1 "Left inguinal hernia, showing the first stitch taken for the closure of the internal ring from below upward, in order to reform the inguinal canal.

2 "Left inguinal hernia, showing the manner of closure of the internal ring, with the double continuous tendon suture. The needle is rethreaded for withdrawal.

3 "Represents the free dissection of a right inguinal hernia.

a. The spermatic cord elevated upon a hook.

b. The posterior fold of the relaxed transversalis fascia lifted between the thumb and finger a little below the opening of the large internal ring, ready for the introduction of the needle carrying the suture for the first stitch. When the tissues (of the posterior wall) are less relaxed they are elevated upon a hook.

4 "Represents the introduction of the needle threaded with the suture. The loop is left loose, to be pulled through and unthreaded. The needle when unthreaded is to be threaded with the longer opposite end of the suture and withdrawn, carrying the suture with it, thus completing the first stitch.

"Diagrammatic illustrations of the author's method of coapting structures by means of the double continuous animal sutures.

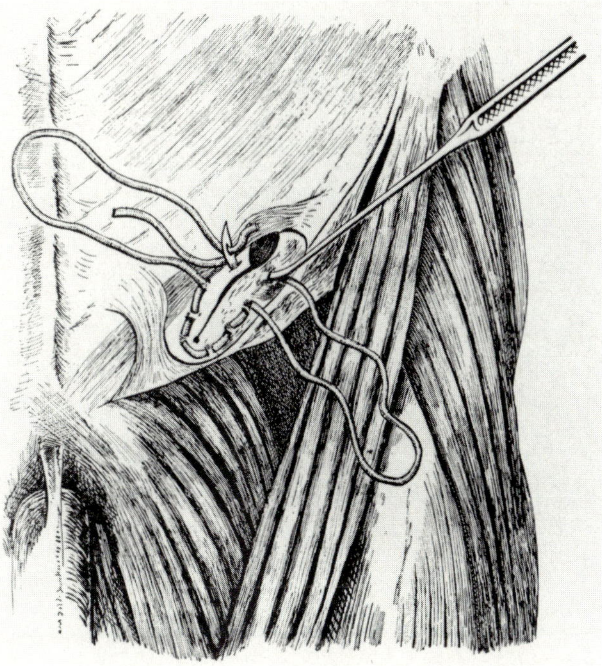

2

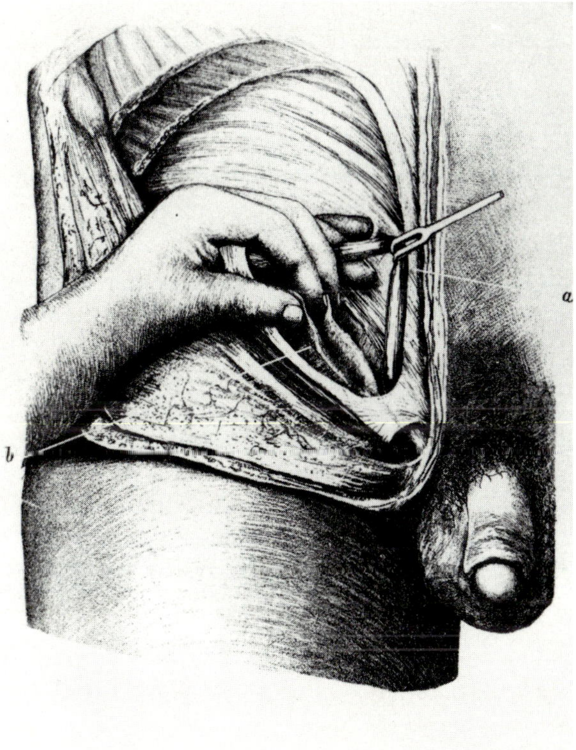

3

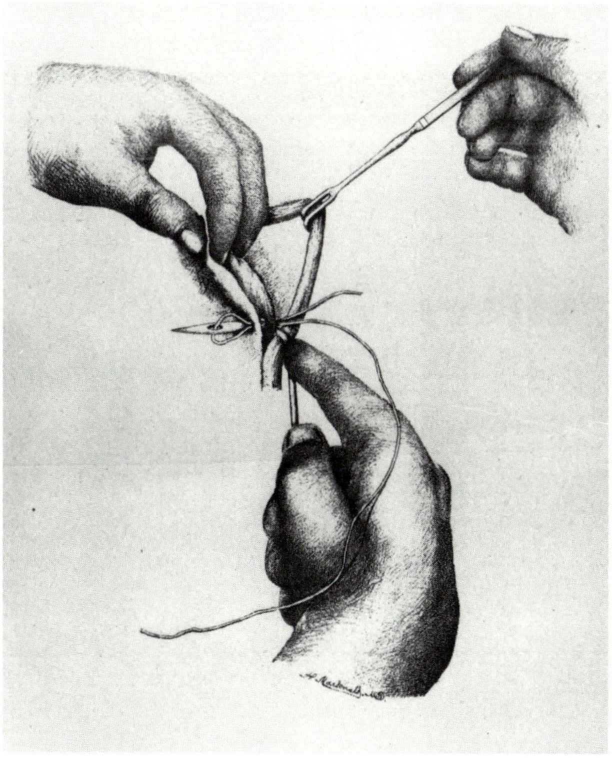

4

HENRY O. MARCY (1837–1924)
Continued

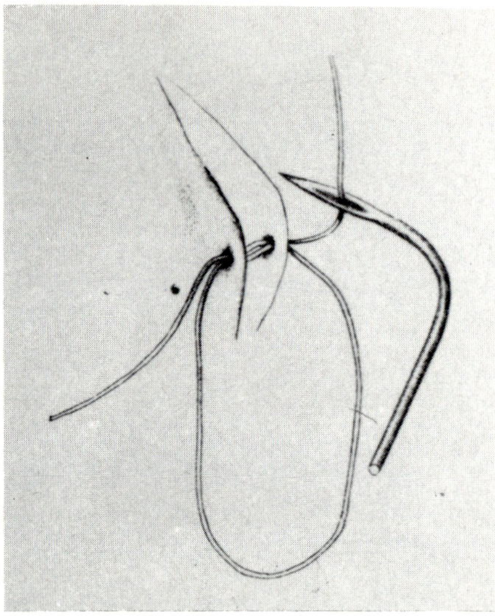

5

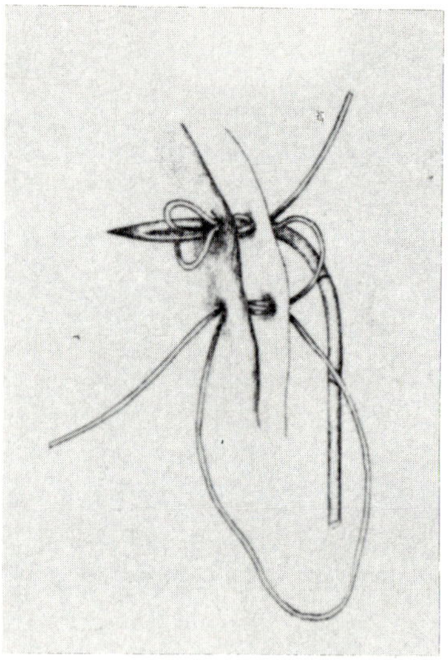

6

5 "The needle having been withdrawn to complete the first stitch, shown as a loop, is still threaded with the end of the suture and ready for its second insertion. This should be a quarter of an inch from the first stitch.

6 "The needle, having pierced the tissues for the second stitch, is ready to be unthreaded, and then to be threaded with the opposite end of the suture and withdrawn.

7 "The end of the suture which had been carried through with the needle at its second insertion is unthreaded, and the needle, rethreaded with the opposite end of the suture, is ready for withdrawal, and this will complete the second stitch.

8 "The stitches are completed and loosely drawn to better exhibit the method of continuous suturing. When the sutures are drawn taut, the parts are evenly coapted and firmly held in position without undue pressure.

9 "Shows the peritoneal sac sutured evenly across at its base and resected. The deeper structures forming the posterior wall of the canal have been coapted by a deep double continuous tendon suture closing the internal ring quite upon the elevated cord.
a. Spermatic artery.
c. Inguinal canal.
m. Structures posterior to the inguinal canal.
i. Former site of the external ring.
p,p. Peritoneum.
s. Spermatic cord.
v. Vas deferens.
w. Superior border of the abdominal wall.
l,s,1. First layer of sutures, including only the peritoneum.
l,s,2. Second layer of sutures, coapting and intrafolding the transversalis fascia, closing and elevating the internal ring."

REFERENCES

1. Marcy, HO: A new use of carbolized catgut sutures. Boston Med Surg J *8*:316, 1871.
2. Marcy, HO: The radical cure of hernia by the antiseptic use of the carbolized catgut ligature. Trans AMA *29*:225–305, 1878.
3. Marcy, HO: The cure of hernia. JAMA *8*:589–592, 1887.
4. Marcy, HO: *The Anatomy and Surgical Treatment of Hernia.* New York: D. Appleton and Company, 1892.

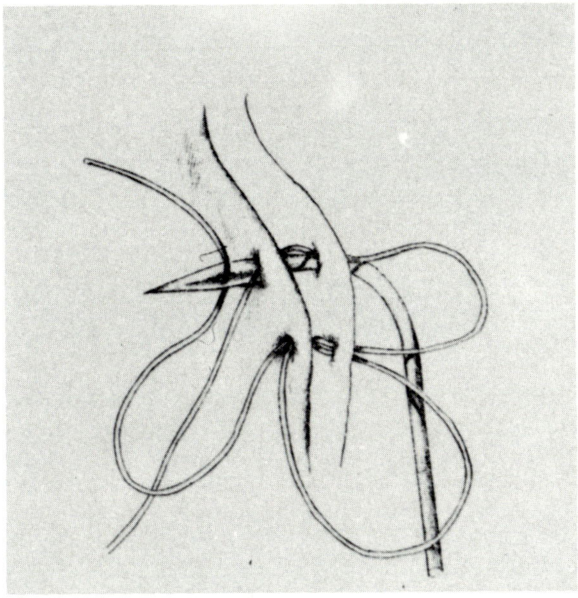

7

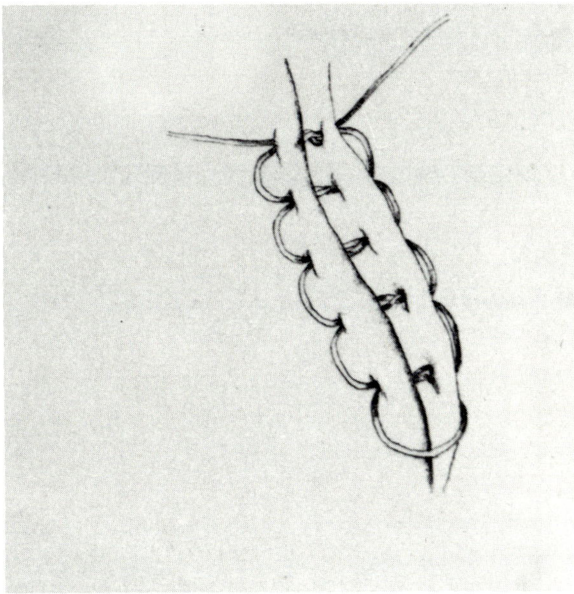

8

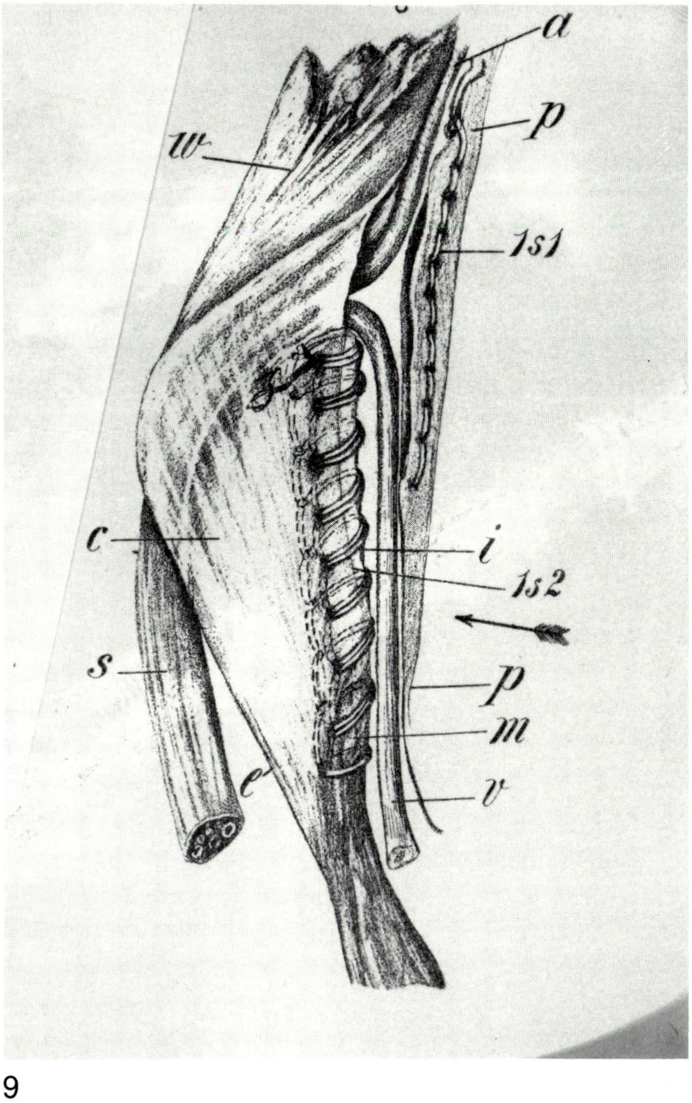

9

EDOARDO BASSINI
(1844–1924)

Plate CV

In the first sentence of his classic article on the treatment of inguinal hernia, Bassini apparently had some qualms relative to its publication when he stated: "Considering all that is written about the radical treatment of the inguinal hernia up until now, it can be somewhat risky to try to publish more about this subject."[1]

Before this publication in German, Bassini had written two preliminary articles in Italian.[2, 3] He was 40 years old when, on December 23, 1884, he performed for the first time the operation that bears his name. Previously, however, he had either observed or performed a variety of the surgical techniques that were being commonly used in the repair of inguinal hernias, and was disturbed by the high incidence of recurrence. This stimulated an ardent interest in the study of the anatomy of the inguinal region during operations and in cadaver dissections. His observations demonstrated the need to establish the inter-relationship of anatomic and physiologic principles in the surgical repair of inguinal hernias.

Imbued with these principles and convinced of the "necessity of another operation method," Bassini stated, ". . . I thought this could be done by a reconstruction of the inguinal canal as it is found under normal physiologic circumstances, namely; . . . a canal with two openings, one abdominal and one subcutaneous; with two walls, one in back and one in front, and through the middle of which the spermatic cord traverses obliquely."[1]

Bassini separated the new method into four parts. In the first part, under deep anesthesia and strict antisepsis, the skin overlying the inguinoscrotal hernia is incised to expose the aponeurosis of the external oblique muscle.

In the second part, starting at the subcutaneous inguinal ring, the aponeurosis of the external oblique muscle is split up to the abdominal hernial ring to form two flaps. By blunt dissection the spermatic cord and neck of the hernial sac are lifted in toto on the index finger. Also by blunt dissection the hernial sac is isolated from the spermatic cord up to the level of the hernial ring. The sac is opened, its contents are reduced, and the neck of the sac is tied with a simple ligature. The hernial sac is then resected a half-centimeter below the ligature (**1**). When the hernia is large and the neck of the sac is wide, a suture ligature is added to reinforce the closure of its neck.

In the third part, the spermatic cord is retracted superiorly toward the abdominal wall. The lateral (inferior) flap of the aponeurosis of the external oblique muscle is retracted downward and its medial (superior) flap upward. In this way the groove formed by Poupart's ligament may be seen, and the posterior (shelving) border of this ligament is freed to its deepest point. The lateral border of the rectus abdominis muscle and the three-part layer—formed by the internal oblique muscle, the transverse (transversus abdominis) muscle and the vertical fascia of Cooper (transversalis fascia)—are freed from the overlying aponeurosis of the external oblique muscle and the underlying subserous adipose connective tissue. This permits the approximation, without difficulty, of the cut three-part layer to the lower isolated border of Poupart's ligament, using interrupted sutures of silk that start 2 to 3 cm from the border of "the triple musculo-aponeurotic layer." This is done "over a distance of 5–7 cms from the pubic bone," and the spermatic cord is displaced about 1 centimeter toward the anterior superior iliac spine (**2**). In this illustration, however, a continuous suture is depicted, rather than interrupted sutures as stated in the text.

When this step is completed, the internal or abdominal opening ("ring") is restored and a "new" posterior wall of the inguinal canal is formed. In the fourth part of the operation, the spermatic cord is placed on the newly formed "floor" of the inguinal canal and covered by the suture union of the overlying cut margins of the aponeurosis of the external oblique muscle (**3**). This is done with a continuous suture that is being loosely inserted for clarity of exposition. Later, when this suture is drawn taut, a snug closure of the external (subcutaneous) ring about the exit of the spermatic cord is obtained. The skin margins are then sutured and a wound dressing is applied. A drain is used only in longstanding large hernias in which the dissection and isolation of the sac has been difficult.

On December 23, 1884, the operation was initiated and continued as a clinical study through July 31, 1889. During this period a total of 262 operations were performed on 227 patients. The shortest duration of follow-up, from the date of operation to the date of publication of the article, was nine months; the longest, five years and four months. Interestingly, for all 227 patients there is a thumbnail sketch pertaining to the related clinical data. A summary of the statistical data pertinent to these patients is presented.

EDOARDO BASSINI (1844–1924)
Continued

THE BASSINI OPERATION FOR INGUINAL HERNIA:
DECEMBER 23, 1884–JULY 31, 1889

I	Number of patients	227	
	Number of operations	262	
	Nonincarcerated ("free") hernias		251 (96.0%)
	Incarcerated hernias		11 (4.0%)
	Strangulated—1 (9.1%)		
			262 (100.0%)

II	Nonincarcerated ("free") hernias	251
	Number of patients	216
	Men	206 (95.0%)
	Women	10 (5.0%)
	1 girl, 9 yrs old	

Types of Hernia			*Location of Hernia*		
A. Acquired		196 (78.0%)	Right side	115	(53.0%)
B. Congenital		55 (22.0%)	Left side	66	(31.0%)
Funicular	13 (23.7%)		Bilateral	35	(16.0%)
Testicular	42 (76.3%)			251	(100.0%)
		251 (100.0%)			
C. Indirect		232 (92.0%)			
D. Direct (Hesselbach's)		19 (8.0%)			
		251 (100.0%)			

III

Age Groups

Age (years)	*Number of Patients*	Percent
0–9	21	10.0
10–19	43	20.3
20–29	53	25.1
30–39	37	17.5
40–49	26	12.3
50–59	23	11.0
60–69	8	3.8
Total	211	100.0
Age not stated	5	
Grand total	216	

Youngest 13 months; oldest 69 years.

THE BASSINI OPERATION FOR INGUINAL HERNIA: DECEMBER 23, 1884–JULY 31, 1889 *Continued*

IV Morbidity and Mortality Study

A. Nonincarcerated ("free") hernias

Number of Patients	Morbidity	Mortality
216	11* (5.0%)	1† (0.5%)
Number of Operations		
251	11* (4.4%)	1† (0.4%)

B. Incarcerated hernias — 11 pts.

Morbidity/mortality

Number of patients — 2 (18%)

1. Urosepsis and pyemia.
   Gross intraoperative contamination.
   69-year-old old man. Died 21 days postoperatively.
2. Septic shock: preoperative and postoperative.
   Gangrenous loop of small bowel.
   39-year-old man. Died 4 hours postoperatively.

V Follow-up Study

A. Nonincarcerated ("free") hernias

Number of patients (250 operations)	215‡
Lost to follow-up	4
Available for study (246 operations)	211
Number of recurrences (Operative recurrence rate: 2.8%)	7§ (3.3%)

B. Incarcerated hernias

Number of patients	11‖
Available for study	9
Number of recurrences	1 (11.0%)
Original hernia: direct	

*Wound infections: "Omissions in the antiseptic treatment of the wounds."

†69-year-old man, 15 days after operation. Necropsy: pneumonia. Wound healing per primum.

‡One of original 216 patients died postoperatively.

§In 5 patients (bilateral hernia—2 patients).

‖Two patients died postoperatively.

EDOARDO BASSINI (1844–1924)
Continued

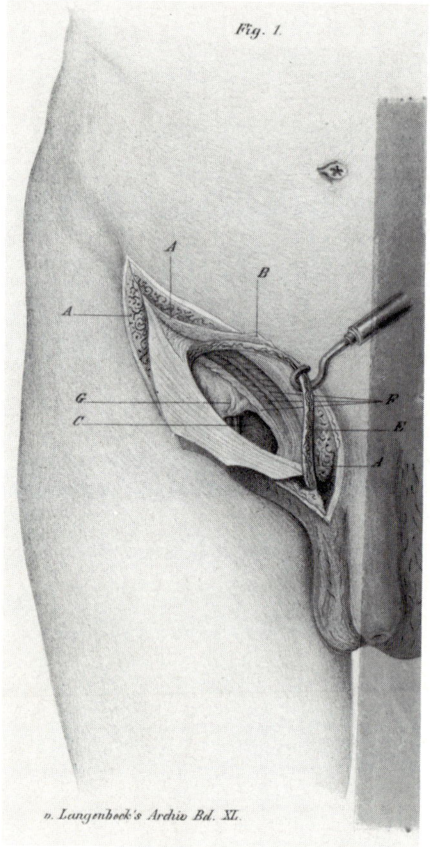

1

1 The following illustrations and legends are from Bassini's classic article. "Shows the first part of the third stage of the operation.

A, A, A The subcutaneous fat and fascial layers.

B The 'medial' (superior) part of the divided external oblique aponeurosis.

C The under or preperitoneal fatty areolar tissue layer.

D There is no letter D in the illustration. If there were, however, it would be the label for the posterior ('shelving') border of Poupart's ligament, which is visible.

E The spermatic cord pulled up.

F Three fold layer; musculus obliquus internus, M. transversus, Fascia verticalis Cooperi.

G Epigastric vessels.

2 "Shows the end of the third part of the operation. That means the suture of the musculoaponeurotic 'three fold layer' to the posterior ('shelving') border of Poupart's ligament.

3 "Represents the 4th stage of the operation: the spermatic cord is put back in its place; on top one can see the divided edges of the aponeurosis of the obliquus externus up to the spermatic cord's outermost location in the inguinal canal. The continuous suture is also shown although it is better to use interrupted sutures. The letters always indicate the same parts."

Bassini's description of the operation and the complementary illustrations are in complete uniformity and preclude any misinterpretation by the reader. Unfortunately, in Marcy's publication (see previous section) the lack of such uniformity makes it difficult to determine the specific anatomic tissue layers that are sutured together in the restoration of the obliquity of the inguinal canal. It is believed, therefore, that in the repair of an inguinal hernia, credit should be given to Bassini as the first surgeon to practice complete division of the fascia of the posterior wall of the inguinal canal.

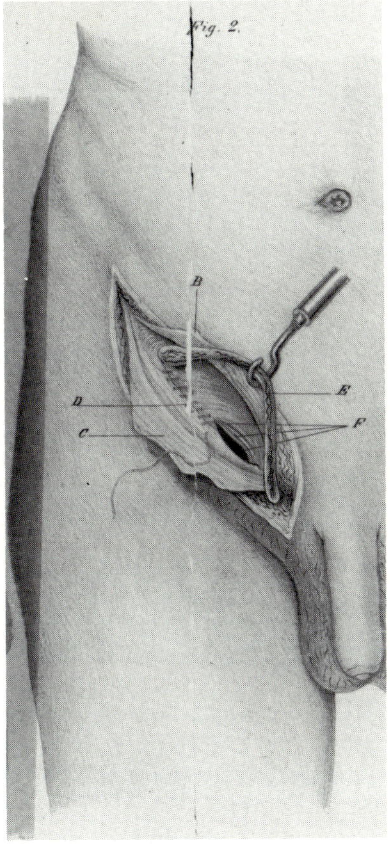

2

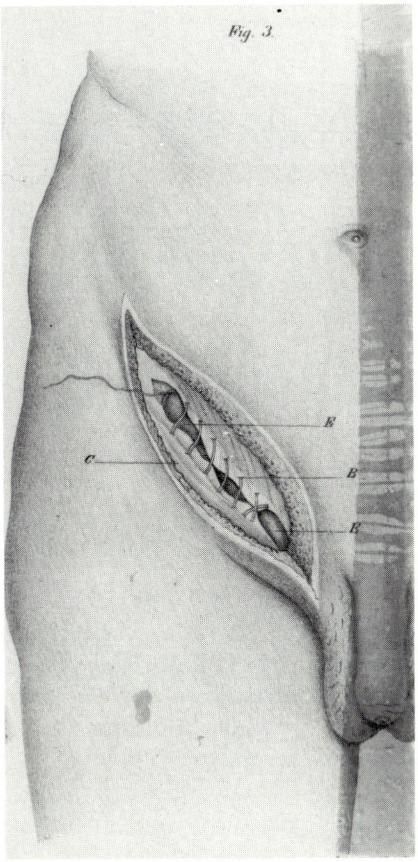

3

The ultimate tribute is that of Halsted: "Bassini unquestionably has the priority." He later wrote, "Indeed, I have not seen a single paper since Bassini's which contributed anything new."[4] Moreover, the continued failure to refer to the original source remains the primary cause for the perpetuation of errors in the many and varied "Bassini operations" that are performed.

Currently, the classic operation of Bassini is frequently stated to be a "one-layer Shouldice repair" of an inguinal hernia. This warrants a clarification. In the original operation described by Shouldice,[5] the attenuated fascia of the posterior wall of the inguinal canal was not divided, as was routinely practiced by Bassini. Instead an inversion imbrication in continuity was done. In his second publication, eight years later, Shouldice reported for the first time the division of the fascia of the posterior wall of the inguinal canal and its sutured reconstruction.[6] This technique, with minor modifications, remains the basic anatomic feature of the Shouldice operation.

On the basis of historical fact, disparate "Bassini" and "Shouldice" operations undoubtedly will continue, with disparate results. Prevention of them and of further perpetuation of errors will be best accomplished by the educational practice of routinely referring to the original articles of the respective authors.

REFERENCES

1. Bassini, E: Üeber die Behandlung des Leistenbruches. Archiv. für klinische Chirurgie *40*:429–476, 1890.
2. Bassini, E: Nuovo metodo per la cura radicale dell'ernia inguinale. Atti Congr Assoc Med Ital (XII Congress) *2*:179–181, 1887. (Full report published in Padua, 1889.)
3. Bassini, E: Sopra 100 casi di cura radicale dell'ernia operata metodo del-autore. Archiv Atti Soc Ital Chir *5*:315, 1888.
4. Halsted, WS: An additional note on the operation for inguinal hernia. In *Surgical Papers by William Stewart Halsted,* Vol. 1. Baltimore: Johns Hopkins Press, 1924, pp 306–308.
5. Shouldice, EE: Surgical treatment of hernia. Ontario Med Rev *12*:43–69, 1945.
6. Shouldice, EE: The treatment of hernia. Ontario Med Rev *20*:670–683, 1953.

WILLIAM STEWART HALSTED (1852–1922)

Plate CVI
Plate CVII

William Stewart Halsted was born in New York City on September 23, 1852, the son of William M. Halsted Jr. and Mary L. Halsted (née Haines). He graduated from Yale College in 1874 and in 1877 received his medical degree from the College of Physicians and Surgeons in New York City. The same year, he was appointed as House Surgeon in the New York Hospital.

One year later, in September of 1878, he departed for Europe where he stayed for a period of two years, returning to New York in September 1880. During this stay he visited the outstanding Surgical Clinics in Germany, Austria, and Switzerland, where he made lifelong friendships with many of the noted European surgeons. He also became fluent in the use of the German language.

Upon his return to New York, he received surgical appointments in numerous hospitals and established a friendship with Dr. William H. Welch, a pathologist, who was a member of the Faculty of the Bellevue Medical College. In 1884 Welch was appointed Professor of Pathology at The Johns Hopkins Hospital, which was not to open until May of 1889.

In December of 1886 Welch invited Halsted to come to Baltimore, where he stayed until April 1887. During these five months he worked daily in Welch's laboratory, carrying out animal experimental studies. One of these studies, on the end-to-end anastomosis of the intestines, was published in 1887.[1] In this study he demonstrated the anatomic importance of the "submucous coat" or layer as the essential "holding power" for sutures in an intestinal anastomosis.

In May of 1889 The Johns Hopkins Hospital was opened, and Halsted was appointed its first Surgeon-in-Chief. In 1892, on the opening of the medical school, he was appointed the first Professor of Surgery in The Johns Hopkins University. He held these two appointments continuously for 33 and 30 years, respectively, until his death on September 6, 1922. He is buried in the Greenwood Cemetery in Brooklyn, New York.[2]

Dr. Halsted's surgical interests were protean. In the two volumes of the *Surgical Papers by William Stewart Halsted*,[3] he left a surgical legacy to past, present, and future generations of surgeons. In reading these papers one can only marvel at the extent and excellence of his scholarly pursuits. The "man himself" is eloquently portrayed in the eulogy given by Dr. Rudolf Matas.[4] Finally, Dr. William H. Welch, in his introduction to MacCallum's biography of Halsted stated: "We his colleagues of the medical faculty, always regarded Halsted as embodying the highest ideals of the university professor, of the scientific investigator, and of the clinical teacher and surgeon."

THE HALSTED I OPERATION

On November 4, 1889, at the meeting of The Johns Hopkins Hospital Medical Society in Baltimore, Halsted presented five patients on whom he had performed operations for the radical cure of hernia. A report of this presentation was published in January of 1890 in the first issue of The Johns Hopkins Hospital Bulletin.[5]

The patient group comprised two men aged 20 and 48 years, respectively, with large reducible inguinal hernias, and three boys, one seven years and two eight years of age. In two the hernias were small; in one it was large.

The first operation, on June 13, 1889, was performed on a boy with a large congenital right inguinal hernia. The fifth operation was performed on October 12, 1889, on a boy with a small inguinal hernia. At the time of the report in January of 1890, the shortest period of follow up was about three months and the longest approximately seven months.

In this operation, the skin incision begins at the external abdominal ring and ends one inch or less (in children) to the inner side of the anterior superior spin of the ilium. It is then deepened through the underlying musculoaponeurotic structures to the level of the peritoneum. The vas deferens and the internal spermatic vessels are mobilized to the lateralmost end of the incision and held in a retractor.

The hernial sac is opened and dissected from the surrounding tissues. The redundant portion of the sac is excised, and its remaining walls are approximated with quilted sutures. The vas deferens and spermatic vessels are transplanted to the lateral angle of the wound. Using interrupted sutures of strong silk, the musculoaponeurotic structures of the abdominal wall, between the skin and the peritoneum, are then sewn together from the crest of the pubes to the lateralmost angle of the incision.

The cord is placed on top of the one-layer mass closure and emerges about one inch to the inner side of the anterior superior iliac spine. The skin incision is closed over the cord using interrupted buried sutures of fine silk. One or two short gauze plugs are used as drains.

WILLIAM STEWART HALSTED (1852–1922)
Continued

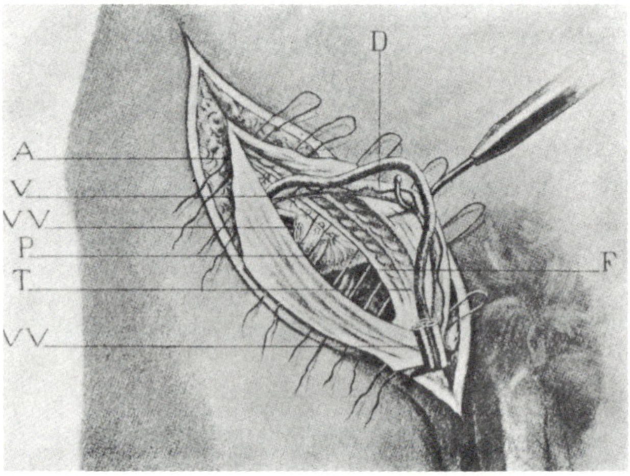

1

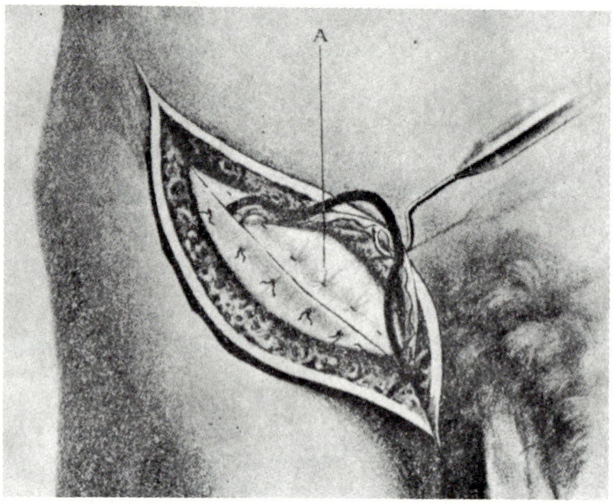

2

The gauze plugs are removed on the seventh day and the patient is permitted out of bed on the 21st day.

The two figures reproduced here illustrate the Halsted I operation.[6]

1 A high ligation and excision of the redundant hernial sac has been done (P). The vas deferens and the "thinned out" internal spermatic vessels, held in a hook, are retracted upward (D), and the quilted untied deep mattress sutures of heavy silk ("six or eight") are inserted.

Superiorly (F), these sutures pass through the aponeurosis of the superior leaflet of the external oblique muscle, the internal oblique and transversus abdominis muscles, and the transversalis fascia; and inferiorly, through the transversalis fascia, Poupart's ligament, and the fibers of the aponeurosis of the external oblique muscle.* The stumps of the excised veins (VV) and the conjoined tendon (T) are depicted.

2 The mattress sutures have been tied, and the two outermost or lateral sutures pass through the deep muscles on each side of the transplanted cord to form a snug, but not tight, closure about its exit. The cord is laid on the aponeurosis of the external oblique muscle (A) and the skin closed with buried interrupted sutures of fine silk.

Comparisons are frequently made between the Bassini and the Halsted I operations, although there is a difference. The essence of the Bassini operation is the transplantation of the spermatic cord onto a "new" floor of the inguinal canal, formed by the suture of the "three fold layer"—the internal oblique and transversalis (transversus abdominis) muscles and the "vertical fascia of Cooper" (transversalis fascia)—to Poupart's ligament. The "roof" of the canal is formed by the suture of the cut margins of the aponeurosis of the external oblique muscle over the transplanted cord. Accordingly, there is a two-tier reconstruction of the whole of the inguinal wall, with the cord transplanted between the tiers.

---

*Although not labeled in the illustration, the inclusion of these structures, inferiorly, is indicated by the free strands of the mattress sutures that emerge beneath the inferior leaflet of the aponeurosis of the external oblique muscle (A).

In the Halsted I operation the inguinal musculoaponeurotic wall superiorly—comprising the aponeurosis of the external oblique muscle, the internal oblique and transversus abdominis muscles, and the transversalis fascia—is sutured inferiorly en bloc to the transversalis fascia, Poupart's ligament, and the aponeurotic fibers of the external oblique muscle, as a single-layer reconstruction of the full thickness of the inguinal wall. The transplanted cord has its exit through the lateralmost muscular portion of the single layer reconstruction and is covered by the subcutaneous tissue and skin.

When Halsted performed his first radical operation for the cure of an inguinal hernia, he was not aware of Bassini's operation until Bassini's publication in German in 1890.[7] Previously Bassini had published two articles in Italian, but these lay fallow until his report in 1890. In fact, Halsted referred to an article published by Bassini in Italian in 1889 but remarked that "The month was not stated."[8] Bassini, in 1887, presented the first report of his "new method" for the radical surgical cure of inguinal hernia.[9] Seventy-two operations were performed in 64 patients (63 men and one woman), eight of whom had bilateral operations. This presentation was published in a short abstract but appeared in 1889 as a complete report. This was the year Halsted had mentioned, yet Bassini had reported these operations two years earlier. Interestingly, the title of the operation as listed by Halsted is the same as the title in the published abstract, except in the latter the word "operativo" is not included. In his second publication in Italian in 1888, Bassini presented a report of his first 100 patients who were operated upon for the radical cure of inguinal hernias.[10]

During the three and a half years from June 13, 1889 through January 29, 1893, 82 operations were performed in 81 patients (one of whom had a second operation four months later for the repair of a recurrent hernia).

An interesting part of this clinical study was the fact that 23 (28%) of the patients were children whose ages ranged from 14 months to nine years. Since children in these age groups are an exceedingly transient population for follow-up studies, it is not surprising that 11 were lost to follow-up. Furthermore, in the subgroup of children 14 months to four years of age, seven of the 11 were lost to follow-up.

In the remaining 12 children, the follow-up study ranged between five months and two and a half years, with six of the 12 being followed for less than one year. Because of the high propensity for further losses in these children, the number of children available for evaluation would most likely be minimal or even none.

Also of interest is the fact that in 17 of these 23 children the hernias were small, in four they were large, and in the remaining two the size was not recorded. The predominance of small hernias in these children is of surgical significance since in 14 of the 17 children so classified, the classic Halsted I operation was done. This included the "thinning of the cord" by excision of segments of the accompanying veins. In retrospect, this would seem to represent not only an unduly radical operation but a concomitant high potential for the complication of testicular atrophy. In fact, it was this specific complication that later resulted in its omission in all the operations in children and selectively in those performed in adults. However, because of the large number of children lost to follow-up and the high potential for a continuing greater loss, the exact number who may have had atrophy of the testicle is unknown.

WILLIAM STEWART HALSTED (1852–1922)
Continued

THE HALSTED II OPERATION

In 1903 Halsted introduced his modified technique (Halsted II) for the radical cure of inguinal hernias with the statement, "The present operation has evolved by degrees and stands for the experience of 14 years derived from more than 1000 operations for the cure of inguinal hernia; features of the old . . . have been dropped and new ones . . . added."[11]

One of the new features was the nontransplantation of the cord, permitting it ". . . to lie . . . undisturbed in its bed and to trust to the suture of the internal oblique muscle to Poupart's ligament . . . to effect a cure." Another feature was the use of the cremaster muscle because of its strength and attachment to Poupart's ligament.

Its use was in those patients in whom the lower part of the canal was unprotected because of a fascial deficiency in the conjoined tendon. Although the cremaster muscle was more frequently sutured to the undersurface of the internal oblique muscle, in selected instances it was sutured over this muscle. As Halsted remarked, its use in this manner conformed with ". . . one of the great principles in Surgery; there is no tension."

Bloodgood had observed the great variation in width of the conjoined tendon in relation to the incidence of direct recurrences at the lower angle of the wound. To prevent this complication he recommended transplanting the rectus muscle by division of the rectus sheath posteriorly rather than anteriorly (as previously practiced by Wölfler[12]) and bringing the belly of the muscle behind the internal oblique muscle for its suture to Poupart's ligament.

This technique was used in 12 patients, but the follow-up period was too short to properly evaluate the results. Halsted questioned its use, however, since he feared that the contraction of such a strong muscle as the rectus would disrupt its sutured attachment to Poupart's ligament.

When the veins of the spermatic cord were large, which was the usual finding, they were excised with "great care" to avoid extravasation of blood into the surrounding tissue. This practice however, was ultimately abandoned.

The figures reproduced here illustrate the Halsted II operation.[11]

3 A series of untied mattress sutures of fine silk have been inserted through the internal oblique muscle, well back of its free border, to engage the muscle bundles of the lower flap of the cremaster muscle. When these sutures are tied, the cremaster will be approximated to the undersurface of the internal oblique muscle.

4 The mattress sutures are tied and their strands cut. A series of untied catgut sutures, to unite the internal oblique muscle and conjoined tendon to Poupart's ligament, are inserted. If tension on the suture line is present, "relaxation cuts" are made in the anterior rectus sheath.

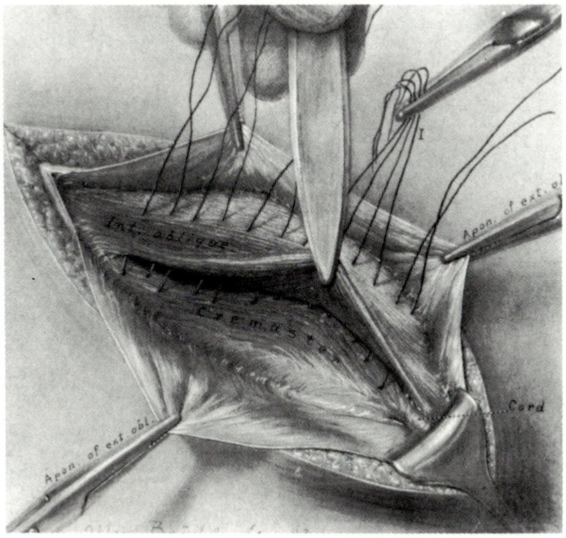

3

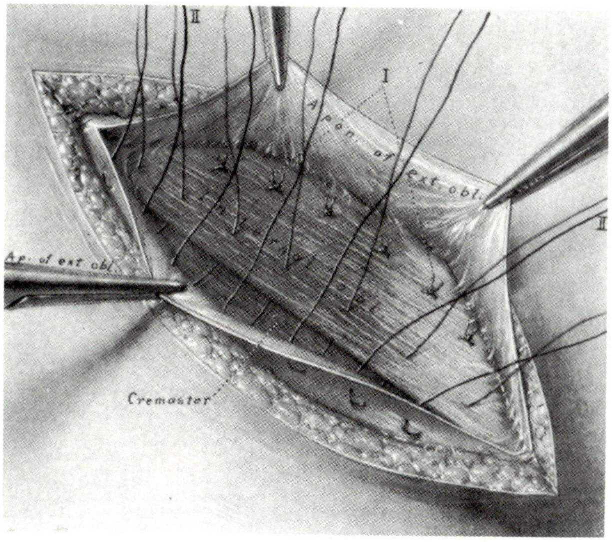

4

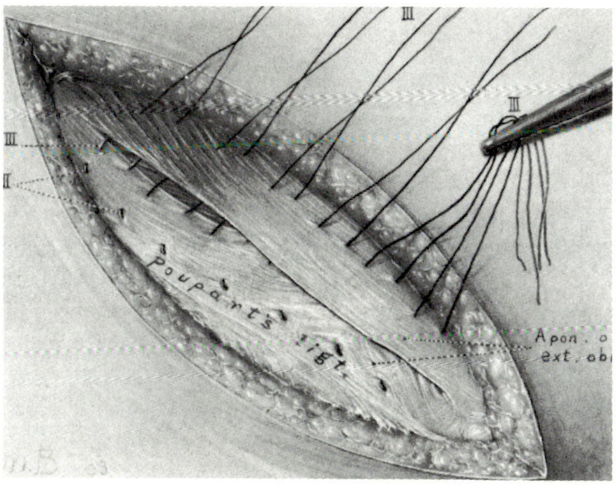

5

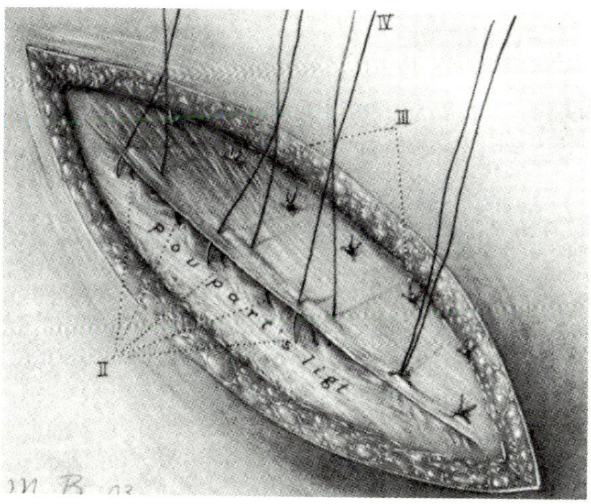

6

5 A series of interrupted silk mattress sutures are inserted to imbricate the inferior leaflet of the aponeurosis of the external oblique muscle, beneath its superior leaflet.

6 The imbrication sutures have been tied and their strands cut. The interrupted mattress sutures of silk are inserted and tied in sequence to approximate the free cut margin of the superior leaflet of the external oblique aponeurosis to its inferior leaflet. This completes the musculoaponeurotic reconstruction.

WILLIAM STEWART HALSTED (1852–1922)
Continued

7 Sagittal view depicting the completed four "steps" in the anterior repair of an inguinal hernia.

8 The use of a turned-down flap of the anterior sheath of the rectus muscle for the closure of the lower part of the inguinal canal, when weakened by an attenuated or absent conjoined tendon, is demonstrated. This technical maneuver was originated by Halsted, who first used it in 1899.

The skin wound is closed with a continuous buried suture of silver wire and covered with five or six layers of silver foil. The wire is withdrawn in two weeks, but the patient is kept in bed for 18 to 21 days.

In contrast to the Halsted I operation, in which the transversalis fascia was an anatomic essential of the hernial repair, in the Halsted II operation this structure is neither mentioned in the text nor labeled in any of the illustrations. In fact, the anatomic site of the transversalis fascia—the innermost layer of the anterior abdominal wall—is not exposed, since in this operation the untransplanted cord is permitted ". . . to lie . . . undisturbed in its bed." Of necessity, therefore, the Halsted II repair is anterior to the hernial defect or "hole" in the fascia of the posterior inguinal wall.

The use of the cremaster muscle in this "new repair" is difficult to understand. Muscle bundles, regardless of their size and apparent strength, have exceedingly poor holding power for sutures. The repetitive muscle contractions during their daily use create tissue tension and a tendency for the sutures to tear through their sites of attachment.

It is also apparent that Max Brödel exercised his "artistic license" in the representation of the internal oblique muscle, since it is never seen as such in the operating room. Halsted apparently anticipated such a comment when he stated, "The drawing . . . possibly exaggerated . . . the size and extent of the internal oblique muscle as well as the cremaster."[11] Furthermore, the suturing of the internal oblique muscle to Poupart's ligament does not conform to the admonition to suture only white fascia to white fascia rather than red muscle to white fascia.

The imbrication of the aponeurotic layers of the external oblique muscle to strengthen the hernial repair has not been supported by the later studies of Farris and colleagues[13] or Dunphy.[14] In his experimental studies in rabbits, Farris demonstrated that the distraction force required to disrupt the on-end fascial closures was consistently greater than that required to disrupt the sutured imbricated layers, which indicated poorer healing in the latter. Similarly, Dunphy demonstrated experimentally that the on-end suture of freshly cut margins of fascia evoked a much greater fibroblastic response and better healing than when the fascial layers were approximated by sutured imbrication.

A fitting conclusion to these comments is Halsted's translation of Billroth's prophetic statement: "If we could artificially produce tissues of the density and toughness of fascia and tendon, the secret of the radical cure of hernia would be discovered."[15]

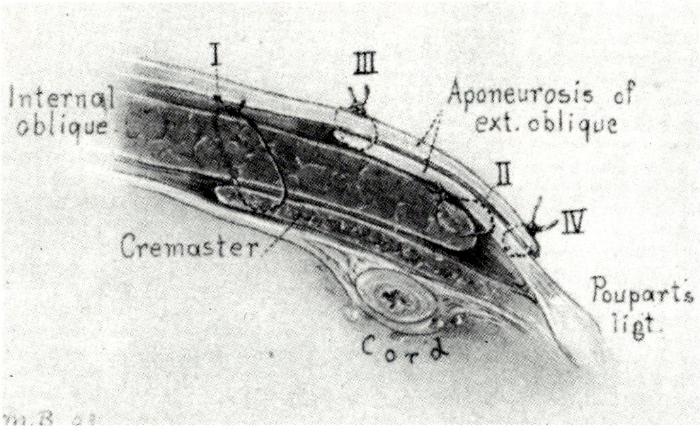

7

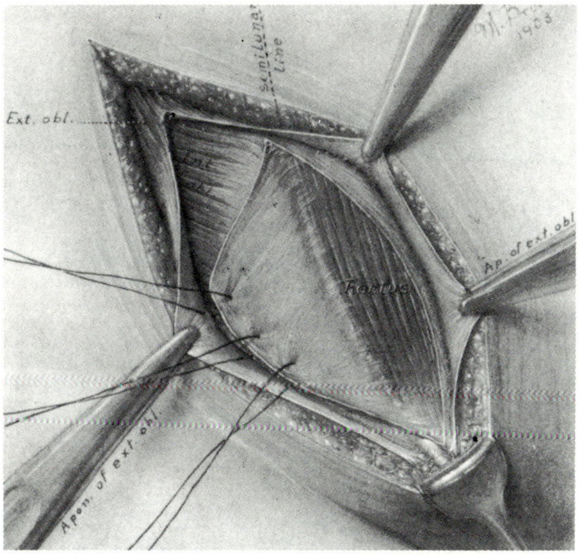

8

REFERENCES

1. Halsted, WS: Circular suture of the intestine. An experimental study. Am J Med Sci *94*:436–461, 1887.
2. Biographical information from MacCallum, WG: *William Stewart Halsted, Surgeon.* Baltimore: Johns Hopkins Press, 1930.
3. Halsted, WS: *Surgical Papers by William Stewart Halsted* (2 vols.). Baltimore: Johns Hopkins Press, 1924.
4. Matas, R.: William Stewart Halsted, 1852–1922. An appreciation. Johns Hopkins Hosp Bull *36*:2, 1925.
5. Halsted, WS: The radical cure of hernia. Johns Hopkins Hosp Bull *1*:111–112, 1890.
6. Halsted, WS: The radical cure of hernia in the male. Ann Surg *17*:542–556, 1893.
7. Bassini, E: Ueber die Behandlung des Leistenbruches. Archiv für klinische Chirurgie *40*:429–476, 1890.
8. Halsted, WS: An additional note on the operation for inguinal hernia. In *Surgical Papers by William Stewart Halsted* (Vol. 1). Baltimore: Johns Hopkins Press, 1924, pp. 306, 308.
9. Bassini, E: Nuovo metodo per la cura radicale dell'ernia. Atti Congr Assoc Med Ital (XII Congress) *2*:179, 1887. (Full report published as *Nuovo metodo per la cura radicale dell'ernia inguinale.* Padua: Prosperini, 1889.)
10. Bassini, E: Sopra 100 casi di cura radicale dell'ernia operata metodo del-autore. Archiv Atti Soc Ital Chir *5*:315, 1888.
11. Halsted, WS: The cure of the more difficult as well as the simpler inguinal ruptures. Johns Hopkins Hosp Bull *14*:208–214, 1903.
12. Wölfler, A: Zur Radical operation des freien Leistenbruches. In *Beitrage zur klinischen Festschrift f Billroth, T.* Stuttgart: F. Enke, 1892, pp. 552–603.
13. Farris, JM, Smith, GK, and Beattie, AS: Umbilical hernia: An inquiry into principles of imbrication and a note on the preservation of the umbilical dimple. Am J Surg *98*:236–242, 1959.
14. Dunphy, JE: On the nature and cure of wounds. Moynihan Lecture. Ann R Coll Surg *26*:69–87, 1960.
15. Halsted, WS: *Surgical Papers by William Stewart Halsted* (Vol. 1). Baltimore: Johns Hopkins Press, 1924, p. 271. (Original from Czerny, V: *Beitrage zur Chirurgie.* Stuttgart: Ferdinand Enke, 1878, p. 13.)

INDEX

Note: Page numbers in *italics* refer to illustrations; page numbers followed by t refer to tables.